UNDERSTANDING CHILDREN AND YOUNG PEOPLE'S MENTAL HEALTH

Edited by

Anne Claveirole RGN, RMN, RNT, L es L. MSc, Cert Ed, PhD

*Lecturer/Researcher in Children and Young People's
Mental Health
School of Nursing, Midwifery and Social Care
Edinburgh Napier University
Edinburgh
Scotland*

Martin Gaughan RMN, RNLD MPhil, PG Cert (TLHE), BSc (Hons)

*Lecturer in Children and Young People's Mental Health
School of Nursing, Midwifery and Social Care
Edinburgh Napier University
Edinburgh
Scotland*

WILEY-BLACKWELL

A John Wiley & Sons, Ltd., Publication

Wiley-Blackwell is an imprint of John Wiley & Sons Ltd, formed by the merger of Wiley's global Scientific, Technical and Medical business with Blackwell Publishing Ltd.

Registered office
John Wiley & Sons Ltd, The Atrium, Southern Gate, Chichester, West Sussex, PO19 8SQ, United Kingdom

Editorial office
John Wiley & Sons Ltd, The Atrium, Southern Gate, Chichester, West Sussex, PO19 8SQ, United Kingdom

For details of our global editorial offices, for customer services and for information about how to apply for permission to reuse the copyright material in this book please see our website at www.wiley.com/wiley-blackwell.

This book is published in the following electronic formats: eBook 9780470973172.

Designations used by companies to distinguish their products are often claimed as trademarks. All brand names and product names used in this book are trade names, service marks, trademarks or registered trademarks of their respective owners. The publisher is not associated with any product or vendor mentioned in this book. This publication is designed to provide accurate and authoritative information in regard to the subject matter covered. It is sold on the understanding that the publisher is not engaged in rendering professional services. If professional advice or other expert assistance is required, the services of a competent professional should be sought.

Library of Congress Cataloging-in-Publication Data

Understanding children and young people's mental health / edited by Anne Claveirole, Martin Gaughan.
   p. ; cm.
  Includes bibliographical references and index.
  ISBN 978-0-470-72345-6 (pbk. : alk. paper) 1. Child psychiatry. 2. Child psychopathology. 3. Adolescent psychiatry.
4. Adolescent psychopathology. I. Claveirole, Anne. II. Gaughan, Martin.
  [DNLM: 1. Mental Disorders. 2. Adolescent Psychology. 3. Child Psychology. WS 350 U548 2011]
  RJ499.U477 2011
  618.92'89—dc22

                2010013939

A catalogue record for this book is available from the British Library.

Set in 10/13.5 pt TrumpMediaeval-Roman by MPS Limited, A Macmillan Company

1 2011

CONTENTS

Notes on Contributors   ix
Foreword   xiii
Acknowledgements   xvii

Introduction   1

1 Setting the scene   4
Anne Claveirole
    1.1   Introduction   4
    1.2   Social context   5
    1.3   Children and young people's mental health   13
    1.4   'Every Child Matters': What can we do to help?   20
    1.5   Conclusion   27

2 The family   29
Duncan Tennant and Anne Claveirole
    2.1   Introduction   29
    2.2   What is 'normal' family functioning?   30
    2.3   The family life cycle   33
    2.4   Family structure   37
    2.5   Recent developments: narrative approaches
        to family therapy   39
    2.6   Attachment and family therapy   41
    2.7   Parenting support and education   42
    2.8   Conclusion   44

3 Psychosocial development   46
Geraldine Jones
    3.1   Introduction   46
    3.2   Theories of development   47
    3.3   Infant attachment   47
    3.4   Adolescent identity formation   51
    3.5   Adolescent self-esteem   54
    3.6   Adolescent reasoning ability   55
    3.7   Adolescent egocentrism   56
    3.8   The psychological impact of puberty   57
    3.9   Adolescent brain development   58

3.10 The value of contextual theories in explaining
development of children and adolescents 59
3.11 The PVEST model 60
3.12 Conclusion 63

4 Self-harm 64

Martin Gaughan
4.1 Introduction 64
4.2 What is self-harm? 65
4.3 How common is self-harm? 66
4.4 Vulnerability and resilience 68
4.5 Promoting resilience 69
4.6 Models of self-harm 71
4.7 Assessment 74
4.8 Intervention 76
4.9 Informal support 77
4.10 Promoting positive behaviour 77
4.11 Self-help 78
4.12 Making access easier 79
4.13 Talking therapies 80
4.14 The personal impact of working alongside
children and young people who self-harm 83
4.15 Conclusion 84

5 Depression 87

Martin Gaughan
5.1 Introduction 87
5.2 Defining depression 88
5.3 Prevalence 90
5.4 Vulnerability 91
5.5 Assessment 93
5.6 Symptoms of depression in children and young people 95
5.7 Protective factors and promoting resilience 98
5.8 Interventions 99
5.9 Cognitive–behaviour therapy 99
5.10 Interpersonal psychotherapy for
depressed adolescents 100
5.11 Medication 101
5.12 Psychodynamics 103
5.13 What else helps? 104
5.14 The family 105
5.15 Conclusion 105

6 Suicide 108

Martin Gaughan
6.1 Introduction 108
6.2 What is suicide? 109
6.3 How common is suicide? 109
6.4 Vulnerability 111
6.5 Resilience 115
6.6 Risk assessment 117
6.7 Models of assessment and intervention 118
6.8 Applied suicide and intervention skills training 120
6.9 Skills-based training on risk management 121
6.10 Intervention 122
6.11 Prevention 125
6.12 Postvention 127
6.13 Conclusion 128

7 Child abuse and child protection 132

Julie Hendry and Marlene Macinnes
7.1 Introduction 132
7.2 Definitions of child abuse 133
7.3 Incidence and prevalence 136
7.4 Risk factors 137
7.5 Policy 139
7.6 Assessment 139
7.7 Prevention 144
7.8 Interventions 145
7.9 Conclusion 147

8 Eating disorders 149

Gavin Cullen
8.1 Introduction 149
8.2 What are eating disorders? 150
8.3 How common are eating disorders? 153
8.4 What causes eating disorders? 154
8.5 Resilience factors 158
8.6 Assessment 159
8.7 Interventions 161
8.8 Psychological support 161
8.9 Conclusion 163

9 Early onset psychosis 165

Martin Gaughan
9.1 Introduction 165
9.2 Time to change? 166

9.3   Prevalence   167
9.4   Vulnerability to psychosis   168
9.5   Early and very early onset psychosis   171
9.6   Phases of psychosis   172
9.7   Prevention and early intervention   173
9.8   Assessment   174
9.9   Interventions   177
9.10 Drug treatment   178
9.11 Effectiveness of medication   179
9.12 Side effects   180
9.13 Talking therapies   182
9.14 Promoting resilience, staying well and recovery   184
9.15 Involving the family   186
9.16 Conclusion   188

10 ADHD   **191**
Lorna Jones and Anne Claveirole
10.1   Introduction   191
10.2   What is ADHD?   192
10.3   The experience of ADHD   192
10.4   ADHD as a diagnostic category   194
10.5   Prevalence   195
10.6   Risk factors   196
10.7   Resilience: factors affecting outcome   200
10.8   Assessment   201
10.9   Interventions   205
10.10 Conclusion   213

11 Autistic spectrum disorders   **217**
Gillian Marshall-McConnell and Anne Claveirole
11.1   Introduction   217
11.2   Definition and classification   218
11.3   Prevalence   222
11.4   Risk factors/causation theories   223
11.5   Associated problems   226
11.6   Development   230
11.7   Assessment and diagnosis   233
11.8   Management of care   234
11.9   Conclusion   238

12 Misuse of substances   **239**
Liz Brodie and Jayne Reed
12.1   Introduction   239
12.2   Substance use and substance misuse   240

12.3　Prevalence　241
12.4　Patterns of use and misuse in children and young people　242
12.5　Vulnerability and resilience　244
12.6　Environmental and family factors　245
12.7　Early intervention and recognition　246
12.8　Assessment　246
12.9　Intervention　249
12.10　Conclusion　254

References　256
Index　305

Dedication

I would like to dedicate our book to my mother and father — Anne

To Babs, for being so kind and supportive, and Kirsty for being everything a father could wish for — Martin

NOTES ON CONTRIBUTORS

Liz Brodie
RMN, MA (Hons), PGDip Drug and Alcohol Studies, PG Cert (TLHE)
Lecturer in Mental Health
School of Nursing, Midwifery and Social Care
Edinburgh Napier University
Edinburgh
Scotland

Anne Claveirole
RGN, RMN, RNT, L es L., MSc, Cert Ed, PhD
Lecturer and Researcher in Children and Young People's Mental Health
School of Nursing, Midwifery and Social Care
Edinburgh Napier University
Edinburgh
Scotland

Gavin Cullen
RMN, BSc in Mental Health Practice, PG Certificate in CBT
Senior Charge Nurse
NHS Lothian Child and Adolescent Mental Health Services
Royal Edinburgh Hospital
Edinburgh
Scotland

Martin Gaughan
RMN, RNLD, MPhil, PG Cert (TLHE), Bsc (Hons)
Lecturer in Children and Young People's Mental Health
School of Nursing, Midwifery and Social Care

Edinburgh Napier University
Edinburgh
Scotland

Julie Hendry
RMN, PGDip Child Care and Child Protection
Mental Health Practitioner
Co-ordinator in Child Sexual Abuse Team
NHS Lothian Child and Adolescent Mental Health Services, Edinburgh
Scotland

Geraldine Jones
BA (Hons), BSc (Hons), MSc Occupational Psychology, DEd Pscyh
Member of the British Psychological Society
Lecturer in Developmental Psychology School of Life, Sport
    and Social Sciences
Edinburgh Napier University
Edinburgh
Scotland

Lorna Jones
RN (Mental Health), BSc (Hons) Neuroscience, BSc Mental Health
    Nursing, NMC Registered Specialist Practitioner (Mental Health)
Independent and Supplementary Nurse Prescriber
Team Leader/Community Nurse Specialist in ADHD Team
NHS Lothian Child and Adolescent Mental Health Services
Edinburgh
Scotland

Marlene Macinnes
MA (Hons), BSc (Hons), MSW, Dip SW, Certificate in Child
    Protection Studies
Social Worker, NHS Lothian Child and Adolescent Mental
    Health Services
Edinburgh
Scotland

Gillian Marshall-McConnell
MA Professional Development – Disability Studies, PGCE Special Needs
Independent Consultant Related Qualifications and Assistant
Director for the Scottish Society for Autism

Glasgow
Scotland

Jayne Reed
RN (Mental Health), BSc Nursing with Health Studies, MSc Adolescent
    Addiction Studies
Senior Community Mental Health Nurse (Young People and
    Substance Use)
NHS Lothian Community Drug Problem Service
Edinburgh
Scotland

Duncan Tennant
RMN, RGN, MSc, UKCP Registered Family Therapist
Senior Specialist in Systemic Psychotherapy at the Department of
    Psychiatry at St John's Hospital, NHS Lothian
Livingston, West Lothian
Scotland

FOREWORD TO UNDERSTANDING CHILDREN AND YOUNG PEOPLE'S MENTAL HEALTH

During the last 20 years or so, spurred in many ways by Rutter's epidemiological study in the mid-1970s, the whole subject of children's mental health has risen quite extraordinarily on the political agenda. Before then, the emphasis of concern amongst those working closely with children largely rested upon children's social and economic welfare, their education and protection. The idea of 'children's mental health' sat uncomfortably in people's minds – the word 'mental' being so firmly associated with illness that to put it alongside that of 'children' was tantamount almost to stigmatising them all. Gradually, however, there has occurred a significant shift in thinking in social policy. The mental health of children is now seen as of crucial importance, and the promotion of children's mental health at large is now viewed as necessary as the prevention and treatment of specific mental health problems.

Two reasons for this stand out. The first has to do with a growing realisation that so many of the social ills that worry us all – criminality, violence, drug and alcohol misuse, dysfunctional families, child abuse – have much to do with the mental health of those involved. The knowledge that we have gained, during the course of the twentieth century and more recently, of child development and family functioning has brought home to us the fact that we can so readily make sense of many of these problems and indeed anticipate them. The other has to do with a growing recognition that some of the pressures of our contemporary society are bearing heavily on the minds of our children, so much so that their mental health is in jeopardy. The inexorable pace of technological and cultural change in our times in an ever widening global context is making the task of growing up increasingly difficult. It is also making the art of parenting all the more challenging. Most of the evidence that we now have testifies to the fact that we have a mounting child mental health problem on our hands.

It is in the midst of this frankly alarming context that we welcome the arrival of this book. It sets out to help us understand what is going on in the minds of children and young people today and in their parents and carers. It lays out the social, cultural and family predicaments in which children are living and then takes us through some of the different kinds of muddle and trouble and anxiety and terror that different kinds of children suffer at different times of their lives. Throughout, it holds in mind the sheer complexity of children's mental health problems, the sheer interdependence of so many factors that influence the course of their development. Children struggle through life with different endowments, different experiences of attachment to their parents, different shapes and sizes of families. Children from different ethnic backgrounds have to make their way against particular resistances and obstacles in our society. And boys and girls go through different mental experiences as they deal with their different bodies and the expectations placed upon them by other children and adults.

It is indeed a confounding world of difference, something that clearly defies clean categorisation or certain diagnosis and treatment. In relation to most of the mental health problems and disorders, there is an almost insurmountable difficulty in arriving at a consensus about definition. And because of this, prevalence rates of child mental disorders vary widely.

However, despite such complexity, all is not lost – for in the face of it, therapeutic endeavours of all kinds abound. It is an endearing characteristic of most therapists and carers that, in the face of adversity and often long odds, they carry an abiding hope that they can make things better for the children and their families who come their way. However damaged or thwarted children may be, therapists and carers work to help them to become 'what they are capable of becoming' and to be as flexible and as resourceful as they can be under the circumstances in which they live. It may be that they do not fully succeed, that minimising harm may be as much as can realistically be achieved in some cases, but at least they try to bring about positive change.

How they go about doing this is a story in itself. The ways of therapy are diverse and in many ways baffling. Whatever may be asserted by some therapists, the fact is that little is known for sure from research about which therapeutic techniques work best with which kind of children from which kind of environment at which point in time. However, what can be said with some conviction is that no therapy can work without nurturing a consistent and reliable therapeutic relationship in which the child can feel safe enough to communicate his or her difficulties. There is much to be said too for those therapies that excite a curiosity in children to explore their selves and behaviour, as well as those that can bear the paradoxical and complicated nature of so many mental health problems in children and families. For example, what tolerance do therapists have in making sense of the young teenager who damages her body 'in an attempt to preserve the integrity of the mind' (p. 112)? And how far can they give due consideration to those who have the everyday responsibility of caring and parenting and teaching children in difficulty with themselves and others?

The authors of this book need to be congratulated on tackling the many various issues and problems that any study of child mental health involves. Their writing is direct and straightforward, they provide us with useful facts and they give us a measured and unbiased analysis of the variety of views and perspectives that abound in this field. Their chapters, moreover, are organised in such a way that they leave us with little doubt where we are going and what we are supposed to do. They set us activities which we are expected to carry out and introduce us to the relevant literature and resources.

All in all, the book generates a sense of critical enquiry within us and reminds us that the promotion and treatment of children's mental health is everybody's business. In this day and age (to pick up the first few words of the Introduction to this book), children's mental health is now truly seen as a major public health issue. The Scottish Executive's title for its report on child abuse (2002a) captures the gist of it all: *It's Everyone's Job to Make Sure I'm Alright*. And it can be said that it is the job of this book to go some way in making sure that this happens.

Peter Wilson
Psychotherapist and former Director of YoungMinds

ACKNOWLEDGEMENTS

We would like to thank the library staff at Comely Bank Campus who under the excellent leadership of Sheena Moffat have been so helpful and supportive over the years: Margarete Case, Cathy Coventry, Margaret Green, Julie McGregor, Agnes Miller, Cluny Nixon, Brenda Prior, Val Robertson, Simon Ward and of course Sheena Moffat herself.

We would also like to thank the young people with whom we have worked over the years: you have been an inspiration to us. Finally thanks to all our colleagues in the mental health team at Edinburgh Napier University and in the NHS Child and Adolescent Mental Health Services: most of our ideas have come to maturity through discussions with you.

INTRODUCTION

In this day and age, children and young people face challenges unknown to those of previous generations. They have to perform educationally, socially and interpersonally. They are expected to look good and called upon to make consumer choices. They negotiate relationships using methods and media unheard of 20 years ago, from text messaging to online networking. Their behaviour is recorded, examined and made public through 'YouTube' and 'Bebo'. They are available 24 hours a day via mobile phones and the Internet. As technology develops, they will have to accommodate further changes. For some young people, the hurdles are made greater by adversity, whether poverty, physical, learning or developmental disability, trauma, immigration, asylum seeking or refugee status. Children and young people face these unprecedented challenges under the scrutiny of the public and the critical eye of the media.

As society changes, family life is exposed to turmoil. Many children and young people have to make sense of and adapt to the changes imposed by separation, loss, divorce and the reconstitution of families. Those looked after by local authorities have to adopt new rules and negotiate different ways of being, with new adults in their lives, sometimes in institutional settings. In refugee and asylum seeking families, they have to adapt to a new culture, in unfamiliar surroundings, often in poverty. This book is about the mental health challenges children and young people face and how we, adults, can work alongside them to help them face and overcome such challenges.

What is remarkable is that most children and young people are able to cross the choppy waters and emerge into adulthood relatively unscathed. However, there is also growing concern about changing trends in their mental health, with new risk factors for all, and particular ones for some,

Understanding Children and Young People's Mental Health, first edition. Edited by Anne Claveirole and Martin Gaughan. Published 2011 by John Wiley & Sons Ltd. © 2011 John Wiley & Sons Ltd.

of developing problems. The mental health of children and young people receives increasing attention. More than ever before, their emotional and psychological well-being has become the subject of research, with a new focus on the early years.

In this book we have brought together practitioners and academics who are specialists in the theory and practice of children and young people's development and mental health to write about particular areas of interest and expertise. Our aim is to inform and challenge the reader with its content, and to encourage further exploration of the subject. We hope that, while it starts from a UK perspective, this text will be of interest to people working in other English-speaking countries.

The initial chapters focus on the context of children and young people's lives: twenty-first century society (Chapter 1) and the family (Chapter 2); Chapter 3 examines individual psychosocial development at two crucial moments of a child's life, infancy and adolescence. In Chapters 4–12, we have chosen to present particular mental health difficulties which children and young people may have to face; not every category of problem is there, nor do we believe that children and young people's problems can be neatly packaged. We recognise that there is a need to focus on those children and young people who have complex needs and do not fit easily into diagnostic categories. Children and young people with learning disabilities, those looked after and accommodated, refugees and asylum seekers, ethnic minorities and those young people whose developing sexuality takes them beyond expected social norms are neglected groups whose mental health issues can be overlooked. Standard interventions are not suitable for everyone and may need to be adapted to engage and support children, young people and families who differ from the mainstream, live on the margin of society or are viewed as 'different'. The chapters on mental health challenges highlight some of the complex problems children and young people face and we intend them to be read as information resources, to encourage reflection and an examination of values, attitudes and thoughts.

Much of the writing in this book is about relationships. The relationships children and young people have in the home are the bedrock of mental health, from the earliest bond between mother and child to the growing bonds between all family members – which must lead us to pause and reflect on the needs of those who do not have families, or those who live in chaotic families, and consider the different and sometimes challenging environments in which children and young people develop. The relationships young people have at school and with significant adults in their local environments are also crucial. Thinking about how we, as health and social care staff, engage young people, and their families/carers is central to working alongside children and young people.

At the time of writing, a number of key strategies which embrace newer ways of constructing mental health are being proposed in England and Scotland. In England, the Department of Health (2009) is consulting on 'New Horizons' – a mental health strategy with a whole population approach which lays the foundation for community ownership of mental health issues. For more than a decade, the Scottish government has been at the forefront of development in proposing that mental health be mainstreamed and that everyone take responsibility for ensuring that children reach their full potential. It is encapsulated in *Towards a Mentally Flourishing Scotland* (Scottish Government, 2009). We hope *Understanding Children and Young People's Mental Health* will contribute to increasing awareness of children and young people and that it will promote reflection on the mental health issues that affect them.

Chapter 1

SETTING THE SCENE

Anne Claveirole

School of Nursing, Midwifery and Social Care, Edinburgh Napier University, Edinburgh, Scotland

1.1 Introduction

In this chapter, we will examine the context in which the mental health problems of children and young people emerge: our western society and its recent developments; the globalisation process and its impact on our culture; what children and young people's mental health is, what endangers it, what protects it and how we can promote it; what mental health problems are, how we might prevent their occurrence as well as intervene to resolve, or at least improve, them. We take a child to be under 18 years of age.

> **Learning outcomes**
>
> After studying this chapter, you should be able to:
>
> 1. Reflect on the present social conditions of industrialised countries, such as the one you live in, with regard to community, individualism, trust and well-being.
> 2. Appreciate the impact of social conditions in industrialised countries on some indicators of children and young people's well-being.
> 3. Define mental health in younger people and discuss the difference between mental health problems and mental disorders.
> 4. Be aware of current trends in children and young people's mental health difficulties and have some understanding of their evolution.

Understanding Children and Young People's Mental Health, first edition. Edited by Anne Claveirole and Martin Gaughan. Published 2011 by John Wiley & Sons Ltd. © 2011 John Wiley & Sons Ltd.

5. Recognise the difference between risk, protective, precipitating and maintaining factors in the lives of children or young people who have mental health problems or mental disorders.
6. Understand and critique current national mental health-promoting strategies aimed at influencing the mental health of children, young people and families.
7. Critically examine your service's own assessment procedures and reflect on its treatment practices regarding the therapeutic relationship with and participation of children, young people and their parents.

1.2 Social context

Global context

Globalisation is a recent word which refers to the growing interdependence of individuals and nations. Cultural, economic and political changes in one corner of the globe affect everyone's environment, economy and politics: we are increasingly aware of living in one world, linked by active networks of information and communication.

Throughout this world, societies have changed more rapidly in the last hundred years than at any time in history. Pre-modern societies (hunting–gathering, pastoral or agrarian) have been disappearing, leaving just a few in remote areas of the earth, undermined by modernisation. Previously traditional countries like India and China are becoming industrialised and their populations urbanised. In the nations of Europe and North America, the rate of technological development has led to radical changes in social structures and lifestyles. These changes have taken place over an extremely short time:

> *The Englishman of 1750 was closer in material things to Caesar's legionnaires than to his own great-grandchildren* (Landes 1969 in Fulcher and Scott 2007).

The way nations weather such changes has an impact on national communities and individuals: the families, children and young people who are the focus of this book. When, in 1989, the United Nations issued the Convention on the Rights of the Child (United Nations 1989), their intention was to lay down international norms of well-being for all children regarding their entitlements to protection, education and, in proportion to their growing maturity, self-determination. Most states of the world signed this convention because they recognised that children's successful growth and development is the key to a society's well-being and its future, and that it cannot be left to chance.

Yet, as we take stock, global development does not appear fully to support the goals of the convention. Disparity of wealth throughout the world has increased: over 21% of the world's population still lives on less than a dollar a day (Bellamy 2005), and more than 80% live in countries where income differentials are widening (United Nations 2007). Although many poor countries signed the convention, their struggle to invest in health, education and social welfare remains acute and often fails. In wealthy ones, there is growing awareness that childhood is being shaped by forces which are often at odds with the best interests of children (UNICEF 2007).

This English-language text will focus on children and young people's mental health in English-speaking industrialised countries, taking the UK where it is published, as its starting point. However, immigration brings into these countries the influence of many other cultures on child development, child care and family life, and this must be taken into account.

Rich industrialised countries

In the UK, the Centre for Economic Performance (CEP) at the London School of Economics reviews evidence from the social sciences, particularly psychology and economics, to make policy recommendations to the government (http://cep.lse.ac.uk/_new/about/default.asp). As part of its programme of research, the CEP has investigated mounting evidence that well-being has been static since the Second World War in spite of unprecedented economic growth (Layard 2005). Whereas people are richer, work less, have longer holidays, travel more, live longer and are healthier, they are not happier, and the correlation between income and well-being stops at a certain average gross domestic product (GDP); evidence of this exists for industrialised countries like Japan, North America and those of the European Union (Layard 2005). Moreover, levels of clinical depression, alcoholism and crime, which show a considerable increase in the same period in the same countries (Rutter and Smith 1995), confirm that wealth does not mean happiness. Layard (2003) defines happiness as 'feeling good' and 'enjoying life' and unhappiness as 'feeling bad and wishing things were different'. Another indicator of this surprising state of affairs is a recorded increase in mental health problems across all age groups but particularly among young people (West and Sweeting 2003, Collishaw et al. 2004).

In the same vein, recent findings from an extensive public consultation regarding society today, conducted in the UK by the Joseph Rowntree Foundation (JRF), show a strong consensus of views among respondents that shared values have declined, communities break up, individualism is high and poverty is corrosive in our otherwise affluent society (JRF 2008). Layard's research (2005) found something similar: in 1999 less people thought others could be trusted (29%) than in 1990 (44%) or in 1959 (56%). Autonomy, self-determination and individual freedom are currently held as core social values; however, when individuals come to think that making the most of their own life is their primary duty, ahead of community concerns and looking after each other, a balance is lost and individualism sets in (Layard 2005), which is the opposite of trust and mutuality. Yet trust plays an important part in social well-being. In an analysis of the findings of the annual life satisfaction survey Gallup World Poll taken in 130 countries (Gallup Organisation 2007), the economist John Helliwell (2003) draws attention to the fact that trust is closely linked to life satisfaction. Trust in neighbours, the police, colleagues and employers is rated as highly valued so that the way people relate to each other and the extent to which they engage in helping others correlate strongly with their satisfaction with life. Helliwell (2008) suggests that this should be more regularly monitored in global and national surveys and used for planning in organisations, businesses and communities.

✎ **Activity**

Look up Helliwell in this chapter's Recommended Reading section and go to the recommended website.

Read one of Helliwell's papers, make notes of the main messages and take time to reflect on the issues.

Children and young people face pressures which are not dissimilar to those of adults: growing economic inequality, pressure to consume, family break-up, competition with peers and focus on achievement; new technologies and media which expose them to new activities and pleasures but also to dangers and difficult choices (Layard and Dunn 2009). If they do not do well, their future may be compromised. A successful adult life in the complex economies of industrialised countries requires a high level of education and skills, yet many young people do not complete their secondary school education and do not have the qualifications that will enable them to access employment (European Commission 2008). UNICEF (2007: 39) raises concerns about 'the changing ecology of childhood' in rich countries because the social context there, marked by economic instability, individual priorities and rumbling discontent, does not prioritise the nurturing of children and young people.

Impact on children and young people's well-being

The Good Childhood Inquiry commissioned by the Children's Society (Layard and Dunn 2009) suggests that children and young people experience childhood in a different way to previous generations. The report mentions some of the changes which have brought this about:

- Information technology: children have access to previously unimaginable levels of information;
- Demographics: children regularly interact with different cultures, languages, faiths and traditions (some schools service populations where up to forty languages are spoken);
- Family break-ups and both parents working;
- School examinations and pressure for good results;
- Highest level of relative poverty for 50 years and an increased lack of social mobility.

Such concerns about children's well-being are paradoxical because, like adults, children have better lives than ever before: better health, better education, better homes, more holidays away and more money and possessions, including access to technology for communication, music and entertainment.

How do children and young people fare in our English-speaking industrialised countries? In 2007 UNICEF, the United Nations' arm concerned with children's welfare, published an overview of children's well-being in countries of the Organisation for Economic Cooperation and Development (OECD), using as much data as were available and comparable in each country. The OECD is a group of 30 industrialised nations founded in 1948 to develop economic and social policy. All its member states are based on representative democracy and have a free market economy; together they account for two-thirds of the world's goods and services (UNICEF 2007). In the report, each country is scored on six dimensions of well-being broadly corresponding to sections of the United Nations Convention on the Rights of the Child (1989): material well-being, health and safety, education, family and peer relationships, behaviours and risks, and subjective well-being (see Table 1.1). By well-being UNICEF means the following:

> When we attempt to measure children's well-being what we really seek to know is whether children are adequately clothed and housed and fed and protected, whether their circumstances are such that they are likely to become all that they are capable of becoming.

Above all we seek to know whether children feel loved, cherished, special and supported within the family and community, and whether the family and community are being supported in this task by public policy and resources (UNICEF 2007).

The UNICEF report shows the UK and USA faring poorly on almost all measures of child well-being. The average score of these countries puts them at the bottom of a league of 21 rich nations for which enough comparable data were available. Ireland and Canada are in the middle third of the table; no suitable data were available for Australia or New Zealand (see Table 1.1). Findings from the UNICEF 2007 report are summarised here together with comments from a 2009 report on child well-being and

Table 1.1 Summary of the Findings of a UNICEF (2007) Report Regarding Six Dimensions of Child Well-being in 21 Rich Countries

	Average Ranking	1*	2*	3*	4*	5*	6*
Netherlands	4.2	10	2	6	3	3	1
Sweden	5.0	1	1	5	15	1	7
Finland	7.3	3	3	4	17	6	11
Spain	8.0	12	5	16	8	5	2
Switzerland	8.0	5	9	14	4	10	6
Denmark	8.2	4	4	8	9	12	12
Norway	8.3	2	8	9	10	13	8
Belgium	10.0	7	12	1	5	19	16
Italy	10.0	14	6	20	1	9	10
Ireland	10.2	19	19	7	7	4	5
Germany	11.2	13	11	10	13	11	9
Greece	11.8	15	18	17	11	7	3
Canada	12.0	6	14	2	18	17	15
France	12.5	9	7	15	12	14	18
Poland	12.5	21	16	3	14	2	19
Czech Republic	12.7	11	10	11	19	8	17
Austria	13.7	8	20	19	16	15	4
Portugal	14.0	16	15	21	2	16	14
Hungary	14.5	20	17	13	6	18	13
United States**	18.0	17	21	12	20	20	–
UK	18.5	18	13	18	21	21	20

Source: Adapted from UNICEF (2007).
These 21 OECD countries had sufficient comparable data to be included in the table; nine others (Australia, Iceland, Japan, Luxemburg, Mexico, New Zealand, the Slovak Republic, South Korea and Turkey) did not.
*Each number denotes a dimension of well-being: 1: Material well-being; 2: Health and safety; 3: Educational well-being; 4: Family and peer relationships; 5: Behaviour and risks; 6: Subjective well-being.
**The overall ranking for the USA is determined by its average rank over five of the six indicators; insufficient data being available for the 'Subjective well-being' category (see report p. 26).

Top third	Middle third	Bottom third

poverty in Britain, which addresses similar issues (Child Poverty Action Group, CPAG, 2009).

The effort to measure and monitor child well-being is recent. The available data still vary across countries. This UNICEF Report Card (2007) is more detailed and complete than previous ones but there are still gaps and inadequacies. One of these is the prevalence of data regarding mainstream children (those who live at home and go to a standard school) over data about vulnerable and excluded children: those with disabilities, those who do not go to school, those from ethnic minorities, refugees and children brought up in institutions. However, efforts are now being made to develop representative indicators of child well-being and to collect comparable data across the world.

Indicator 1: material well-being

Poverty was assessed by combining indicators of relative income poverty, unemployment and deprivation. It is well documented that poverty affects child well-being in multiple ways, particularly if it is prolonged (Bradshaw and Mayhew 2005). Children brought up in poverty are more vulnerable to poor health, learning and behavioural difficulties, underachievement, low aspirations, teenage pregnancy, low skill levels, low-paid jobs and unemployment. This does not mean that many children brought up in poverty as it is defined here will inevitably experience these negative outcomes but it does mean that poverty is a serious disadvantage.

In 4 of the 21 countries considered, less than 5% of children live in relative income poverty (a certain percentage below national median income); in 9 countries, less than 10% do; but in the UK, Ireland and the USA more than 15% of children live in poverty. In March 1999, the UK government committed itself to eradicating child poverty by 2020 and there has been progress (Bradshaw 2005); the CPAG argues that policy is going in the right direction, but that it needs to take much more radical action (CPAG 2009). Layard and Dunn (2009) find that child poverty in Britain is at an unacceptably high level for such an economically advanced nation.

Some countries score better on child well-being than other wealthier nations (the Czech Republic for instance). This leads UNICEF (2007) to state that no 'obvious relationship' (p. 3) exists between child well-being and a nation's GDP per head of population. The CPAG report, however, maintains that a relationship does exist, although countries can buck this trend (CPAG 2009). A relationship is evident between social inequality and well-being: more equal societies score higher on well-being (CPAG 2009).

Indicator 2: health and safety

The health and safety of children in today's developed countries has improved considerably and quickly, taking the rate of children dying before the age of five in Europe from 20% to 1% in a century. Nevertheless, there are differences between countries: this is the UK's strongest indicator (nearly reaching the mean score of the 25 countries entered) and the USA and New Zealand's poorest; Ireland is in the bottom third.

Indicator 3: education

This was measured through achievements in reading, maths and science, the proportion of children staying in school beyond the age of 15 and the ratio of those not in education, employment or training between the ages of 15 and 19. It is an important measure of child welfare: much of children's lives are spent in school and the outcome of their studies is likely to have an impact on their future. In OECD countries, the ordinary business of life (work, home, finance, citizenship) requires increasingly complex skills. Those who leave education too soon will be at increasing disadvantage, risking exclusion and marginalisation.

Twenty-four countries are listed: Ireland does well on this measure, the USA is midrange and the UK scores poorly. Both the USA and UK have a substantial proportion of citizens without general education or vocational competence (Layard and Dunn 2009). Poland, with a low GDP per capita, scores very well.

Comparable data across countries were only found for young people aged 15 and over. However, with regard to the UK, the Children's Society reports that literacy and numeracy in primary schools increased in the 1990s but the standard of individual schools varies greatly in relation to social deprivation (Layard and Dunn 2009).

Indicator 4: family and peer relationships

This is a dimension of life important to children and young people but it is difficult to measure and the data are more limited than for other indicators. It is particularly relevant here because the quality of relationships has a bearing on children's mental health, as we will see in the next section.

This indicator was measured through family structure (percentage of single parent and stepfamilies), family relationships (percentage of children eating with their parents more than once a week and spending time talking to them) and peer relationships (percentage of 11- to 15-year olds finding their peers kind and helpful).

The USA and the UK have the highest level of single and step-parent families. The CPAG claims that no association exists between this and child well-being (CPAG 2009) but the UNICEF report links it to greater risk to well-being. Family break-up has been shown to increase the proportion of academically underachieving children and children with emotional problems by about 50% (Pryor and Rogers 2001) but most parents underestimate this (Layard and Dunn 2009).

In many countries, children seem to eat with their parents several times a week but a much smaller number report talking regularly to their parents, with only 3 out of 21 countries above 70%. The USA, the UK and Ireland are in the top half of the table. However, just over 40% of children in the UK regard their peers as being 'generally kind and helpful', which is the bottom of the league.

Indicator 5: behaviours and risks

This section of the report uses data on health (eating breakfast and fruit every day, taking exercise, being overweight) for which most countries do not stray far from the average, apart from Poland which is much better than average and the USA which is much worse because of high obesity levels. Risk behaviours consist of smoking, drugs and alcohol misuse, sexual risk-taking and teenage pregnancy. The UK does particularly badly here: it is at the bottom of the table and considerably worse than the next nearest country. The USA and Canada, while better, are in the bottom five countries. Experience of violence is the last measure: it includes all forms of violence: bullying, fighting, abuse and indirect experience of violence such as domestic abuse. In 2003, UNICEF reported that in some industrialised nations, 6.5% of children experienced serious maltreatment (UNICEF 2003).

Indicator 6: subjective well-being

Here the focus is on children's own perception of their health, school life and personal well-being. Overall, countries seem to differ significantly, the lowest ranking being the UK. Canada is below average, Ireland over average and insufficient data is available for the USA. Between 5% and 10% of young people said they felt out of place, left out of things, awkward or lonely.

The findings reported by UNICEF make clear that economic success does not imply well-being for a nation's children. It is interesting to measure the wide variations in child well-being across industrialised nations highlighted in the report against the collective commitment of the

United Nations Convention on the Rights of the Child. Complementing national research with evidence culled from comparisons with other similar nations may make the impact of transnational factors clearer and help us isolate factors of success.

 Activity

Read the UNICEF Report Card 7 on Child Well-being in Rich Countries (UNICEF 2007) which you can find on the Internet.

Make a list of the findings which surprise you positively and those which surprise you negatively. Discuss this with a colleague or a friend and compare your views.

1.3 Children and young people's mental health

Well-being and mental health

Well-being, which we have just defined and discussed, is a broader concept than mental health but the two are related: impaired mental health impacts on children's overall well-being and lack of well-being of whatever kind acts as a risk to mental health. In this section we shall examine what being mentally healthy means for children and young people, what factors in their lives may endanger their mental health and, conversely, what factors may protect their mental health and promote resilience. Some young people develop mental health problems or disorders: we shall define these terms and discuss current trends, what some see as a worrying increase in the prevalence of mental ill health amongst children and young people.

Good mental health is more than the absence of diagnosable mental health problems; it relates to and is interdependent with general well-being. In a young person, good mental health involves the capacity to develop in the following dimensions:

■ Physically, emotionally, intellectually and spiritually;
■ Intra-personally, it means finding an identity, a sense of mastery over self and life, and being resilient; it includes confidence, positive self-esteem and assertiveness; the ability to play and learn and finding pleasure in doing so; a sense of purpose and belonging, and a grasp of the difference between right and wrong;
■ Inter-personally, it comprises becoming aware of others and empathising with them and the ability to enter into and sustain mutually satisfying personal relationships (Health Advisory Service, HAS, 1995)

A large number of personal, physical, behavioural, social, economic, cultural and environmental determinants contribute to mental health and mental well-being (World Health Organization 2004b, Cattan and Tilford 2006).

Mental health problems are difficulties and disabilities experienced in the areas outlined in this definition. They may arise from genetic or environmental factors; the latter may be personal to the child, originate in the child's family or in the wider context.

Risk and protective factors

The origin of mental health difficulties in children and young people is complex and multifactorial. Factors which predispose a child to developing mental health problems – risk factors – are negative dimensions in the child's life, such as a poor self-esteem, an ill parent or living in poverty. The more risk factors there are, the greater the stress on the child. Positive factors, on the other hand, are strengths which protect a child from mental health problems or mitigate the effect of stress, like a high self-esteem, a secure attachment or a supportive social network. Risk and protective factors can be classified into three categories: those belonging to the individual child's biological and personality make-up, those from the child's family and those from other social environments (see Table 1.2). The family makes a prominent contribution to children's well-being in its own right, but it also facilitates their access to positive opportunities outside the family and plays a part in mitigating the negative effects of other social environments (Sameroff 2006).

The balance of risk and protective factors adds up like a balance sheet which, if the negatives are too high, can take a young person over a stress tolerance threshold. This model goes some way towards explaining the causal pathway of mental ill health but the picture is somewhat more complex. Carr (2006) stresses the presence of precipitating factors, such as an illness, bereavement or incident of bullying, which trigger the onset of a problem or exacerbate it. Maintaining factors perpetuate a problem instead of promoting its resolution (see Table 1.2).

Some risk factors have been shown to be predictive of mental health problems on their own. For example, in a study investigating the simultaneous impact of child, family and neighbourhood factors on diagnosed psychiatric disorders, Ford et al. (2004) found that children with a physical illness, a low intelligence quotient (IQ) or reading difficulties were more likely than most to develop a mental health problem. Other factors have been shown to be independently linked to specific disorders. Ford et al. (2004) again showed that parents with

Table 1.2 Factors Influencing Children and Young People's Mental Health

	Risk Factors (predispose a child to developing problems)	Precipitating Factors (Usually Life Events) (trigger the onset or recurrence of problems)	Maintaining Factors (perpetuate problems once they have started)	Protective Factors (support a child's mental health under stress)
Personal	■ Genetic handicap ■ Difficult perinatal history ■ Early ill health ■ Low intelligence ■ Difficult temperament ■ Poor self-esteem	■ Illness/Injury ■ Changing house or school ■ Loss of a friendship ■ The advent of a new developmental phase (e.g. adolescence)	■ Biological factors ■ High anxiety ■ Early life difficulties ■ Maladaptive and immature coping strategies ■ Cognitive distortions about self, others and the environment ■ Learning difficulties	■ Good physical health ■ Intellectual ability ■ Easy temperament ■ High self-esteem ■ Positive adjustment
Family	■ Insecure attachment ■ Chronic family stress ■ Poor parenting ■ Parental substance misuse and mental health problems ■ Family conflict and violence ■ Parental separation ■ Institutional upbringing ■ Abuse and neglect	■ A birth or bereavement ■ Parental separation ■ Parent becoming unemployed ■ Abuse	■ Difficult parent–child relationship ■ Insecure attachment ■ Family ill health, stresses and conflicts ■ Parental separation ■ Abuse and neglect	■ Secure attachment ■ Responsive parenting ■ Good parental adjustment ■ Clear/direct communication ■ Good parental relationship ■ Father involvement

(Continued)

Table 1.2 (Continued)

	Risk Factors (predispose a child to developing problems)	Precipitating Factors (Usually Life Events) (trigger the onset or recurrence of problems)	Maintaining Factors (perpetuate problems once they have started)	Protective Factors (support a child's mental health under stress)
Environmental	■ Lack of social support ■ Deviant peer group ■ Negative school experience ■ Community problems ■ Low socio-economic status	■ Sudden adverse community conditions	■ Socio-economic disadvantage ■ Contextual stresses at school or in the community	■ High social support ■ Low community stress ■ Positive school ■ Supportive peer group ■ High socio-economic status

common mental health disorders were more likely to have children with anxiety or behavioural problems; being older, poor general health and adverse life events were strongly associated with depression whereas lone parenting and adverse life events correlated with anxiety and neuro-developmental disorders. However, some factors were not independently associated with mental disorders, such as school and neighbourhood disadvantage, social class, household income, parental employment or marital status and family size. This means that their role in the causal pathway is less significant than that of independently linked factors.

However, other studies suggest that it is also the accumulation of factors rather than one factor on its own that is the most detrimental (Rutter *et al.* 1975, Rutter 2006). From studies using different risk factors, there is compelling evidence that the more risk factors there are, the worse the outcome is for the child, no matter which risk factors are involved (Sameroff 2006). Risk factors tend to cluster so that children often experience many and recurring risk factors (such as poverty, lone parenting, lack of social support and so on). Multiple risk factors affect children's IQ as well as their mental health.

Resilience

A child with more positive factors is likely to show greater resilience in the face of stress than a child who has fewer of them. Resilience is a concept akin to positive mental health and social competence but Rutter (2006) stresses its interactive nature: resilience is present when a child comes out relatively well of negative experiences. Resilience does not simply equal the balance between risk and protective influences (which would be similar for all children); it takes into account children's individual variations in response to the same stresses. Not only are there many contributors to children's mental ill health, but individual children react to the same contributors in their own specific way.

The more precise our knowledge about the causal pathways of mental health problems and disorders is, the better targeted our health and social care interventions can be.

Problems and disorders

In studies of children and young people's mental health, a distinction is often drawn between mental health problems and mental disorders. We must bear in mind that 'disorder' is a term many young people dislike because of its psychiatric connotations and stigmatising effect (Street and

Herts 2005). The distinction is nevertheless useful to make sense of statistical data.

The term 'mental disorder' (World Health Organization 1992) implies a 'clinically recognisable set of symptoms or behaviours associated in most cases with considerable distress and substantial interference with personal function' (Meltzer *et al.* 2000: 1). The term 'mental health problem' is broader and includes 'a very broad range of emotional or behavioural difficulties, which may cause concern or distress' (Health Advisory Service 1995: 15). It can be helpful to think of problems and disorders as being on a continuum.

With regard to trends, it has been estimated that around 20–25% of children and young people have mental health problems at some time during their childhood (Mental Health Foundation 1999, Jané-Llopis and Braddick 2008). Statistics based on mental disorders are more conservative (see Table 1.3). After analysing the 2004 census data for children aged 5–16 in Britain, Green *et al.* (2005) reported a prevalence of mental disorders of about 10% (see Table 1.4). Five to 10-year-old boys had almost twice as many mental disorders as girls, due to the high ratio of conduct disorders, Autistic Spectrum Disorders (ASD) and Attention Deficit Hyperactivity Disorders (ADHD) amongst boys; in the 11–16 age group, boys still had more mental disorders than girls for the same reasons but proportionally less so because of the rise in emotional disorders (particularly anxiety and depression) amongst girls. The chances of a child developing a mental disorder increased with being a boy, being older, being white, being part of a reconstituted family and coming from a low socio-economic background.

Fonagy *et al.* (2002) and Green *et al.* (2005) highlight a convergence of research results that indicate higher rates of mental disorders in adolescents than in children. This is partly due to the increase in psychotic

Table 1.3 Prevalence of Mental Disorders for 5- to 16-Year Old Children

Disorder		Percentage
Emotional disorder		3.7
Anxiety	3.3	
Depression	0.9	
Conduct disorders		5.8
Hyperkinetic disorders (ICD-10)		1.5
Less common disorders		1.3
ASD	0.9	
Eating disorders	0.3	
Total		**9.6**

Source: From Green *et al.* (2005). Crown Copyright 2005.

Table 1.4 Prevalence of Mental Disorders by Age and Sex

Disorder	5- to 10-Year Olds			11- to 16-Year Olds			All Children		
	Boys	Girls	All	Boys	Girls	All	Boys	Girls	All
Emotional	2.2	2.5	2.4	4	6.1	5	3.1	4.3	3.7
Conduct	6.9	2.8	4.9	8	5.1	6.6	7.5	3.9	5.8
HKD	2.7	0.4	1.6	2.4	0.4	1.4	2.6	0.4	1.5
Less common	2.2	0.4	1.3	1.6	1.1	1.4	1.9	0.8	1.3
Total	**10.2**	**5.1**	**7.7**	**12.6**	**10.3**	**11.5**	**11.4**	**7.8**	**9.6**

Source: From Green *et al.* (2005). Crown Copyright 2005.

disorders which are very rare before puberty, but not exclusively so since Green *et al.* (2005) did not include psychoses in their analysis. There is evidence that psychosocial disorders are rising in adolescents in Western countries (Rutter and Smith 1995, Collishaw *et al.* 2004). Collishaw and colleagues (2004) compared data collected in Britain by similar methods in 1974, 1986 and 1999 and reported a substantial increase in conduct and emotional disorders, although not in hyperactivity disorders. They stress that the causes for this are not clear but they point to social changes in family structure, economic conditions and youth culture as potentially fruitful directions for further research.

In a West of Scotland study of 15-year olds' psychological distress surveyed 12 years apart (1987 and 1999), West and Sweeting (2003) found that the mental health of this age group appeared to have deteriorated. The most striking result was that the rate of psychological distress had almost doubled for the girls, particularly those of middle-class backgrounds. This suggests the appearance of new stressors. Because the increase in worry coincided with the approach of national examinations, the authors muse that girls' academic success may bring them more stress than confidence, but also that educational stressors come to join other, typically female stressors (the pressure on middle-class girls to be both clever and attractive has often been noted).

A well-known group of young people vulnerable to mental distress comprises those looked after by local authorities, particularly those brought up in institutions. Yet this is a group often excluded from epidemiological data because of its unstable engagement with schools and other social groups where surveys take place. A British study comparing looked-after children and children from private households aged 5–17 found that those looked after by local authorities had a higher prevalence of educational and neuro-developmental difficulties than those from private households; they also had the highest prevalence of most psychiatric disorders. Furthermore, only 9% of those without a psychiatric disorder showed good adjustment (fewer than one in ten), against 47% of children in private households (around one in two) (Ford *et al.* 2007).

In summary, mental health in children and young people means more than the absence of mental difficulties. In most cases when these arise, their causes are complex and include a number of factors, some of which are specific to the child, others attributable to the family and wider environment. Other factors in a young person's life affect the resolution of these difficulties: some help and some hinder a return to mental health.

Statistical analysis of national and international epidemiological data suggests changing trends in children and young people's mental difficulties in industrialised countries. There seems to be an increase in specific disorders, particularly in some social groups such as boys raised in deprived socio-economic circumstances, children raised in the care of local authorities and middle-class adolescent girls. A more systematic collection of epidemiological data in OECD countries in forthcoming years could help us understand what affects children and young people's mental health and how to reverse some downward trends.

   Activity

Think of some children and young people you know who have mental health difficulties of some kind or another.

Can you work out factors which may have increased their vulnerability to mental health problems?

Are there protective and maintaining factors in these children or young people's lives?

Are they within a known at-risk group?

1.4   'Every Child Matters': What can we do to help?

'Every Child Matters' (2003) is the name of a programme of change designed to improve the lives of all children and young people in England and Wales. (see website www.dcsf.gov.uk/everychildmatters/). The report 'It's Everyone's Job to Make Sure I'm All Right' (Scottish Executive 2002a) makes recommendations for better child protection in Scotland. Such titles testify to the good intentions of governments to do the best they can for children and young people. Yet it seems clear that progress remains to be made and that we may even be going in the wrong direction: our culture appears to be causing children and young people growing stress and unhappiness.

As the Scottish report title suggests, it is everyone's job to look out for children. So how can we promote well-being and mental health for all children, prevent mental health problems in vulnerable groups and intervene to support and help those who develop mental health problems and disorders?

Promoting mental health and preventing mental ill health

It is important to improve the conditions of children and young people's mental health for their sake, but also because we know that the quality of people's mental health in childhood affects their mental health in adulthood (Rutter 1996); promoting children and young people's mental health also promotes the future mental health of the population as a whole.

The World Health Organization defines mental health promotion thus:

> *Mental health promotion aims to promote positive mental health by increasing psychological well-being, competence and resilience, and by creating supportive living conditions and environments* (World Health Organization 2004b: 17).

Mental health promotion is a broad umbrella term for activities which aim to address the determinants of health (the risk, protective and maintaining factors discussed earlier) in order to enhance the mental health of the population. These determinants are many: physical, psychological, social and cultural, economic and environmental. They can and must be addressed at both micro-levels (individual, family and neighbourhood) and macro-levels (national and international).

Mental health promotion focuses primarily on positive health and mental well-being for all, but it also includes preventive strategies targeted at groups known to be at risk of mental ill health (e.g. young people brought up in institutions); the quest to live well, even in the presence of mental illness (for instance the 'recovery' approach, inspired by people with lived experience of mental illness), can be seen as an aspect of mental health promotion (Scottish Executive 2003, O'Hagan 2009).

Good health promotion is based on certain principles: Cattan and Tilford (2006) argue that it must be holistic and participatory, respect cultural diversity, promote positive health as well as prevent ill health and target both social structures and individual lives.

How do these generalities apply to children and young people? Earlier in this chapter, we discussed the impact of globalisation on industrialised countries and the consequences of post-war culture on the mental health of these societies. Some of the political and business decisions we make seem to compromise rather than enhance the mental health of children and young people (World Health Organization 2005). Layard and Dunn (2009) stressed the impact of individualism and consumerism. Can health promotion strategies contribute to reversing this process?

In our rapidly changing cultures, a growing number of young people appear to experience an acute sense of alienation and impermanence, to lack cultural certainty and guidelines and to have difficulty finding meaning for their lives and an identity for themselves (Arnett 2002). However, current research also points to what may help these young people: positive mental health is associated with a sense of belonging, co-operation and trust, sometimes called social capital (De Silva *et al.* 2005, World Health Organization 2004b). So macro-interventions to maintain and enhance social capital would make an impact on the mental health of children and young people (Rowling 2006). There are other key societal determinants of mental health, such as culture, poverty and mental health inequalities. They too need broad social interventions. To have a broad enough impact, these strategies have to be implemented by cross-sector partnerships between the public, private and voluntary sectors, and by collaboration between health, housing, finance and education departments, at local, national and international levels. Currently however, macro-interventions are much less common than micro-interventions, and evidence of their efficacy is scarce (Cattan and Tilford 2006).

At present, health promotion strategies are more likely to be targeted and preventive than broad and universal; yet addressing mental health risk factors by encouraging change in target individuals and families can be unfair. Rowling (2006) expresses concern at the current emphasis on individual resilience as central to good mental health, and on social and emotional learning programmes (such as emotional literacy or parent training) as key interventions to support it, good as those may be, because this approach expects individuals and families to provide for their own health whereas several major determinants, such as health inequalities, are outside their control.

Socio-economic status, gender, disability and ethnicity all contribute to mental health inequalities. If not redressed in childhood, inequalities in health are likely to extend into later life (Tilford 2006). Poverty has an impact on every aspect of children and young people's well-being, regardless of whether definitions of absolute or relative poverty are used; therefore reducing poverty is essential to improving children's mental well-being (CPAG 2009). Several wealthy countries come off badly in the UNICEF (2007) report, yet this can be reversed if the welfare of children is given priority in policy making: the CPAG (2009) recommends urgent investment in low-income families.

Tilford (2006) recommends local policies to implement socially supportive, inclusive environments for schools and youth groups and broader interventions nationally, such as child-friendly policies, child-inclusive legislation, participative and inclusive practices and resource allocation to support them. This includes support for parents, teachers, youth and community workers and health and social care staff because children's environments need to be physically and emotionally safe and the carers are key to achieving this aim (Rowling 2006).

With regard to targeted health promotion, Rowling (2006) recommends focus on the life events we know to undermine children and young people's mental health: conflict and violence in relationships, families, communities and nations (such as bullying, domestic violence, racism, street warfare, wars and natural disasters) and loss, such as parental separation, death and bereavements. Layard and Dunn (2009) lay particular emphasis on reducing conflict in family life:

> *Nothing is more important than this: if parents gave more priority to maintaining their feelings for each other, this would do more for children than much of the rest of what they do for their children* (Layard and Dunn 2009: 27).

To summarise, promoting mental health comprises both strategies aimed at whole populations and preventive schemes targeting specific groups. The wider determinants of health, such as culture, poverty and health inequalities, need a combination of both to be effective – although currently the targeted, preventive approaches are more common. To redress some of the unwanted effects of the lifestyle of rich nations on children, young people and families' mental health, a determined and internationally collaborative effort will be necessary.

 Activity

Identify a current national health-promoting or public health strategy aimed at influencing the mental health of all children, young people and families.

- Find the policy document that launched it and its rationale.
- Use existing scientific and professional literature to critique this strategy.
- Do the same with a current preventing scheme targeted at a specific at-risk children or young people's group.

Assessing and intervening

Those in the best position to recognise the presence of mental health difficulties in children and young people are in the community: carers in families, schools and health centres; parents, teachers, general practitioners (GPs), nurses, educational psychologists, youth workers and social workers; it is important that they are trained to identify signs of mental health problems.

When a young person develops symptoms of distress, any of these carers may refer a child to Child and Adolescent Mental Health Services (CAMHS); these services will use their expertise to assess the problem and suggest possible interventions. In this section, general points only will be considered because the assessment of, and possible interventions for, specific problems are the object of other chapters.

A comprehensive assessment will involve several members of a multi-disciplinary team. In order to understand the problem and its possible determinants, a fulsome picture of the family's environment needs to be available: the assessors must enquire about socio-economic conditions, ethnicity, neighbourhood, employment, school and other factors of potential significance in the environment. The family's origin and membership (one or two parents, own, step, adoptive or foster children); the child's relationships (with the main carers and other adults, with peers, at home, school and in other settings); the young person's learning abilities and environment; the family's links with the neighbourhood and the parents' ability to cope are all relevant information.

Although a child or adolescent may be the 'identified patient' the young person's difficulties may be one way of drawing attention to problems in the family or with other family members, such as relationship problems between the parents or a sick sibling.

Children and young people entrusted to the care of a local authority often belong to complex networks made of their family of origin as well as other carers, such as a social worker. Some do not live with a family but in a residential setting. Assessing the links between these systems of care and the contribution they make to the child's support and/or difficulties is important (Claveirole et al. 2006, YoungMinds 2006).

When the assessing team has reviewed the child's problems and the factors which have contributed to them, there comes a point when a working hypothesis of what is happening, why it is happening and how it might be helped can be formulated:

> *A formulation is a mini-theory that explains why the presenting problems developed, why they persist, what protective factors either prevent them from becoming worse or may be enlisted to solve the presenting problems* (Carr 2006: 135).

It is desirable for the formulation to make sense to the family, to other carers, the referrer and the young person, as well as to the assessing team. If the formulation does not make sense to them, they are unlikely fully to co-operate with the intervention. From the formulation, an intervention plan can be devised.

Important aspects of all interventions (see also Claveirole *et al.* 2006)

Consultation and participation

Children and young people are entitled to participate in their assessment and treatment, to give their views of what is going on in their lives and to share their feelings about it (United Nations 1989). For this to happen, they need the support of trusted adults who put enough time aside to listen to them and explain what is happening. Information has to be age appropriate to be understood. With good communication, even young children can think about what is going on and share what they would like to see happening (Street and Herts 2005).

Research has shown (Claveirole 2005) that parents whose children are receiving mental health care, particularly when difficulties have been long-standing, need a great deal of help and support from professionals. They want to be listened to and understood, to be advised about the management of their child, to have mental health problems and their treatment explained to them, and to be involved in decisions regarding the young person. There is also evidence that they do not always get this.

Families' experience is that their son's or daughter's mental health problems can seriously disrupt their lives. Parents feel vulnerable and guilty that they have not, somehow, protected their child or that they have perhaps caused the problems. Siblings also need support to understand and cope with what is happening. This means parents and carers need to be involved from the assessment stage onwards. This is not always easy and it takes time.

Informed consent

Children, younger ones in particular, can be brought to a consultation by their parents without understanding why, or what it means. Although parents can consent on behalf of young children, children of all ages need to know who you are, why they are seeing you and what the purpose of the meeting is. They must give their own consent to it. So when you meet a child or a young person for the first time, it is important to check what they know and what they understand about their presence in the service and to go on involving them from then on.

The consent children and young people and their families give to the therapeutic process is not a static thing and it may need ongoing discussion. It is the basis of all collaborative work.

The therapeutic relationship

Children and young people are likely to behave towards staff members in the way that they have been used to behaving with adults close to them. In this way (rather than by telling you directly), they reveal a lot about their inner world, their ability to trust and the kind of anxieties they have. This can be put to therapeutic use by helping the child or young person make sense of the way they relate.

Attachment theory suggests that children need to establish a secure bond with their primary carers in their early childhood in order to have the confidence to explore the world around them (see Chapter 3). Children's natural attachment needs make separations sensitive times which have to be handled with age-appropriate care. Young children need to have their carers close by them much of the time and they need access to familiar comforting objects to help them manage absence. However, these needs do not stop with early childhood: older children and adolescents need health care staff to be mindful of the importance and uniqueness of interpersonal relationships. This applies to family carers but it also applies to the therapeutic relationships between staff and children or young people. If a child trusts a member of staff, issues of attachment, separation and loss within that relationship deserve attention. Children and young people must have key staff members to relate to who are available, consistent and predictable; they need time to attach and time to separate from significant workers, therefore beginnings and endings must be managed sensitively.

It is important to remember that young children's perception of reality can be very different from that of adults and to remain open to children's way of thinking and the strength of their feelings. They may not be what we would expect.

When a child or young person comes to be referred to a specialist service because mental health difficulties have developed, generic standards of good practice apply to their assessment and treatment as well as the more problem-specific approaches which will be discussed in other chapters.

✎ **Activity**

Think of a specific child with mental health difficulties that you know.

■ Has a comprehensive assessment been carried out?
■ What is your evidence for thinking this?

If you work with children or young people who have mental health problems, examine how your work setting takes care of therapeutic relationships with (a) children or young people and (b) their parents.

1.5 Conclusion

The mental health of children and young people depends on many factors: personal, psychological and social. Some personal factors are genetic in origin but many determinants of mental health are cultural, and some contemporary risk factors are highlighted in this chapter. Trends in the mental difficulties presented by children and young people today appear to be changing and, for some groups at least, to be worsening. The Children's Society report (Layard and Dunn 2009) proposes in its conclusion a number of social changes to improve the conditions of children and young people's lives, such as valuing social relationships over the pursuit of individual success, promoting social values of trust and respect, reducing educational failure, working towards the elimination of child poverty and supporting family stability and parenting skills.

Recommended reading

Carr, A. (2006). *The Handbook of Child and Adolescent Clinical Psychology: A Contextual Approach*, 2nd edition. London: Routledge.

Cattan, M. and Tilford, S. (2006). *Mental Health Promotion: A Lifespan Approach*. Berkshire: Open University Press, McGraw-Hill Education.

Claveirole, A., Gaughan, M., Hindle, D. and Wrate, R. (2006). *New-to-CAMHS Teaching Package*. HeadsUpScotland, Scotland: National Project for Children and Young people's Mental Health. Available at http://www.nes.scot.nhs.uk/mentalhealth/publications/documents/NewToCAMHS-FINAL.pdf.

Helliwell, J. F. (2008). *Life Satisfaction and Quality of Development*. National Bureau of Economic Research (NBER Working Paper 14507, November 2008) Canada: University of British Columbia. Available at www.econ.ubc.ca/helliwell/.

Layard, R. and Dunn, J. (2009). *A Good Childhood Searching for Values in a Competitive Age*. London: The Children's Society, Penguin.

UNICEF (2007). *Child Poverty in Perspective: An Overview of Child Well-being in Rich Countries Innocenti Report Card 7, UNICEF*. Florence, Italy: Innocenti Research Centre. Available at http://www.unicef.org.uk/publications/pdf/rc7_eng.pdf.

Chapter 2
THE FAMILY

Duncan Tennant[1] and Anne Claveirole[2]

[1]*Department of Psychiatry, St John's Hospital, Livingston, West Lothian, Scotland*
[2]*School of Nursing, Midwifery and Social Care, Edinburgh Napier University, Edinburgh, Scotland*

2.1 Introduction

The family is the natural environment in which children and young people grow up. It is the smallest social unit and it is entrusted with raising the next generation. Families play an important part in promoting the mental health of children and young people: this becomes immediately apparent when we know that children brought up in institutions are among the most at risk of developing mental health problems (Ford *et al.* 2007). However, some families struggle to give children the attention, support and control they need and the well-being of these children suffers. Conversely, a child's difficulties, with autistic spectrum disorder say, or attention deficit hyperactivity disorder, often have a detrimental effect on other family members. Therefore, it is important to take the family into account when trying to understand children and young people's mental health.

In this chapter we will explore how families function, how they develop over time and what their structure looks like. To do this, we will use frameworks and concepts drawn from the practice of family therapy. Then we will discuss ways in which health and social care staff can work with families to support them or to help them change in order to be more effective protectors of children's mental health.

For general texts on working with families, you might want to refer to, among others, Whyte (1997), Wright and Leahey (2000) or Carr (2000).

Understanding Children and Young People's Mental Health, first edition. Edited by Anne Claveirole and Martin Gaughan. Published 2011 by John Wiley & Sons Ltd. © 2011 John Wiley & Sons Ltd.

Learning outcomes

After studying this chapter, you should be able to:

1. Discuss what 'normal' might mean with regard to family life, family functioning and structural aspects of the family.
2. Explain why it is important to see family life in a multi-generational perspective and analyse the phases of the family life cycle using your own life as an example.
3. Explore more recent developments in the theory and practice of working with families.
4. Understand the importance of attachment theory in understanding the family.
5. Contrast the behaviours which parent education programmes aim to encourage in parent and child with the behaviours these programmes aim to discourage.

2.2   What is 'normal' family functioning?

The family therapist Carl Whitaker relates a story of interviewing a normal family in front of a panel of family therapists and 1,500 observers. The overwhelming majority of the audience saw the family as highly dysfunctional and pleaded with Whitaker to provide therapy for them, expressing the fear that the consequences would be dire for all family members if he did not. The family were not offered therapy and several years later were interviewed again by Whitaker who discovered that none of the audience's predictions had come true. This story illustrates the tendency of family therapists to look for dysfunction where it does not necessarily exist. Perhaps a useful place to begin exploring the application of family therapy ideas is with a discussion of what normal and abnormal family functioning means.

In her book on family processes, Walsh (2003) takes up the challenge of defining family normality and this section draws on chapter 1 of Walsh's book. In the context of the unprecedented social changes of recent decades, the patterns of family life have also changed. Walsh (2003: 4) stresses that our concepts must take account of 'the changing views of changing families in a changing world' because what we call normal is a social construction, influenced by culture-based values. There is a danger that by declaring some family processes 'normal' and others 'abnormal', we stigmatise and marginalise those who do not fit these norms.

Functional and dysfunctional

Something functional is something that works; a family that works is a family that carries out its essential tasks, which consist in supporting the growth and well-being of its members, particularly nurturing and protecting those who are vulnerable, such as children and older people (Walsh 2003). This is assessed in the context of the family's own beliefs about what is normal, its stage in the life cycle and other circumstances. Rather than labelling a family as dysfunctional, an alternative is to label a family life *pattern* as dysfunctional. Dysfunctional patterns are associated with signs of distress (Walsh 2003). A pattern may be functional (i.e. work well) for one person or part of the family but costly or dysfunctional for another. For example, the pattern of family activities at the weekend may be highly functional for the children, who have interesting hobbies, but costly for the parents' relationship if the parents do not have enough time to spend together because they ferry the children to their various activities. The interface of the family with other social systems must also be included in any assessment because of their impact on the family's functioning. For example, employment patterns may be functional for the workplace but not for the family if parents have to work late and cannot spend enough time with their children.

The traditional family of the past is a myth

It is often said that current family life has been degraded by social changes and that it compares poorly with that of earlier generations. Walsh (2003) challenges this view of things. There is, she says, a romanticised notion of what the traditional family used to be, based on folklore transmitted through the media and reflecting a longing for a happier, simpler life (Walsh 2003). The multi-generational households of the past did not have an easy time; they were prey to many hazards: unplanned pregnancies, high child mortality and untimely adult deaths meant that intact families were much less common than they are today. In those days, life was more precarious and individual needs were subordinated to the survival of the family. Society and family were patriarchal structures; mothers did less mothering and more work; children were not given a qualitatively different status from adults: they were simply at the bottom of the social hierarchy and were often subjected to hard labour (Walsh 1993).

The nuclear family of modern time is also a myth

The nuclear family model of family life came out of the post-war period in Western democracies and was relatively short-lived; it was mainly white and middle class; although it has been idealised, it is now less common

(Walsh 2003). The postmodern family has replaced it, bringing a greater variety of family styles, with higher divorce rates, lower birth rates and lower standards of living. Two-thirds of families have dual earners and most mothers work. Most divorcees remarry. According to US statistics, divorce and remarriage affect just under 50% of first marriages (Bramlett and Mosher 2001). More people live on their own; young people often take longer to leave the family home for financial reasons, and postpone marriage and parenthood. Many adults live in a cohabiting relationship at some time in their lives; some of these are between same-sex partners. A growing number of couples are multi-racial and multi-faiths (Walsh 2003). Single parent households are common: whereas 1 in 14 children lived in single parent families in 1972, in 2008 it is 1 in 4 (Family and Parenting Institute 2009, Lavis 2010). Even in the current upheaval in family life patterns, however, a loving committed relationship remains seen as the cornerstone of happiness and family life (Walsh 2003). The gap between rich and poor has worsened in the last 20 years (see Chapter 1) and more families live in poverty (National Equality Panel 2010). These negative economic conditions affect the stability and well-being of families, excluding them from full integration into social networks, sometimes leading to conflict and violence, substance misuse, family breakdown and further poverty. Women and children suffer disproportionately (Walsh 2003).

The myth of the proper gender order

The complementary roles of men and women in the family – the 'breadwinner/homemaker' model – used to be functional for society (for the industrial economy of the time), but you could argue that it was dysfunctional for the family because father was peripheral and mother demeaned and overstretched. The nuclear family worsened this situation by increasing the isolation of women. The latter part of the twentieth century saw an increase in mothers having careers yet also keeping the responsibility for 80% of the childcare and domestic tasks (Walsh 2003).

New family challenges

As people live longer, couples are challenged to live together for 50 years or more and families extend over several generations. As they reach their 80s, people increasingly live with chronic illnesses and families have to take on caring responsibilities. Those over 85 are the most vulnerable: about 20% of them may be affected by dementia (Department of Health 2007). New technology and advances in medicine allow us to prolong life at both ends of the lifespan, requiring new ethical questions to be addressed. However, in some impoverished communities, poor health actually shortens the life cycle (Walsh 2003).

/ **Activity**

How does your family compare with the myths of family life described above?

2.3 The family life cycle

The family life cycle is a developmental way of looking at families; it provides a context for the individual development of family members and overlaps with it; it is also influenced by socio-cultural developments outside the family. When working with families, it is important to bring a life cycle perspective to what is happening. Carter and McGoldrick's work with families has been influential and this section is based on it (Carter and McGoldrick 1999). They stress the importance of assessing a family's development and using therapeutic interventions to re-establish its developmental momentum.

The family as a system moving through time

Carter and McGoldrick (1999) remind us that the family is unique in that members can only join through birth, adoption or marriage, and members can only leave through death. Business organisations can fire dysfunctional members or members can resign if they do not like the way the system is operating. Not so with the family. Families have a shared history and a shared future. When the unfolding of the family life cycle is interrupted, signs of distress and dysfunction are likely to appear.

The multi-generational life cycle model

Families comprise the emotional system of three to five generations. Relationships between family members change and the psychological distance between them increases and decreases as they move along the life cycle (Carter and McGoldrick 1999). The multi-generational life cycle model emphasises the connectedness between generations. Family members do not have the option of choosing not to be a part of a family – or not to be shaped by its culture, attitudes, taboos and expectations.

Crises during the life cycle, such as the addition or loss of a family member, cause stress and can give rise to symptoms of dysfunction. The family life cycle varies with cultural groups, even when immigration goes back more than one generation. Carter and McGoldrick (1999) also stress the effect of current events, so that different generations are each under the influence of the historical period through which they have lived (e.g. the Second World War, the 1960s, an economic recession). Each generation has what Carter and McGoldrick (1999) call a 'life-shaping impact' on the next one, while each lives through its own maturational tasks.

Carter and McGoldrick (1999) describe a life cycle model with a horizontal axis (the here and now, as the family deals with problems, stresses and family tragedies) and a vertical axis (family history, which includes family patterns, myths and taboos). Bowen (1978) found that families had a way of reproducing similar patterns of difficulties at the same nodal points over several generations. For example, if the family of origin of one or other spouse had difficulty in dealing with the birth of the first child, there may be problems at the same life cycle stage in the next generation. Where problems on both axes converge, a quantum leap in stress takes place. The addition of social or political stresses, e.g. poverty, will increase stress levels even further.

Families lack a temporal perspective when they are experiencing problems and the use of a life cycle model in therapy can help to restore this perspective of movement through time.

The changing family life cycle

The family life cycle in the late twentieth and early twenty-first centuries differs considerably from earlier versions. For example, the 'empty nest' phase is relatively new and has come because people live longer. Previously the child rearing phase took up the entire adult lifespan. Women now have a young adulthood independent of family, where previously they moved directly from family of origin to marriage.

Stages of the family life cycle

Launching of the single young adult

This is a crucial stage in the family life cycle. Carter and McGoldrick (1999) begin the cycle at this stage because this is when the young adult decides what to take from the family of origin and what to leave behind. Of significance is the fact that it was not previously deemed a necessary stage for women but now is. Carter and McGoldrick view problems occurring when there is no change in the status of the young adult or in the hierarchical order between parent and young adult. The shift to a mutually respectful adult–adult relationship is required in order for separation to take place.

The joining of families through marriage

Current statistics in the UK show that the rate of first marriages has decreased by almost 10% in the last 30 years. However, couples who cohabit are twice as likely to separate as married couples (Family and Parenting Institute 2009, Lavis 2010). Carter and McGoldrick (1999) view the joining of families in marriage as the joining of two social systems, not just two individuals. They highlight the decreasing popularity of marriage, putting this down largely to the poor return on the investment women have made in marriage. Women have traditionally approached marriage with more enthusiasm and been rewarded less than men. Men approach marriage with apprehension and in fact get a better deal out of it than women. Women are afforded a low status yet they often do a greater share of the day-to-day work.

Becoming parents: families with young children

The highest separation and divorce rate is at this stage in the life cycle. Problems related to authority over children, conflict over child care, and the tensions and demands made on dual career couples may provide an explanation for this. However, divorce has increasingly been shown to have a seriously detrimental effect on the welfare of children (Amato and Keith 1991, Pryor and Rogers 2001). Three key factors seem to be at play: the impact on children of conflict between their parents, the impact of the stress caused by divorce on the relationships between parents and children, and the impoverished status of the broken family.

The transformation of the family system in adolescence

At this stage in the life cycle, boundaries must become permeable. Parents no longer can have complete authority and flexibility is required. Adolescents move between dependence and independence. An adolescent can introduce new values to parents and parents rail against these. Therapy involves changing the view parents and adolescents have of themselves and each other. Midlife crisis is common at this stage. It is a point when focus on adolescent difficulties may mask marital problems.

Families at midlife: launching children and moving on

This is the newest and longest phase in the family life cycle. Parents may now launch their children 20 years before they retire. Greatest number of exits and entries to the family occur at this stage and parents frequently experience emptiness and depression, particularly women. Consolidation of the marital relationship is required if it is to survive and parents may hold onto the last child to avoid divorce.

Major variations in the family life cycle

Divorce and remarriage

Emotional pressure peaks

- when the decision to divorce is made
- when it is announced to family and friends
- when money and custody issues are discussed
- when physical separation takes place
- when actual legal divorce takes place
- when there is contact about money or children
- when each child graduates, marries, has children or is ill
- as each spouse remarries, moves, becomes ill or dies.

Mourning and dealing with hurt are major features at each of the above stages. As in other transitions, complete cut-offs are harmful. Therapy includes enabling those involved successfully to face and negotiate the challenges of each transition.

The life cycle of poor families

Carter and McGoldrick (1999) point out that tertiary education elongates the interval between generations. When young people start working straight after their school years without further education, the unattached young adult phase is directly followed by families with children (this may involve three generations living together if the young couple cannot afford/ find a house). In very deprived households, there is little prospect of further education or steady employment, and adulthood starts with having a child, often very young.

Cultural variations

Family cultures can be varied and this must not be ignored. The therapist must encourage families to carry out the transitions appropriate to their ethnic background.

In summary, the concept of the family life cycle implies that families, like individuals, develop in time. Generations are linked, and family membership is different from membership of most other organisations.

Carter and McGoldrick (1999) analyse in detail each phase of the family life cycle and the way in which it has changed over the years. They suggest that one way of supporting families in crisis is to help them see the developmental dimension of what is happening to them.

 Activity

Select a time in your life and think about the implications of the life cycle model for your own family. Ask yourself the following questions:

- What stresses were present at that time?
- Who was most and least affected by them?

How were relationships affected by the transitions faced at this stage in your family life cycle?

Select a different stage in your life and ask yourself the same questions, comparing your perspective in the two examples.

2.4 Family structure

Minuchin (1974) provided some useful ideas for thinking about families in relation to family structure. He suggested that transactional patterns regulate family members' behaviour (for instance, mother instructs son – son obeys and this defines the relationship). The family structure presented here is the basic framework of structural family therapy, but these concepts are widely used in other contexts.

According to Minuchin, family patterns are maintained by *two systems of constraint*. The first is *generic*. This refers to universal rules governing family organisation such as:

- There must be a power hierarchy: parents and children are on different levels of this hierarchy.
- There is a complementarity of function between husband and wife: they are interdependent and working as a team.

The second system of constraint is *idiosyncratic*. This involves mutual expectations of individual family members, the result of years of negotiation both explicit and implicit, often around daily events. These operate on 'automatic pilot'. Reasons for them may be forgotten but the patterns remain.

Change beyond a certain range is resisted. Preferred patterns are kept as long as possible. Deviations by individuals result in pressure to conform (such as inducing guilt).

Systems, subsystems and boundaries (see Minuchin 1974, Chapter 3)

The structural model, like most other family therapy models, relies heavily on concepts borrowed from systems theory (von Bertalanffy 1968). Subsystems are the various constituents of the larger family system. One such subsystem is the parental subsystem, another is the sibling subsystem.

Boundaries define who is included in and excluded from the various subsystems, which in turn rules how people relate across boundaries. For example, a mother may reinforce the boundary which separates the parental and sibling subsystems by not allowing one sibling to discipline another.

The structural model posits that the boundaries between subsystems must be clear for interpersonal skills to develop. Effective functioning of the parental executive subsystem requires no interference from children or grandparents. Effective peer relationships require non-interference from parents.

The structural model describes a continuum from disengaged (too rigid) to clear (normal) and enmeshed (diffuse) boundaries between subsystems. Enmeshed families are viewed to be costly to individuals in that their autonomy is compromised due to over-involvement with family members. At the disengaged end of the continuum, only extreme stress in an individual is noticed by other family members. Enmeshed families are extremely involved with each other over the slightest problem. Disengaged family members fail to collaborate to solve even major problems.

The spouse subsystem

The task of the spouse subsystem is to achieve complementarity and mutual accommodation. It must develop patterns whereby each spouse loses part of their separateness in order to gain interdependence. A clear boundary around this subsystem is necessary. It should not be crossed inappropriately, nor should it be too rigid. It should operate as a haven from the outside world and other parts of the family system.

The parental subsystem

This subsystem emerges with the arrival of the first child and needs boundaries which allow the child access to both parents without crossing the boundary into spouse functions. As the child comes into contact with extra-familial influences, parents must accommodate to these. The parental subsystem must provide nurturance, guidance and control. The structural model suggests that the levels of these must change to support age appropriate autonomy of children, but stresses that parents require authority over children.

The sibling subsystem

The task of this subsystem is to enable children to learn to compete, to cooperate and to negotiate. Children learn quickly to accommodate to the adult world, but they have more difficulty in peer relationships with regard to sharing, negotiating, competing, etc. Boundaries around this subsystem must be clear in order that children have privacy and learn to be independent.

Family adaptation

The structural model is similar to the family life cycle model in that it views the family as a social system in transformation and transition. It also views pathology and dysfunction as a failure of the family system to adapt to change.

   Minuchin's analysis of family structures provides some very useful ideas to think about families, such as transactional patterns, boundaries, systems and subsystems and the way they relate to each other in the overall family group. As the family system has to adapt and change, it sometimes fails to cope. This is when it needs help (Minuchin 1974).

  Activity

Analyse the structure of your current family or family of origin to describe:

- Systems and subsystem
- Boundaries
- Some transactional patterns

2.5 Recent developments: narrative approaches to family therapy

The narrative approach developed by White and Epston (1990) has been highly influential in recent family therapy practice (see also White 1993, 2007). Some of the features of this approach, drawn together by Freedman and Combs (1996), are outlined in the following sections.

Externalising conversations

These involve separating the person from the problem and are usually begun by an exploration of the effects that the presenting problem has on family members. A problem that has lasted a long time and survived every effort the family has made to solve it is demoralising and family members tend to think that it demonstrates negative qualities about their family, a family member or a family relationship. When the family comes for help, they may describe themselves, or a child, only in terms of the problem, having lost sight of the bigger picture. Michael White (1990: 39) calls this a 'dominant story of family life', but there are always feelings and experiences that have been excluded from this dominant story. The separation of the person from the problem allows the opportunity to explore alternative stories and ways of addressing the problem.

Alternative stories

As family members separate from the problematic aspects of their lives, it becomes possible to raise awareness of alternative, less problematic aspects which they may have lost sight of.

Development of an alternative story

By exploring and linking together examples of problem-solving from the past, an alternative and preferred story of family life can be developed through use of the following types of question:

- Can you think of any examples in the past where you have been able to take a united front?
- Is there anything about your relationship in the past which may have predicted this kind of success?

The narrative approach provides a useful way of working with families: it offers a way of uncovering the family's pre-existing resources and mobilising these. An advantage of this approach is that it provides an anti-dote to the tendency of some earlier models to pathologise family relationships. The use of externalising conversations is a particularly helpful component of this approach.

 Activity

Visit the Dulwich website and read a paper or book chapter by Michael White. Make notes about what strikes you regarding this approach to working with family.

2.6 Attachment and family therapy

The importance of a secure base

John Bowlby's last book (1988) focused on the concept of a secure base. The importance of early attachment was discussed in chapter 2. Suffice to say that the attachment figure provides a secure base from which the infant can explore in the knowledge that the carer is available when protection is needed. As the child grows up, other attachments are formed, and in these new relationships a reciprocal secure base is provided by each person for the other.

The family as a secure base

John Byng-Hall (1995: 104) defines a secure family base as '. . . a family that provides a reliable network of attachment relationships which enables all family members of whatever age to feel sufficiently secure to explore relationships with each other and with others outside the family'. The development of this secure base is a family responsibility; it means being aware that these attachment relationships must be protected and it guarantees that family members will be helped if they need it.

Attachment and relationships

Sustaining the parental relationship is important because the existence of a secure base is undermined by disharmony between parents (Gordon *et al.* 2001). Research shows that the growing attachment between a young infant and its mother is more likely to deteriorate if the mother does not have a partner. Support to mother can also come from a wider group of adults. Community research shows that adults are more likely to get on well with neighbours if their children are securely attached (Belsky *et al.* 1989 in Byng-Hall 1995).

Situations that undermine the secure family base

Byng-Hall (1995) outlines a number of circumstances which undermine the secure family base including the following:

■ Loss or fear of loss of an attachment figure. This is common in the case of badly managed marital breakdown.

- Attachment figure capture. Examples of this include a clingy child attached to a parent to the exclusion of other children, or a partner who blocks the children's contact to the other partner.
- Turning to an inappropriate attachment figure: for example, one parent not acting as an attachment figure for the other who turns to a child instead, thus undermining his/her role as a parent to that child.

Attachment issues in family therapy

Byng-Hall's approach involves the therapist providing a temporary secure base to enable the exploration and modification of the family's attachment network, with the aim of enabling the family eventually to 'secure its own base'. He emphasises the importance of the therapist's availability throughout the process of therapy. He will usually make contact with the family soon after a referral in order to demonstrate his availability and pay close attention to ensuring that he engages warmly with each member of the family at the first session. He will then begin with weekly sessions, then fortnightly/monthly, then every 3 months. This may mean that the family attends for 10–12 sessions spread over 1–3 years. This allows a relatively brief therapy in terms of number of sessions while still providing a long-term secure base.

The application of attachment theory to understanding and working with families provides another important dimension to this work. Byng-Hall's framework provides a very useful way to ensure that attachment issues are central to work with families.

2.7 Parenting support and education

There is evidence that parenting has become more stressful and demanding since the 1970s (Nuffield Foundation 2009). Parenting programmes have been increasingly used in recent years because they have been shown to help parents who struggle with bringing up their children. The hope is that these children will be spared potential mental health problems, or alternatively, that problems which begin early, like conduct disorders, may improve (Richardson and Joughin 2002).

There are many possible reasons why some children get a disadvantaged start in life, such as economic and environmental disadvantage, single and teenage parenthood or the state of health, education and experience of their parent(s). Children looked after by local authorities are known to have higher rates of mental health problems (Ford et al. 2007). So do children of those who misuse drugs and alcohol or who are involved in crime (Rutter and Smith 1995). Parents' own experience of parenting and attachment has a significant influence on the way they parent their children (Main *et al.* 1985) and parenting programmes aim to support them.

The number of at-risk families is a significant minority. Increasingly, there has been a concern on the part of the government to intervene early in the parenting process so that children can have a 'good enough' start in life. The SureStart programmes, delivered in England and Wales as part of Every Child Matters (http://www.dcsf.gov.uk/everychildmatters/about/), include such schemes targeted at disadvantage groups.

This preventative approach requires collaboration to take place between the agencies that have contact with young families such as social workers, health visitors, general practitioners, the health and social services, nurseries, child-minding personnel and schools. Parenting support programmes have to be sensitive to families' needs and find ways of listening to children and parents. There are many such programmes. Some focus on prevention and early intervention (Sanders *et al.* 2003, Whitehead and Douglas 2005), others target emotional and behavioural problems and child protection (Puckering 2004, 2007), whereas yet others specialise in working with children whose behaviour is out of control (Webster-Stratton and Herbert 1994, Richardson and Joughin 2002). Voluntary agencies as well as local health centres and outpatient departments can be in the best position to deliver them. Finances need to be set aside for the purpose because this approach is not cheap – although addressing difficulties early saves money on health and social care bills later – and the returns are slow.

In the last part of this unit, we will highlight the aims of such programmes, describe some of their approaches and discuss their most important components.

Aims of parenting programmes

1. To offer support and guidance
2. To help parents find ways of reducing stress at home
3. To promote positive parenting through the use of good communication skills
4. To teach children more effective social skills, problem-solving skills and anger management skills
5. To reduce out-of-control behaviour in young children and the associated risk of later conduct disorders

Effective parenting skills include consistent limit setting and clear behaviour expectations; child-centred behaviours such as playing with the child, listening to him/her, praising him/her, smiling, touching, cuddling; reinforcing the child's satisfactory behaviour by commenting on it and praising it; decreasing the frequency with which parents direct their children's behaviour or criticise it.

In order to teach these skills, the programmes are careful not to criticise parents but to praise what they do well. This in itself is a model for the parents to follow with their own children.

In some groups the emphasis is on teaching, in others it is on the mutual support parents bring to each other. Many programmes are based on techniques of behaviour modification in warm and non-judgemental relationships with the helpers. Often parents eat together and give feedback to each other on the homework they have had to do since the last session. Videos of play time or meal time at home can be brought in and analysed individually. Many programmes are for parents of children under age 5, some go up to 8. Some will work with the children separately, others will not.

Such programmes have the disadvantage that they are fairly intensive and therefore expensive; and they only reach a small proportion of the families who need them.

2.8 Conclusion

This chapter has focused on the life of the family. It is tempting to build a blueprint of what a normally functioning family is like and to diagnose dysfunction in those who do not fit it, but the truth is that families come in many shapes and sizes. The function of the family is to offer a secure base to its members and to nurture and protect those who are vulnerable. Some families struggle to achieve this and may need support and intervention. Assessing a family's place in its life cycle and the way its members' relationships and roles are structured can help us make sense of what is going on. Some families with young children are known to be at risk of not coping well with their children's developing needs. Parenting programmes are increasingly used, both to anticipate difficulties in vulnerable families and to intervene early when problems have already started (such as out-of-control behaviour). Working with the family should form an integral part of any therapeutic intervention involving children.

Recommended reading

Barker, P. (2007). *Basic Family Therapy*, 6th edition. Oxford: Blackwell.

Carr, A. (2000). *Family Therapy: Concepts, Process and Practice*. London: Wiley

Walsh, F. (2003). Conceptualisation of normal family processes. Chapter 1. In: Walsh, F. (ed) (2003). *Normal Family Processes*, 3rd edition. New York: Guildford Press.

Whyte, D. A. (ed) (1997). *Explorations in Family Nursing*. London: Routledge.

Wright, L. M. and Leahey, M. (2009). *Nurses and Families: A Guide to Family Assessment and Intervention*, 5th edition. Philadelphia, PA: FA Davis.

Chapter 3

PSYCHOSOCIAL DEVELOPMENT

Geraldine Jones

School of Life, Sport and Social Sciences, Edinburgh Napier University, Edinburgh, Scotland

3.1 Introduction

During childhood and adolescence, young people have to cope with a myriad of challenges. The psychological effects of the development of cognition, identity and physical maturation in childhood and adolescence are play out in a complex interrelationship between the individual and their environment. In this chapter we will discuss the psychosocial development of children, particularly attachment in infancy, and the development of adolescent identity. Mental health difficulties can occur during childhood, in the transition between childhood and adolescence, or during adolescence. It is important to remember that for all the individuals in these three categories there is an additional burden of having to cope with normal adolescent developmental issues. These developmental issues will be discussed in this chapter. The chapter ends with a discussion of a recent contextual model of identity development which explains the psychological impact of risk and stresses in the lives of children and adolescents. Before discussing attachment, we will consider how different theoretical perspectives within psychology affect how we perceive development.

Learning outcomes

After reading this chapter, you should be able to:

1. Evaluate Bowlby's (1969) attachment theory and the internal working model.
2. Critically evaluate Erikson's theory of identity formation.

Understanding Children and Young People's Mental Health, first edition. Edited by Anne Claveirole and Martin Gaughan. Published 2011 by John Wiley & Sons Ltd. © 2011 John Wiley & Sons Ltd.

3. Analyse the concept of adolescent egocentrism.
4. Understand the psychological impact of puberty and its timing.
5. Evaluate the contextual critique of the organismic theories of psychosocial development.
6. Apply a case study to Spencer *et al.*'s (1997) contextual PVEST model.

3.2 Theories of development

In the past 30 years, child developmental psychology has altered its theoretical approach. There has been a challenge to the assumptions previously made that were based on organismic and mechanistic models of development (Lerner *et al.* 1989). Organismic models, like Freud's (1938) psychodynamic and Piaget's cognitive theories, assumed that development would follow a normative path: one person's development would be much like another's (Pepper 1942). For an up-to-date psychodynamic approach to the development of children and young people, see Hindle (1999). The mechanistic model assumed that once certain factors were in place, there would be a predictable developmental change (Pepper 1942). For example, the behaviourist theory is mechanistic in that it suggests that development is the result of learning experiences. Organismic and mechanistic approaches have been challenged by a contextual dynamic analysis of the person in their environment which suggests that potential development will be relatively plastic rather than normative (Lewis 1997). Plasticity in development is the ability to be flexible and adapt across the lifespan.

In the light of new evidence about the flexibility of development, we need to critique existing theories. In the next section, Bowlby's (1969) organismic theory of attachment will be critiqued from a contextual perspective.

3.3 Infant attachment

Bowlby (1969) identified that children need to feel attached to people in their lives in order to develop trust and to have a secure base from which they can explore and learn. Bowlby (1969) used psychodynamic principles and developed them on a scientific basis (Holmes 1993). Previously, psychodynamic research used an understanding of the inner world and fantasy as a method of investigation, but Bowlby (1944, 1951) looked at actual deprivations that children had suffered due to insufficient attachment (Bowlby 1944). Bowlby (1979) found that sustained trauma like hospitalisation or poor parenting caused problems of insecure attachment which resulted in poor mental health and other long-term difficulties. The characteristics of secure and insecure attachment will be outlined next.

Secure attachment

Secure attachment in an infant is characterised by a mutual synchrony which is initially monitored by the mother (Harrist and Waugh 2002). Synchrony is where there is a reciprocal co-ordination of mutually regulated actions (Harrist and Waugh 2002). A securely attached older child might feel anxious or in need of support if they are in new situations. This social referencing to the parent involves making eye contact, looking for cues which will signal whether it is safe to explore or withdraw back to the caregiver's secure base. The parent–child interaction is a continuous monitoring of distance regulation (Ainsworth *et al.* 1978).

If the responsive figure is unavailable or is inconsistent, a child will develop fear and anxiety which will promote attachment-seeking behaviours and after prolonged experience of unresponsive parenting insecure attachment. Ainsworth (1979) identified two types of insecure attachment: avoidant and ambivalent/resistant. Main and Solomon (1986) later identified a third insecure attachment category called disorganised.

Insecure attachments

1. In *avoidant* attachment, the child has to put up a defence against a carer who is rejecting so that they do not repeatedly feel rebuffed. The child may relate to strangers and his/her mother in similar ways and tends to snub any caring overtures that his/her mother does make. There may be a mismatch between maternal response and the activity of the child. For example, the mother may intrude when the child is playing happily and ignore them when they are upset and need attention.
2. The *ambivalent/resistant* attachment strategy involves submissive clinging to the carer or alternatively a role reversal where the child looks after and cares for the mother. On reunion with their mother, the ambivalent/resistant child may be angry with their mother, needing attention but resistant to any attempt to comfort them. Mothers may ignore their baby's signals or be unpredictable in how they respond.
3. The third pattern of insecure attachment is *disorganised* where the child has no consistent coping strategy. This is only seen in very rare cases of severe pathology, e.g. the result of sexual abuse (Main and Solomon 1986).

Ambivalent, avoidant and disorganised coping strategies are ineffective ways that the child tries to maintain attachments. The insecurely attached child develops persistent primitive feelings of abandonment and resentment which result in anxiety and maladaptive behaviour (Holmes 1993). Their exploration, development and emotional growth are restricted. The mother should be able to act as an auxiliary emotional regulator for the child. If the mother does not, then the child will be overwhelmed with feelings of loss, separation and anxiety with which they cannot easily cope with (Bowlby 1979).

Belsky and Nezworski (1988) found that all socio-economic groups have the same proportion of attachment types, with about 65% secure, 20% avoidant and 15% ambivalent/resistant depending on the sample. However, the proportion of avoidant and ambivalent/resistant attachment rises with mothers who have a depressive illness or in families where there is proven physical or sexual abuse. With depressed mothers, 40% of children were insecure avoidant. In abusive families, 50% were avoidant and 30% disorganised, with only 10% classified as secure (Belsky and Nezworski 1988).

When the carer is not present, the attachment relationship is represented in the child's mind by the internal working model (IWM) that produces an effect when the child thinks about themselves and their caregiver (Bowlby 1973).

The Internal Working Model (IWM)

The IWM acts as a guide to attention, memory and future behaviour throughout childhood and into adulthood. In adulthood the IWM, to some extent, determines:

- What individuals remember about their childhood (George *et al.* 1985)
- The ability to form satisfactory adult intimate relationships (Brennan *et al.* 1998)
- Parenting ability with one's children (Van Ijzendoorn 1995)
- How individuals perceive themselves (Klohnen and Bera 1998)
- How individuals attribute the behaviour of others in ambiguous situations (Bowlby 1973).

Bowlby (1969) identified that the healthy IWM is subject to constant revision. Even when there might be plenty of evidence to suggest that change would be the adaptive route, children with a fixed unhealthy IWM can end up with negative core assumptions which they are unable to revise in the light of experience. The barriers and defence mechanisms engaged in by the insecure child are not always accessible to conscious awareness (Holmes 1993).

Bowlby (1951) tended to think of the child as passive in their loss as if they were reactively moulded by events that occurred in their lives. The contextual theory suggests that attachment is an interactive understanding of oneself and all active relationships and therefore is not determined by one relationship (Lewis *et al.* 2000). The contextual view is that other supportive family members can successfully replace the role of a parent. Also, there are individual differences in how people cope with life events with some being more resilient than others (Beckett 2002).

Contextual theorists point out that attachment is not necessarily as determined as Bowlby anticipated (Cassidy 2000). Lamb *et al.* (1985) suggested that attachment will only remain consistent if the environment remains stable, so we should not assume continuity of attachment. Other researchers reported further evidence to support a contextual critique of Bowlby's (1969) attachment theory. Lewis *et al.* (2000) found that being securely attached as an infant did not offer ego protection if the children's parents got divorced. Attachment type at one year old did not predict maladjustment in adolescence, but divorce of one's parents did (Lewis *et al.* 2000). Weinfield *et al.* (2000) found that there was no attachment continuity from infancy to adolescence in the changeable environment of a high-risk sample. As Lamb *et al.* (1985) pointed out, if security in attachment does not predict competency in dealing with difficult life events in adolescence and adulthood, then the IWM is not as stable and does not function in the way Bowlby (1969) predicted.

To conclude the topic of attachment, the secure infant becomes a flexible resourceful child. The avoidant child tends to be over-controlled. The ambivalent child is under-controlled. Bowlby (1969) identified that the childhood IWM becomes the narrative for the level of social, emotional and cognitive competence that the adult has in life although this has been challenged by recent contextual evidence (Lewis *et al.* 2000).

There are many studies that support Bowlby's theory by reporting:

- Continuity of attachment (Waters *et al.* 2000)
- Adults choose the same attachment type intimate partner (Owen's *et al.* 1995)
- Parents bring up children to have a similar attachment types to themselves (Simpson *et al.* 1992, Fraley and Shaver 1998)
- There is even intergenerational transmission of attachment type over three generations (Benoit and Parker 1994).

However, all but the most fixed IWMs can be altered as a result of individual differences, experiences of new intimate relationships, therapy and reflection (Cassidy 2000). The contextual approach challenges Bowlby's (1969) conclusion that continuity of attachment is due to a fixed IWM suggesting rather that stable environmental circumstances create contexts which maintains attachment (Lewis 1997).

In adolescence, as in childhood, the attachment system becomes more active in times of illness, tiredness or increased anxiety. Anxiety can be caused by the development of identity in adolescence as we will discuss in the next section. In adolescence, a process of separation from parents takes place (Marcia 1980) within the confines of their IWM of attachment. Erikson's (1968) psychodynamic organismic theory identified this separation from parents as one task towards achieving identity formation. Erikson (1968) found that there were eight transition points across the lifespan with identity formation being the fifth.

Short note on the distinction between the terms childhood and adolescence

In the following discussion the term adolescence is used. When Erikson introduced his work on identity formation the distinction between childhood and adolescence was clearer than it is today. Children now mature earlier compared to thirty years ago. In the past children were presumed to suffer less stress and anxiety and have a much more limited role in society than they do today. Much psychological research has been conducted under these assumptions including some reported in the next few sections of this chapter. Today we understand the real difficulties children and younger people have as outlined in the following chapters of this book. Now development is viewed as a continuum. Also, it is understood that some people develop earlier than others. Considering the earlier maturation of children the following topics may be as relevant to late childhood as they are to early adolescence.

3.4 Adolescent identity formation

Erikson's (1968) psychodynamic organismic theory predicted that adolescents were vulnerable to a crisis transition during which separation from parents and individuation took place. The individuation process is when the adolescent has to find their own way in the world by intra-psychic restructuring into a cohesive view of oneself (Frosh 1991). A contextual critique of Erickson's (1968) theory would suggest that a predictable outcome of an identity crisis in adolescence is exaggerated (Lewis 1997). Steinberg (1990) found that 85% of adolescents have reasonably good relationships with their families. The majority of adolescents are well adjusted and can manage the changes in their identity, physical maturation and developing cognition without too much disruption to their relationships if their family is cohesive and adaptable (Mullins *et al.* 2004, Smetana *et al.* 2006). Marcia (1987) and Erikson's (1980) concept of identify achievement has been criticised for considering identity as a single global concept rather than involving domain-specific identities for occupational, religious, political and other affiliations (Groossens 1995). Adolescence is a significant transition however identity is conceptualised (Buchanan *et al.* 1990, 1996), as it involves a restructuring of one's self-concept.

The adolescent self-concept is made up of a psychological understanding of their social and sexual selves (Offer 1969, Offer *et al.* 1992). This psychological understanding is based on whether adolescents have control over their impulses, can create and maintain emotional health and come to terms with their body image. So, for during adolescence and continuing into adulthood, the coping self is constructed around ideas about self-reliance, self-confidence and mental health (Meeus *et al.* 1999, Birman and Trickett 2001). Maintaining a stable self-concept is more difficult during adolescence when individuals need to investigate different alternatives in order to define their personal life choices (Marcia 1966, 1994).

Marcia (1966) found that there are four categories of identity formation (outlined in the following sections) as defined by Erikson (1968): identity diffusion, foreclosure, moratorium and identity achievement (Fig. 3.1). Adolescents may go from one category to another but not necessarily.

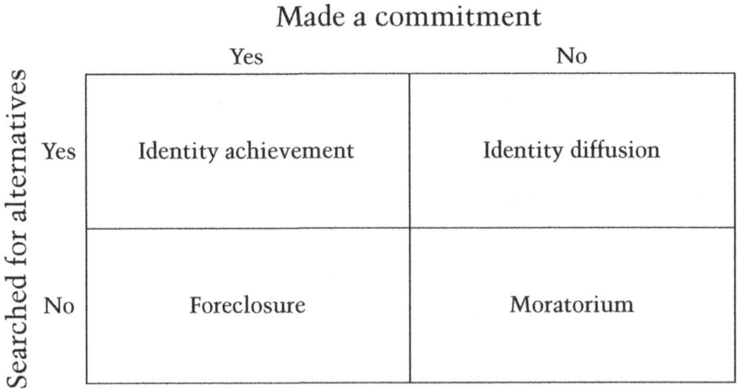

Figure 3.1 Diagram of identity categories based on whether alternatives have been investigated and commitments have been made.

Identity diffusion

In *identity diffusion*, there is no commitment made to a life choice but also no exploration of alternatives, although there may have been some exploration in the past. Many identity diffused adolescents have low ego development, low moral reasoning ability, cannot cope with complex reasoning and are unable to cooperate with others appropriately. Identity diffused individuals have the highest levels of psychological and inter-personal problems.

Foreclosure

Foreclosed individuals have not explored alternatives but have made a firm commitment. Foreclosed adolescents are more likely to have an authoritarian personality, be socially stereotypical, have an external locus of control, poor social skills and be dependent on others but are less likely to be anxious.

Moratorium

Moratorium adolescents go through what is most like the classic concept of an adolescent identity crisis. People in the moratorium status are more likely to have self-doubt, disturbed thinking, impulsivity, have conflict with parents and increased physical symptoms compared to other identity classification types (Kidwell *et al.* 1995).

Identity achievement

Identity achievement describes adolescents who have explored alternatives and made a commitment. They may have had a crisis in the past but that crisis has been resolved. 'Identity achieved' adolescents have the highest level of ego development (Meeus *et al.* 1999) in that they are good at rea-soning about moral decisions, have an internal locus of control and high self-esteem. Identity achieved adolescents are also better at performing under stress and are good at forming intimate relationships.

We find that there is a correlation between adolescents in the *moratorium* and *identity achievement* statuses with more positive personal characteristics than those who are going through identity diffusion or foreclosure (Kidwell 1995). Moratorium and identity achieved adolescents also tend to have good study habits, good behaviour, and low alcohol/drug consumption (Marcia 1994). Parents can accommodate an easier adoles-cent identity transition process.

Parental influence on identity formation

Relationships with parents which allow free expression of independent thought while maintaining close relations facilitate greater ego and identity development (Youniss and Smoller 1985), better psychosocial competence, less depression and more mature moral reasoning (Grotevant and Cooper 1985, Hauser *et al.* 1991 Walker and Taylor 1991, Allen *et al.* 1994). Authoritative homes are more conducive to the development of psychological competence than authoritarian, permissive or rejecting homes (Steinberg 2001). Parental influence is found to be important for some future–oriented aspects of identity (occupational), but peer support is more important for relational identity commitment and exploration (Meeus *et al.* 2002).

Added difficulties can arise if the parent cannot offer support to their adolescent children, or in some cases they can sabotage a young person's psychosocial development (Shulman and Scharf 2000). This situation may escalate when the adolescent has to deal with a developmental task with which the parent has unresolved issues from their own development. Shulman and Scharf (2000) suggested that stress can be reignited in the parent and have a trans-generational exponential effect on the adolescent. Overly intrusive psychological parental control can lead to internalising and externalising problems in the adolescent which in turn leads to further behaviour control and parental monitoring (Kuczynski 2003). High psychological control involving control over the thoughts and feelings of the adolescent undermines optimal development (Barber 1996, 2002). Searching for one's identity will affect an adolescent's self-esteem which will be discussed next (Meeus *et al.* 1999).

3.5 Adolescent self-esteem

Rosenberg (1965) investigated self-esteem with a sample of 5,000 17 and 18 year olds, and found that 20–30% of adolescents had low self-esteem. Low self-esteem adolescents were characterised as feeling incompetent in social relationships, believing that they were misunderstood and not respected. They suffered depression, anxiety and had poor school performance. By comparison, high self-esteem adolescents felt that their personal attributes included self-confidence, hard working, leadership potential and good impression management skills.

Both high and low self-esteem adolescents desired success in their work life after school, but those with low self-esteem did not expect to succeed and had unrealistic expectations (Rosenberg 1965). As you can see in

Box 3.1 Stability of Adolescent Self-esteem

Hirsch and DuBois (1991) found that there were four different paths of self-esteem
stability in the age range between 12 and 14 years.

1. 35% of adolescents had consistently high self-esteem
2. 15% had consistently low self-esteem
3. 25% had a steep decline
4. 5% had a small but significant increase

Block and Robins (1993) found that boys were over-represented in the increasing
self-esteem pathway and girls were over-represented in the declining path.

Box 3.1, 25% of adolescents have a steep decline in self-esteem between
the ages of 12 and 14. This study was also replicated with 12–16 year olds
with similar results (Zimmerman *et al.* 1991). Harter (1990) found that
satisfaction with one's physical appearance contributed most to overall
self-esteem, followed by social acceptance by peers. Harter (1990) reported
that one participant commented 'what's really important to me is how I
look. If I like the way I look then I really like the kind of person I am'.

There are many random events or risks that adolescents encounter which
can alter their self-esteem. These events can be non-normative, in that they
do not happen to everyone in an age group, like divorce and bullying. If the
adolescent is able to deal with one non-normative or normative event at a
time, then they may be able to cope with the adolescent transition more
easily (Coleman 1978). How the adolescent copes with transitions will be
affected by four further aspects which we will discuss in turn.

1. The adolescent's cognitive or reasoning ability
2. The timing of puberty
3. Adolescent brain development
4. The context in which the young person grows up

3.6 Adolescent reasoning ability

Higher-order reasoning develops during adolescence (Kuhn 1991) and may
lead to an increased interest in possible identity development, changes in
self-concept (Damon and Hart 1988), interpersonal understanding (Selman
1980) and a development in moral judgements (Colby and Kohlberg 1987).
Development in cognition and reasoning ability does not end with childhood or even when we become adults (Shayer *et al.* 1976) but is

significant in adolescence. Elkind (1967) identified that there are cognitive reasoning errors that adolescents are particularly prone to make. Elkind (1967) described these inconsistencies as egocentrism: when one focuses on one's own ego and centres on one factor at a time.

3.7 Adolescent egocentrism

Piaget (1952) found that there were advances in perspective taking after the age of 12 years, i.e. the ability to step outside oneself and anticipate the reaction of others. Elkind (1967) found that adolescents overuse this newly acquired skill of perspective taking, creating egocentrism which distorts their image of the world in two ways: imaginary audience and personal fable.

Imaginary audience

Imaginary audience is when the young person is so focused on themselves that they believe they are and the centre of everyone's attention and behave as if they are on stage with an admiring or critical audience. Rankin et al. (2004) found that, although public self-consciousness which is associated with appearance decreases from 13 to 18 years of age, private self-consciousness increases over this time.

Personal fable

Elkind (1967) described how an adolescent can have an inflated opinion about their own importance, feeling that they are special and unique. Personal fable can be either positive or negative. Young people can sometimes live in a fantasy immersed world which can lead to increased risk-taking (Keinan et al. 1984). Halpern-Felsher and Cauffman (2001) found that adolescents were not as skilled as adults in making decisions about risk because of a lack of experience. Jacobs and Ganzel (1995) pointed out that adolescents must consider the potential consequences of their decisions from inconsistent, limited knowledge. Greene et al. (2000) found that 11–25 year olds with high personal fable and high sensation-seeking scores took more risks with drug use, delinquency, alcohol consumption and, particularly, risky sexual behaviour compared to other adolescents.

Elkind (1967) found that egocentrism declined over the adolescent years. As well as increased risk-taking, the potentially negative consequences of egocentrism can be extreme anxiety, acute embarrassment and rumination. Girls are at particular risk of co-rumination with friends which might explain why girls are more prone to internalising maladaptive strategies than boys even though they have good intimate relationships with friends (Rose 2002). Positive consequences from the development of perspective taking can be an increased self-understanding and an improved quality in friendships.

Egocentrism in reasoning is not an optimal tool for logical thought with which to face the difficulties involved in puberty. We will next consider the psychological effect of maturational pubertal changes, the timing of these changes and the context within which these changes occur.

3.8 The psychological impact of puberty

Girls mature about 2 years earlier than boys. The onset of the first period (menarche) is spread over a longer time period for girls than is the onset of puberty for boys. Adolescents have to deal with these physical changes at a time when identity is being formed and when initial identity is tied to physical attributes (Harter 1990). Some studies have shown that adolescents are psychologically unprepared for puberty (Stein and Reiser 1994, Moore 1995). Many studies provide evidence that girls and boys, but particularly girls, are dissatisfied with their body (Richards *et al.* 1990, Balding 2005, Palmqvist and Santavirta 2006, Ricciardelli *et al.* 2006). Dissatisfaction with body image increases if they have poor parental support (Buchanan *et al.* 1996), negative affect, a concern about their diet, depression, and they pay too much attention to appearance discussions with peers and media messages (Sinton and Birch 2006). On a more individual level, there are far-reaching issues about the timing of maturity.

The timing of maturity

When girls enter puberty earlier than their peers, they may encounter problems (Brooks-Gunn and Reiter 1990). With the onset of puberty, girls tend to put on body fat and find breast development embarrassing, which leads to poor body image (Silbereisen and Kracke 1993). As well as poor body image, early developing girls are at risk of problems with eating disorders (Brooks-Gunn and Reiter 1990), parental conflict (Steinberg 1988), early sexual experience and earlier experience of drinking alcohol and smoking (Silbereisen and Kracke 1993). Many of these difficulties are caused by socialising with older girls (Silbereisen and Kracke 1993). Early developing girls' many difficulties are exacerbated in certain contexts, e.g. when there is an expectation to have boyfriends and pressure from media presentation of Western culture's ideal body (Richards *et al.* 1990, Caspi *et al.* 1993). Late developing girls have more child-like bodies, like the thin models who are valued by Western society (Berzonsky and Lombardo 1983).

In contrast to girls, many early developing boys have social advantages and are less likely to have an identity crisis (Tobin-Richards *et al.* 1983, Simmons and Blyth 1987). Early developing boys develop greater muscle capacity and are taller which fits in with our culture's ideal male body image. However, early developing boys can take on pseudo-adult masculinity behaviour and become involved in risk-taking and other associated externalising behaviour (Andersson and Magnusson 1990).

Late developing boys can have different problems. They are smaller than their peers, are likely to be bullied and have feelings of insignificance and inferiority (Peterson and Crockett 1985). These problems will be increased if the school and home environment favours pseudo-adult masculinity in adolescence (Andersson and Magnusson 1990). Late developing boys can also have a problem with delayed brain development (Peterson and Crockett 1985) which we will discuss later.

We can see that for optimal psychological adjustment to maturation, there is a central issue about the reciprocal relation between a person and the environment (Richards *et al.* 1990, Caspi *et al.* 1993). Development is easier if a person feels that they fit into their social sphere and that other people also see themselves as fitting in. (Peterson and Crockett 1985, Lerner *et al.* 1989, Alsaker 1996). Studies looking at the long-term consequences of the timing of maturity found that early maturing males did well in school and had more social prestige in their adult life than late maturing males (Mussen and Jones 1957). Early maturing girls were twice as likely to leave school early and more likely to get pregnant at a young age (Brooks-Gunn and Warren 1985).

It has been found that early maturation can be caused by the context in which the adolescent finds themselves (Caspi and Bem 1990). Parent/adult conflict in the household studied when a child was 7 and again at 9 years was predictive of early menarche in girls as was a father-absent household (Moffitt *et al.* 1992). This can be explained by an evolutionary connection between pubertal maturation and parent–child distance (Steinberg 1989) and increased exposure to unrelated males (Johnston *et al.* 1985).

3.9 Adolescent brain development

We now know that there is significant brain development throughout adolescence. Egocentrism may be explained by the fact that development of the frontal cortex, the most important area of the brain for higher-order thinking, is not fully developed until adulthood (Matsuzawa *et al.* 2001).

It is important for us to understand that there are reconfigurations involving the pruning of neurons in the brain which occur as waves of plasticity in brain development (Giedd *et al.* 1999). This is not a linear development. The waves of plasticity, which continue into adulthood, facilitate the reorganisation of the brain resulting in greater efficiency and effectiveness in communication and reasoning ability. While these reconfigurations occur, there can be quite significant and inconsistent alterations in how the adolescent thinks and processes information (Giedd *et al.* 1999).

Health difficulties which create developmental challenges can only be resolved with mature decision-making and a logical reasoning approach. Problems adolescents encounter are made more difficult because of the cognitive limitations that we have discussed and their changing view of self and identity. We find that poor decision strategies are used by adults in unfamiliar tasks, in choices with uncertain outcomes, and in ambiguous situations. The decision-making style of adolescents is similar to adult skill levels, but because they lack experience and information their decision-making is impaired (Jacobs and Ganzel 1993). Social, emotional and identity issues will affect adolescent choices in life as will personal goals, attitudes, values, emotional states and self-belief.

We may wonder why some individuals can be resilient and strong in the face of difficulties in life and why others are grossly affected by circumstances that some people would find easy to deal with. The contextual model of development is a very useful tool to help find answers to these questions.

3.10 The value of contextual theories in explaining development of children and adolescents

Adolescents, as we have discussed, change, develop, interact with their peers and form their identity. Children's formation of early attachments and the pathway of their cognitive, emotional and social development is dependent on the people in and the circumstances of their environment. To what extent does the environment facilitate or block these changes?

If we consider the contextual model of development once more, we can identify:

1. The risks and transitions a child has to cope with and in what environment
2. The impact of losses and gains in family and peer relationships

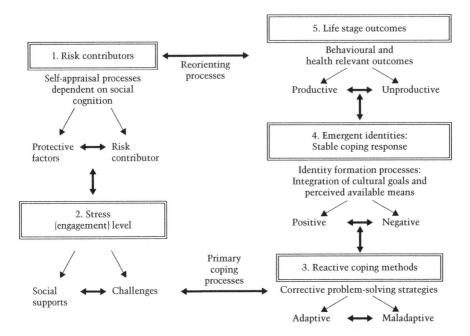

Figure 3.2 PVEST: A cyclical contextual model of development. Adapted from Spencer *et al.* (1997). © Cambridge University Press.

3. The resources a child/adolescent can draw on from non-family groups, e.g. school, helping agencies and societal influence
4. Intergenerational problems

Spencer *et al.* (1997) have modelled this contextual perspective (Fig. 3.2).

3.11   The PVEST model

In Spencer *et al.*'s (1997) PVEST (Phenomenological Variant of Ecological Systems Theory) model we can see that if there is a change in any one factor in a child's life, it will have an effect on everything else. Everything is interdependent. It is common today in applied psychology to consider that an individual's problems can be caused by the context or system (Lewis 1997). If the problem is caused by the context, it cannot be solved by the child or adolescent on their own. Therefore, if we know about the context in detail, then we can also understand what is happening to an individual (Spencer *et al.* 1997).

As you can see, there are five aspects that contribute to identity in Spencer *et al.*'s (1997) model. These five stages occur on a cycle of developmental processes such as biological factors and temperament. This cycle is repeated reiteratively as the child matures. We will now outline the details of the stages and processes in the PVEST model.

1. Net risk/vulnerability level

The harm potential of a net risk (deficient genes, poor background, etc.) will depend on the perception of vulnerability (resiliency). Net vulnerability is the sum of the protective factors (e.g. secure attachment, adult support) and risk contributors (e.g. delinquent friendship group, aggressive temperament) in the individual's life.

Proximal processes
The protective factors and risk contributors are experienced in developmental time through lived experiences called proximal processes.

2. Net stress (engagement) level

A net stress is the actual experience and behaviours which are the results of the perceptions of the previous stage. The experience of the risk is modified by the different supports (e.g. an inspiring teacher, helpful friend) and challenges (e.g. discrimination, negative feedback) that are available.

Primary coping processes
The net stress results in a primary coping method, which is the reactive outcome of the supports and challenges played out over time.

3. Reactive coping strategies

Reactive coping strategies are processes which reduce the potential psychological stress to the individual. The individual thinks through reasons which have caused the events to which they have been subjected to. Dissonance (a perceived difference between the experiences of events compared to how one thought they would be) needs to be reduced to protect the psychological ego. Strategies to deal with the net stress are put in place, which are either adaptive or maladaptive. One approach may be optimum in one situation but not in another, so the outcome is again dependent on the context (the person/environment fit).

Identity formation (secondary coping processes)
Self-appraisal and the perception of the self/environment fit is an important concept at this stage. Secondary coping processes will become more

and more stable over developmental time and contribute to an emergent identity.

4. Emergent identities: stable coping response

Consistent coping strategies from the previous stage lead to a stable identity. This identity is the sum of the genetic, temperament and personality attributes of the individual combined with the outcome of previous stages set in their environmental context. An emergent identity is one's stable perception of oneself (either positive or negative) in the environment which provides psychosocial consistency.

Goal-seeking (tertiary coping and orienting) processes

A positive emergent identity allows a person to look forward with more confidence about the future. If one has a stable view of one's place in the world, it is easier to make plans and set goals. Goals are ways of coping in the environment and are more likely to be optimum if they are the result of a positive emergent identity. Alternatively, goals could be a maladaptive (e.g. deciding to disengage with work) and may lead to an adverse life stage outcome.

5. Life stage outcome

Productive outcomes are good health, stress-free social interactions, adaptive relations with parents, high self-esteem and self-efficacy. Unproductive outcomes are poor health, low self-esteem, feelings of worthlessness and ego fragility.

Reorienting processes

The life stage outcome produces its own dynamics. Depending on what maturational stage the child/adolescent is going through, there will be new risks and stressors. Through a reorienting process, the child/adolescent will engage in risks with a vulnerability level which is influenced by previous stresses, coping strategies and identity.

Spencer *et al.* (1997) have outlined a model of risks, protective factors, stress, challenges and coping strategies which are played out over time in the environment. This cycle represents a model of the way individuals cope with all interactions in their lives. This level of complexity is seen as essential when modelling the developmental context (Lewis 2005). Previous mechanistic and organismic models have been found to be of limited use for applied psychology as they do not take into consideration the complexity of the context (Lewis 1997).

3.12 Conclusion

Attachment, changing cognition, psychological adjustment to changes in physique and identity can be risks or opportunities for the child and adolescent. Spencer *et al.*'s (1997) model shows the complexity of these changes which are played out over developmental time and in a context which may be supportive or alternatively encourage maladaptive approaches. It is important to remember that individuals, made up of genes, temperament and personality, are active in creating their own environments (Plomin *et al.* 1994). However, by setting this active constructive process in context, we can see that some individuals and groups have more options than others.

Recommended reading

Coleman, J. C. and Hagel, A. (2007). *Adolescent Risk and Resilience: Against the Odds.* Chichester: John Wiley.

Coleman, J. C. and Hendry, L. B. (1999). *The Nature of Adolescence.* London: Routledge.

Holmes, J. (1993). *John Bowlby and Attachment Theory.* London: Routledge.

Chapter 4

SELF-HARM

Martin Gaughan

School of Nursing, Midwifery and Social Care, Edinburgh Napier University, Edinburgh, Scotland

4.1 Introduction

Self-harm is the focus of increasing public attention and concern. On the surface, self-harm in children and young people appears to be an increasing problem, and is something adults can find difficult to accept or understand. We are probably better at recognising or acknowledging when self-harm occurs, which in turn has increased our awareness of self-harm. Whether this means there has been an increase in self-harm is open to question, as we do not have data with which to make comparisons. Research, however, seems to indicate self-harm is more prevalent than previously thought (Gunnell *et al.* 2000, Wheeler *et al.* 2008).

In this chapter we will examine definitions of self-harm, how common it is and consider issues of vulnerability and resilience. We will look at reasons young people have for self-harming, as well as examining how we might be able to assist young people who are self-harming. Self-harm engenders different reactions in different people – so we will be looking at our own feelings, thoughts and responses – how we can work with these in a way which is helpful to children and young people.

Self-harm is to some extent culturally determined: what is acceptable in one society may not be acceptable in another. Even within our society, we accept some acts of self-harm more readily than we do others. Excessive alcohol consumption, smoking and skin piercing are more acceptable than overdosing or cutting one's arms. The potential outcome of an act does not determine whether it is viewed as acceptable, and some activities have potentially more dangerous consequences but are more acceptable than

Understanding Children and Young People's Mental Health, first edition. Edited by Anne Claveirole and Martin Gaughan. Published 2011 by John Wiley & Sons Ltd. © 2011 John Wiley & Sons Ltd.

others. From this it may be safe to conjecture that how we feel as individuals about self-harm is influenced by collective as well as individual values and beliefs. These values, attitudes and beliefs will affect how we interact and engage with young people who self-harm.

Learning outcomes

After reading this chapter, you should be able to:

1. Define issues which may make young people and particular groups who are vulnerable to self-harm.
2. Identify issues which may make young people vulnerable to self-harm.
3. Identify groups of young people who are particularly vulnerable to self-harm.
4. Discuss reasons why young people self-harm.
5. Reflect on your own thoughts and feelings about self-harm.
6. Reflect on how a young person who self-harms could be helped.

4.2 What is self-harm?

At first glance finding a definition of self-harm seems relatively simple; there are many similar descriptions which state that self-harm is destruction of body tissue without conscious suicidal intent (Favazza 1989, Schneider *et al.* 1996, Croyle 2007). Self-harm has also been defined as 'self-injurious behaviour with nonfatal outcome' (Fox and Hawton 2004: 16). The difference in definition can depend on the population being studied, e.g. whether it is a hospital based or community sample or whether attempted suicide is being looked at along with self-harm (Madge *et al.* 2008). A number of characterisations have been used for self-harm, such as deliberate self-harm, self-injury, self-mutilation, auto-aggression, along with others. Self-harm can take many different forms, including cutting, burning (Favazza 1989), self-induced vomiting and laxative abuse (Santonastaso 1998). Some of the more severe cases of self-harm such as eye enucleation and amputation of limbs involve people with learning disabilities or young people experiencing a psychosis (Carson *et al.* 1998, Derby *et al.* 1998, Favazza 1998, Shiwach 1998). Lovell (2007) has argued that the term self-injury is often used to refer to people with learning disabilities, while self-harm is seen as relating more to the area of mental health. Despite concerns about the seriousness of self-harm, there is little consensus on what self-harm actually is (Mangnall and Yurkovich 2008). This lack of consensus leads to confusion about what is being studied and may make designing effective interventions difficult.

The National Self-Harm Inquiry (Mental Health Foundation 2006) describes self-harm as:

> A wide range of things that people do to themselves in a deliberate and usually hidden way, which are damaging. (Mental Health Foundation 2006: 5).

The inquiry focused on cutting, burning, scalding, banging, hair pulling and self-poisoning, and did not look at eating disorders, drug and alcohol misuse, and risk-taking behaviours such as unsafe sex or dangerous driving which could also be seen as self-harm.

In this chapter, we have used the term self-harm and avoided the use of deliberate self-harm, because the latter implies a judgement that the harm is intentional and that the young person has control over their behaviour; the term also has the potential to stigmatise young people (Miller and Armstrong 2005). We have chosen to use the term self-harm because it is commonly used in the UK by people working with children and young people and the research community, and is less stigmatising than the other popular term 'deliberate self-harm'. Sutton (2007) sees self-harm as too broad a term and prefers the term self-injury and quotes a definition of self-injury as:

> An expression of acute, psychological distress. It is an act done to oneself, by oneself, with the intention of helping oneself rather than killing oneself. Paradoxically damage is done to the body in an attempt to preserve the integrity of the mind (Sutton and Martinson 2003, cited in Sutton 2007: 1).

This definition refers to direct injury to the body – we have chosen to look at self-harm in a broader context. However, the psychological and emotional processes that occur may be different in children and young people who overdose to those who injure themselves by wounding their body. Sutton and Martinson (2007) remind us of an essential factor that self-harm can reflect a drive for self-preservation rather than self-destruction.

4.3   How common is self-harm?

Each year around 25,000 young people in the UK are admitted to Accident and Emergency departments following an episode of self-harm (Hawton *et al.* 2000). In England, admissions of 14- to 17-year-old males for self-harm rose from 2,195 in 1999 to 2,448 in 2005, while female admissions over the same period rose from 6,597 to 10,052 (Wheeler *et al.* 2008). In Scotland, around 7,000 young people are admitted to hospital each year (Scottish Executive 2002b) and in a study of admissions to Scottish hospitals, Payne *et al.* (2009) found that being of a younger age was a risk factor for readmission to hospital for self-poisoning. In Northern Ireland between the years 2000 and 2005, there was a slight increase in hospital admissions for self-harm from 4,583 to 4,705 and around 280 per 100,000 population are admitted in Northern Ireland each year (Department of Health, Social Services and Public Safety 2006). Girls are up to four times more likely to self-harm than boys (Hawton *et al.* 2006, O'Connor *et al.* 2009) although findings from other studies report more similarity in prevalence rates for males and females (Stanley *et al.* 2001, Muehlenkamp and Gutierrez 2004). Biddle *et al.* (2004) found that males sought help much later than females and were more troubled when they did so. When considering these statistics, the definition of self-harm used and the populations studied need to be taken into account if the statistics are to have relevance.

  Activity

Why do you think that some research identifies females as more likely to self-harm than males? Identify three factors which may contribute to these different rates. Discuss your reasons with a colleague.

While the general perception is that self-harm is on the increase, Goodman and Scott (2005) argue that following an increase between the 1950s and late 1980s, the rates of self-harm have declined. However, others see an increasing incidence of self-harm in young people (World Health Organization 2002, Fortune and Hawton 2005, Tick *et al.* 2008,). In a widely reported and rather alarming headline, Affinity Healthcare (2008) stated that one in three young people in their study had self-harmed; this is in contrast to a study of over 6,000 15-year-old school children which found lifetime self-harm prevalence rates of 13.2% (Hawton *et al.* 2002). The Child and Adolescent Self-harm in Europe (CASE) Study (Madge *et al.* 2008) found overall lifetime prevalence rates in primarily 15–16 year olds of 1.5% for females and 4.3% for males. The rates ranged from 4.05% in The Netherlands to 10.9% in Belgium. Lifetime rates of 10.9% were reported in the cohort from England (6.5% male and 15.3% female). In a similar study in Scotland, O'Connor *et al.* (2009) report lifetime prevalence rates of 6.9% for males, 19.9% for females and 13.8% overall. Madge *et al.* (2008) included thoughts of self-harm in their study, as might be expected thoughts of self-harm at some point in their lifetime were much higher – 9.9% for males and 21.5% for females. O'Connor *et al.* (2009) looked at serious thoughts of self-harm in the previous year and reported 8.5% in males and 19.5% in females.

Parental views are rarely taken into account in research studies. However, in a national survey of mental health in children and adolescents, parents/guardians were asked if their children were self-harming (Meltzer *et al.* 2001). Parents reported self-harm prevalence rates of 0.9% for 5–7 year olds, 1.7% for 8–10 year olds; there is no comparable data from children's accounts for these ages in the study. Parents reported prevalence rates of 1.6% for 11–12 year olds and 2.5% for 13–15 year olds – children reported 4.6% and 6.6%, respectively, for the same ages. It is fairly clear from this survey that parents can be unaware of self-harm when it is occurring.

 Activity

Do you think that self-harm is increasing or declining? Make notes on what has influenced your thinking, e.g. is it research, practice or anecdotal evidence?

4.4 Vulnerability and resilience

Identifying which young people are at risk of self-harm is important if help is to be targeted at the right groups. However, young people do not always fit easily into these groups, and while being in a vulnerable group may be a risk factor it does not mean the young person will self-harm and conversely someone not in an at-risk group may self-harm. The following groups of young people are more vulnerable to self-harm:

- Young people in prison are a particularly vulnerable group (Mental Health Foundation 2006), especially those on remand, which may suggest that isolation, hopelessness and alienation could play a part in the development of self-harm as a coping strategy. Most of these young people however had harmed themselves before they entered prison. In response to a freedom of information request, the Ministry of Justice (2009) cited by Puffet (2009) reported relatively consistent levels of self-harm in the years 2006 (2,062 incidents) and 2007 (1,835 incidents) although the levels of self-harm in the previous decade had increased more than twofold.
- Young Asian women in Britain are thought to be another group vulnerable to self-harm (Bhugra *et al.* 1999, Bhardwaj 2001); it is

conjectured that this may be due to experiencing a clash of cultures. However, Hawton *et al.* (2002) found that Asian girls were less likely to self-harm than their white counterparts.

■ Because of the isolation, victimisation and lack of opportunity available to them to talk about their feelings, Lesbian, Bisexual, Gay and Transgender (LBGT) young people are also vulnerable (King *et al.* 2003).

■ Young people with learning disabilities are a group vulnerable to self-harm, although very often self-harm is seen under the umbrella term of challenging behaviour (Wisely *et al.* 2002, Jones *et al.* 2004).

■ Young people who have been looked after or accommodated present with a disproportionate number of risk factors for suicide and self-harm (Scott and Hill 2006).

Other factors which make it more likely that a young person will self-harm include neglect, bereavement or loss (Ribbens-McCarthy 2005). Loss covers multiple factors such as family breakdown and disruption of important relationships. Drugs and alcohol may also play a part (Hawton *et al.* 2003). While self-harm is not an attempt to kill oneself, young people who do self-harm are more likely to kill themselves than those who do not (Owens *et al.* 2002); and there may be a particular link between repeated cutting of the skin and suicide (Cullberg *et al.* 1988). Trauma and abuse may have been experienced by young people who self-harm, and there may be a link between trauma and self-harm (Fliege *et al.* 2009). This should not be thought of in a simplistic way, rather we should think of all the challenges and affronts to their sense of self which young people may have experienced – whether through the lack of affectional bonds that children with insecure attachment experience, or through the lack of acknowledgement and value of difference that LBGT young people experience (Eisenberg and Resnick 2006).

4.5 Promoting resilience

Promoting resilience in children is a complex task, reliant on understanding the child's inner world, culture and context in which they have grown and are now living. Promoting resilience may involve helping children and young people develop trusting relationships. Teaching children problem-solving strategies may also be helpful (Schmidt and Davidson 2004). Developing techniques and approaches which help a young person identify factors which trigger self-harm may be useful (Slee *et al.* 2007). Assisting a child to develop an educational or vocational identity through which they can feel valued and supported may also promote resilience. Developing children's emotional intelligence may become a protective factor against self-harm. We know that if children are to become resilient, one of the single most important factors is that they are nurtured and parented in a positive way (Webster-Stratton 1992, 1998, Webster-Stratton and Reid 2008). Parenting programmes that promote positive changes in parenting behaviours can therefore be helpful in promoting resilient children; for further information see Chapter 2.

Reasons for self-harm

There are many different reasons why young people self-harm, some of which are outlined in Box 4.1. Managing or coping with difficult emotions may be reasons why young people self-harm. It can also be a way of communicating how they feel. It can be a means of escape or a way of coping with life. Young people use self-harm to take control – often young people perceive a lack of control in their lives and self-harm can be a way of getting some control back, and sometimes young people may not be sure why they harm themselves (Young *et al.* 2007).

Self-harm may be an indication that a child has been sexually abused (Favazza 1992, Allen 1995, Baral *et al.* 1998, Vajani *et al.* 2007). Self-harm can also be a self-punishment (Young *et al.* 2007) particularly for young people who have been sexually abused or young people with anorexia. For children who have been sexually abused, it can be a way of getting back at the abuser. Self-harm paradoxically brings comfort or relief to young people.

Self-harm may be related to coping and problem-solving, in that young people may use self-harm as a strategy for managing. Haines and Williams

---

Box 4.1 Some Reasons Why Children and Young People Self-Harm

- As a release
- To escape
- To 'get back' at other people
- To feel real
- To communicate
- To take away bad feelings
- To feel alive
- To prevent suicide
- To influence others
- Relieving anger
- To get support
- To be in control

(1997) found that people who self-harm engaged in more problem avoidance behaviours than controls and recorded less perceived control over problem-solving options. Kemperman *et al.* (1997) hypothesised that self-harming behaviour has an important mood regulatory function. They found significant mood elevation and decreased dissociation following self-injury, with the dissociation peaking during self-injury.

Having poorly developed social skills may contribute to a young person's self-harm (Laukkanen *et al.* 2009), whereas having close and supportive family/social relationships increases resilience to self-harm and other mental health problems (Daniel and Wassel 2002a). To compound this, low self-esteem (which may be present in young people who self-harm) makes it difficult for young people to engage in reciprocal social relationships.

4.6 Models of self-harm

There are numerous theories around the process of why young people self-harm, some of which are outlined in Table 4.1. Having a theoretical understanding of why young people self-harm can be useful in practice and further study of these models is necessary. We will briefly look at a biological perspective, a psychological perspective and an environmental perspective. It would be simplistic to argue that one model or theory could explain why young people self-harm and it makes sense to think that these different perspectives overlap and influence each other.

Table 4.1 Explanations for Self-Harm

Theoretical Perspectives on Stressors	Functions of Self-harm	Models of Self-harm
Biological perspective	Affect regulation	Behavioural/environmental model
Psychological perspective	Anti-dissociation	The depersonalisation model
Psychoanalytic perspective	Anti-suicide	The interpersonal/systemic model
Cognitive perspective	Interpersonal boundaries	Physiological/biological model
Situational or stressful life perspective	Interpersonal influence	The sexual model/sadomasochism
The social integration perspective	Self-punishment	Affect regulation model
The mental-ill health perspective	Sensation seeking	
McLaughlin (2007)	Klonsky (2007)	Messer *et al.* (2008)

Biological factors

There are a number of biological factors which may influence self-harm. It has been speculated that endorphins and enkephalins may play a role (Winchel and Stanley 1991, Strong 2000). When young people self-harm, endorphins and enkephalins are released which produce feelings of euphoria or reduce stress and provide relief, making self-harm more likely in the future. Some young people may produce endogenous analgesic chemicals which may increase the young person's pain threshold. It is hypothesised that low levels of the neurotransmitter serotonin (which has a role in regulating impulsivity, aggression and mood) may be associated with self-harm by lowering the young person's mood and reducing their ability to regulate their impulsivity, and there is some evidence that this is the case with adults (Mann *et al.* 2001). High levels of serotonin and positive parental relationships may be protective against self-harm (Crowell *et al.* 2008). New *et al.* (1997) have argued that self-harm represents a form of self-directed aggression and may be associated with a decrease in central serotonin (5-hydrotryptamine – 5-HT) function in some people who self-harm. Catecholamines (norepinephrine and dopamine) may play a role as the dopamine system in people with Lesch–Nyan syndrome (which is associated with repetitive self-harm) is impaired (Pascual-Castroviejo and Ruggieri 2008). There may also be changes to the chemistry of the brain following trauma which may make a young person more likely to self-harm. The importance of attachment and raised levels of cortisol in babies who are deprived is also worthy of consideration as a predictor for self-harm. We are however at the early stages of being able to link self-harm to biological markers and we should be cautious at the present time about being able to use biological perspectives to predict self-harming behaviour.

Environmental factors

The environment plays an important part in child development – in particular the family in which a young person is raised. There may be a link between the changes in the brain which occur when children are subjected to deprivation, and the ability to manage and regulate emotions in later life. This ability to manage emotions has a relationship to self-harm, in that the more acutely and quickly distress occurs, the more likely the ability to cope with that distress declines. Children need parents/carers to help them manage and regulate their emotions, and if they do not have the support of parents to manage stress they become unable to regulate their own emotions. Grocutt (2009) sees self-harm as being related to attachment difficulties, and that these problems are often ongoing. Stepp *et al.* (2008) found that adult attachment styles and interpersonal problems played a part in the type of self-harming behaviour.

The implications of a poor attachment and its relationship to the self-regulation of emotions are worthy of continued research.

Psychological factors

Psychological factors can be regarded as mediators in either lessening or increasing the likelihood of self-harm. Increased tension and anxiety are states which often precede self-harm. The psychological state the young person is in influences whether they self-harm. There is evidence that self-harming improves people's mood in the short term (Whitlock 2009). There is an assumption that people who self-harm do it to release tension, which is supported by research (Brain *et al*. 1998, Haines *et al*. 1995). The purpose of self-harm is to regulate the young person's affect – by self-harming they make themselves feel better by reducing anxiety (Favazza 1998). Self-harm can also be seen as an escape from intolerable or uncontainable emotional pain so that the self-harm serves as release and pain is lessened (Sutton 1998). For people who do not self-harm, it can be difficult to understand that something which would create tension in them would calm other people down (Cameron 2007).

Slee *et al*. (2008) argue that self-harm occurs when the young person is either in a depressed mood or experiencing heightened arousal. From a cognitive–behavioural perspective, they see cognitions, distorted thinking and beliefs as important factors leading to self-harm. Thoughts of hopelessness, low self-esteem and self-criticism (among others) are often present in young people who self-harm. When these types of thoughts become dominant, they may prevent young people from being able to arrest their self-harming. Ruminating about problems may be linked to thoughts of self-harm, in that when people ruminate on a stressful event it may cause further distress (Robinson and Alloy 2003, Morrison and O'Connor 2008).

Parental views

Given that parents are often upset and disturbed by their children self-harming, it is surprising that little research has looked at how parents perceive their children's self-harming. Oldershaw *et al*. (2008) looked at a small sample of parents from Child and Adolescent Mental Health Services (CAMHS) in London. They found that parents found their children's self-harm difficult to manage and parents often found themselves tiptoeing round their children following the disclosure of self-harm. Parents described watching and waiting, suspecting that the self-harm was occurring, and either not wanting to ask or not exploring the self-harm. Usually other adults such as teachers confirmed the self-harm. Parents struggled to make sense of their child's self-harm and experienced a range of feelings such as sadness, anger and shock. The self-harm had a negative impact on relationships within some families and a positive impact in others.

 Activity

Spend a few minutes reflecting on how you feel about children and young people who self-harm – you might want to think about a particular child/young person, or children/young people in general. Identify the different feelings you had – are your feelings different now? In what way, if at all, have your feelings changed?

4.7 Assessment

Children and young people's reasons for self-harming are often complex and may not be immediately apparent. If we are to understand why this child or young person is self-harming at this particular time, getting to know the young person and understanding their own view of their internal world is essential. The assessment of young people who self-harm should be carried out with sensitivity and care. Young people may be embarrassed about their self-harming behaviour or consider it a private act. It is important to establish whether the young person had suicidal intent. Many young people who self-harm do not intend to kill themselves (Hawton and James 2005); however, a minority do (Rodham *et al*. 2004). A useful guide to eliciting suicidal intent is to explore the act of self-harm by asking whether the young person feels suicidal, has told anyone they are thinking of committing suicide, has made attempts before and has a plan. Any of these factors is a concern, and the more factors there are the more at risk the young person is. Assessment of suicide in children and young people is discussed in more depth in Chapter 6.

Once you have established the child or young person did not have suicidal intent, an important part of the assessment is getting to know the young person as a whole person before enquiring about self-harm.

Enquiring about self-harm may involve talking with the young person about the meaning of their self-harm. Does the young person self-harm as a release, to make themselves feel real, as an attack on their body because they are disgusted with it, as a way of showing people how bad they feel inside or as a way of getting control over their lives? An understanding of the child or young person's reasoning for self-harm is very important – this may take some time, as young people may be reticent or unsure about talking about these issues. While it *may* be helpful to find out why young people self harm, this may not always be the case and the search for reasons may end up being counterproductive. Young people may not consciously know why they self-harm. Each young person is unique and while there may be factors which are common amongst young people who self-harm, what makes a young person self-harm is unique to the individual.

The length of time the young person has been self-harming, the nature, severity and precipitating factors of the self-harm should be considered. An assessment of the young person's mental state is important as self-harm is often associated with mental health problems such as depression and psychosis (Hawton and James 2005, Harvey *et al.* 2008). Early intervention is obviously important when mental health issues are factors in self-harming. A chain analysis of the events which led to a young person self-harming can be a useful tool for some young people. A chain analysis involves going through the preceding 24 hours outlining what young people did, thought and felt in the lead up to self-harming – in an effort to identify vulnerability or trigger factors.

Young people who self-harm may experience depersonalisation (not feeling real, feeling detached from their body) or derealisation (where the environment feels unfamiliar or unreal); these are both dissociative states. Dissociation is an important factor in self-harm (Klonsky 2007) and the role dissociation plays in a young person's self-harm should be assessed. Dissociation is a defence mechanism, where an unwanted part of or the whole self is split off and detached. Some young people self-harm to allow themselves to feel real, thereby using self-harm to overcome the dissociated self. Other young people become dissociated through the act of self-harm and this can be particularly dangerous as the young person will have less control over themselves when in a dissociated state, making them particularly vulnerable to harm. Alcohol or substance misuse may compound the harm further (Fickl 2007, Evren *et al.* 2008). Dissociation can be connected to abuse in children, when the child finds it incredibly difficult to relate the abuse to themselves and the abuser. This is particularly so when the abuser is someone who is meant to protect the child. The child therefore dissociates themselves from the act and this can become a way of managing difficult or intolerable emotions. Dissociation is an unconscious not a conscious act. For further discussion on dissociation, see Fickl (2007).

/ **Activity**

Sarah is 14 years old, she has cut her arms and you find her alone in a room as she is cutting herself. Make some notes of what Sarah might be feeling and after you have completed that, consider the kind of things you might say to Sarah to acknowledge her feelings.

4.8 Intervention

A number of interventions have been proposed to manage self-harm, and some of these will be outlined in the next section. A minority of young people will need physical or psychological care from a health or social care professional, but the majority who self-harm will not come into contact with services. A range of services therefore need to be provided from self-help to specialist children and young people's mental health services.

Which interventions are most effective and whether the same or different methods should be used for different populations are relatively unclear. Should the same method be used for young people who have self-harmed for the first time, compared to those who have repeated the act? Should the same methods be used for young people who overdose, compared with those who cut? Pattison and Harris (2006) reviewed the evidence for the effectiveness of counselling for children and young people, and found that cognitive–behaviour therapy (CBT), humanistic, interpersonal, psychodynamic and psychoanalytic forms of counselling were effective in helping children and young people who self-harm. Their definition of self-harm included substance misuse, eating disorders, self-injury/harm and suicide.

Engagement of young people at an early stage is essential as some young people find it difficult to engage with interventions. Briefer forms of intervention for some young people may therefore be more helpful than longer-term ones. However, longer-term interventions may provide more containment and be more successful for some children and young people. Despite claims of effectiveness for some interventions, there is a need to tailor interventions to the needs of children and young people. As an example, the evidence for dialectical behaviour therapy (DBT) is expanding but the approach does not suit everyone (Pembroke 2007: 166, Proctor 2007: 109).

Three factors to consider when offering an intervention are consistent support, helping young people communicate and supporting staff (particular in relation to risk-taking and risk management). The importance of risk management should not be underestimated as helping young people manage feelings of self-harm has an impact on adults who are working alongside them. Seeing young people harm themselves can be very distressing; therefore, staff support is not only helpful to the member of staff but also to the young person. We are less likely to push away or reject a young person if we are being supported to make sense of our reactions and feelings. There can be a tendency to want to overprotect and avoid taking risks as the young person's behaviour may already be perceived as being too risky. The importance of intelligent risk-taking should be recognised from the beginning and we should be supported to manage and understand risk. When working with young people, it is therefore crucial to access intervention-related supervision, so that feelings, thoughts and reactions can be processed with the aim of helping both young person and worker.

Different interventions may be more appropriate for particular groups of children and young people or for their developmental stage – children may respond more readily through play therapy. Particular attention needs to be paid to the assessment of children and young people with learning disabilities. Priest and Gibbs (2004) advocate the use of a behaviour problem inventory (Rojahn *et al.* 2002) to assist the assessment of people with learning disabilities. Raghavan and Patel (2005) argue the overlap between mental health problems and self-harming in people with learning disabilities and challenging behaviours is multifaceted; they argue that assessment to establish whether the mental health problem is a factor in the challenging behaviour, or whether there is some other cause, is complex.

Activity

Ahmed is 6 years old, his parents tell you that he regularly bangs his head at home, and has quite marked bruises on his forehead. What might you ask his parents to help you understand what is happening with Ahmed? What more do you need to know and how would you help Ahmed?

4.9　Informal support

There is a tendency to operationalise any form of support or counselling we offer to people, frameworks are placed around our work and these are developed into therapies or interventions which can be researched and their effectiveness evidenced. Some young people do not find these structures helpful and we may need to think of providing help in a different way. Kirk (2007) describes a model of informal support where the emphasis is on flexibility in working with young people and offering a range of informal interventions and locations, such as meeting people in public spaces, going for walks, tenpin bowling and talking about issues the young person might find worrying. This type of approach rather than focusing on counselling or psychotherapy allows a young people to set the agenda and move at their own pace.

4.10　Promoting positive behaviour

There is considerable evidence that promoting positive behaviour in both the home and school environment can have a beneficial effect on younger children (Bauer and Webster-Stratton 2006, Hutchings *et al.* 2007,

Webster-Stratton and Reid 2008). Self-harm can occur in younger children because they may become frustrated and unable to communicate their needs. Similar difficulties may be found in children and young people with learning disabilities. Establishing whether any learning, developmental or neurological difficulties contribute to the child's problems is important. Self-harming behaviour in younger children such as head banging (sometimes referred to as challenging behaviour in the literature) can be helped by the promotion of positive behaviour. Parenting programmes such as those developed by Webster-Stratton (1998) have a strong evidence base for changing parental behaviour and promoting positive family relationships. This involvement of families may be crucial – families may need to be educated about self-harm, as they may have never experienced self-harm before. Families are also an important resource in helping children and young people manage their emotional and social lives. Similarly the thoughtful involvement of carers with children who are looked after and accomodated may be supportive to the child or young person.

4.11 Self-help

Given that the majority of young people do not come into contact with services, help for young people needs to be easily accessible. Self-help books which outline different techniques, strategies, and approaches, such as how to minimise self-harm, manage crises, use problem-solving techniques to help manage thoughts of self-harm, camouflage the skin, may be of help when self-harm initially occurs as well as in the later stages (Arnold and Magill 1998, National Self Harm Network 2000, Schmidt and Davidson 2004). Strategies used by young people to manage their self-harm are numerous, and highlight the creativity which can emerge when young people are faced with challenge; some techniques, which might be helpful, are highlighted in Box 4.2.

Young people are increasingly using online discussion groups to share experiences. The process of online discussion appears to be helpful to some young people, although concern has been expressed that for some these message boards may be downplaying the damage of self-harm and are maintaining self-harm (Rodham *et al.* 2007). Methods of communication are constantly changing; services need to be able to respond to these changes. There are ever-increasing resources available online to offer help or encourage self-help; examples of these can be found at the end of this chapter.

Box 4.2 Some Alternatives to Self-Harm

- Putting ice on your skin
- Distraction
- Listening to music
- Using make-up to create false cuts
- Keeping a journal
- Hitting cushions with a stick
- Exercising
- Chewing a chilli
- Talking to a friend
- Telephoning a helpline
- Doing something creative like artwork
- Drawing over old scars
- Drawing on your arm
- Putting plasters where you want to self-harm
- Shouting – making lots of noise
- Smashing something
- Pinging an elastic band off your wrist
- Using prosthetic skin and cutting it
- Writing
- Creating space between the urge and the act – setting targets to increase the time

---

 Activity

You are at an Accident and Emergency department with Mark a young person you know quite well. He has taken an overdose of Ibuprofen tablets, you don't know how many. When a nurse sees Mark she sighs and says, 'Not again, I've got enough to do tonight seeing people who are really ill'.

How might Mark be feeling?

Why would the nurse say this?

What would you do in this situation?

4.12 Making access easier

Some interventions have been targeted at helping young people gain easier access to services. Cotgrove *et al.* (1995) used a token (green card) with the aim of giving young people immediate access to paediatric services should they require it. Although the results of the study were not statistically significant, it did seem to indicate that the intervention may be helpful in reducing repeated suicide attempts. Harrington *et al.* (1998) found that home-based interventions while not having an effect on the repetition of self-harm reduced the number of children admitted into care. Hawton and

James (2005) argue that home-based treatment programmes may overcome some potential barriers to receiving help. The introduction of Intensive Home Treatment Teams for children and young people's services in some parts of the UK has meant that children and young people can be offered interventions in their home setting; this may go some way to balance the adverse effects a restrictive residential environment can have. Carter *et al.* (2007) report an interesting study which looked at the effect of sending postcards asking how people were throughout the year to adults who had overdosed. While not reducing the number of people who repeated self-harm, it did reduce the number of repetitions and may be of use with young people.

Harm minimisation

An important change in the way that self-harm is managed is the introduction of a harm-minimisation strategy, instead of trying to make them change and stop self-harming, the response is one of acceptance. The young person is not prevented from self-harming but is offered harm-minimisation strategies. Implicit in this approach is the view that self-harm is a way of managing difficult emotions and that by providing acceptance, understanding and giving young people choice and control containment is paradoxically provided (Babiker and Arnold 1997, Hogg 2001, Harrison and Sharman 2005, Pembroke 2007, Shaw and Shaw 2007). However, not all clinicians agree with this approach with some arguing that information on harm minimisation, particularly in self-help guides, may be misinterpreted and cause further harm (Pengelly *et al.* 2008).

In many health care settings, it is common for young people to be asked to sign a contract in which they commit themselves to not self-harming. If they break the contract, a penalty is invoked, sometimes discharge from the service. 42nd Street is a community-based resource reduced based in Manchester for young people who are experiencing stress; they argue that contracts disguise power dynamics between unequal parties, i.e. the young person and the professional. The hidden bargain in the contract is that only when the young person has given up what gives them control, e.g. cutting – will the professionals help. Instead, 42nd Street argues that a young person should be helped to contract with their own empowered self rather than others (Spandler 1996, Arabi *et al.* 2007).

4.13 Talking therapies

Evidence for the effectiveness of the different forms of therapy for children and young people who self-harm is slowly emerging. There are some difficulties in establishing a 'gold standard' regarding evidence in psychotherapeutic approaches (i.e. randomised controlled trial, RCT). There are issues in conducting RCTs where the skill of the person delivering the treatment is a factor and where randomisation may be difficult because of preferences for a particular therapy. These problems are not insurmountable, but they are obstacles, as some modalities (e.g. CBT) may lend themselves to the RCT process more readily than others.

Evidence for the psychodynamic approach relies mainly on small studies, individual case studies or descriptions of treatment approaches (Gardner 2001, Paulson and Everall 2003, Woods 2006). These accounts give useful insights into the complexity of working in a psychodynamic way, and the importance of not giving into feelings of despair and helplessness which can accompany this work. Waska (1998) argues that the psychoanalytic method is the treatment of choice, and that self-destructive behaviours are the sum outcome of unconscious fantasies and these unconscious fantasies can be worked through in therapy. Other analysts argue that changes in mental functioning during adolescence make it possible for the individual to redirect aggression inwards (Newman and Hirt 1983). This is of interest because one of the fundamental tasks of adolescence is the mastery of the revived instinctual drives of which aggression is one (Friedman et al. 1996).

There is an increasing interest in the use of CBT with young people and some evidence that it may be helpful in reducing self-harm. However, most of the evidence is from adult studies and is inconclusive. Slee et al. (2008) report on a study of 90 adolescents and young adults randomly allocated to either treatment as usual (TAU) or TAU plus CBT. The participants were followed up at 3-month intervals until 9 months and the CBT arm self-harmed significantly less than those receiving TAU. There have been criticisms that the conclusions of the study may have been overstated (Kripalani et al. 2008).

Solution focused brief therapy (SFBT) is an intervention which is commonly used with children and young people. Kim (2008) reviewed the effectiveness of SFBT in social work and found it to be effective. The evidence for its use with self-harm in children and young people has yet to be established.

DBT was developed by Linehan (1993a,b) specifically to help people diagnosed as having a borderline personality disorder (BPD) and has been modified for use with young people by Miller et al. (1997). This technique uses cognitive psychotherapy, mindfulness, combined with skills training, family therapy and telephone consultation. The skills taught include teaching young people how to manage emotions problem solve and tolerate distress. Miller and Smith (2008) argue that DBT is the gold standard in terms of effectiveness in the reduction of self-harming behaviour in adults diagnosed with a BPD.

DBT is fairly well established in young people's mental health services. There is evidence that DBT is effective in reducing self-harm in young people with mental health problems (Goldstein *et al.* 2007). Katz and Cox (2002) describe the employment of DBT with a young person who was self-harming, outlining the course and process of treatment and reporting significant reduction in her suicidal ideation. Turner (2000) compared DBT with client-centred therapy (CCT) control condition in young people and young adults and found a significant reduction in self-harming behaviour in those receiving DBT. Katz *et al.*'s (2004) study of 62 young people aged 14–17 years found while there was a reduction in behaviour problems in the DBT group, there was no significant difference in parasuicide events between the DBT and TAU groups. DBT appears to be well accepted by some young people and may be particularly useful for young people in CAMHS. There are however no RCTs in children and young people, although there is evidence from adult studies (Linehan *et al.* 2006).

Group therapies

Groups are particularly important to children and young people; they can be both a challenge and a support. Traditionally, psychodynamic and psychoanalytic techniques have been used in treating young people in CAMHS (Black 1993), although CBT and DBT groups are becoming more prevalent. Projective techniques such as those used in art or other creative therapy groups can be useful particularly in young people who have difficulties with emotional literacy. The artwork can be seen as a symbolic representation of the act of self-harm and via this young people can be helped to express, and eventually control, their feelings around self-harm. Green (2007) described the process of setting up a social action group, where young people were empowered to act collectively to confront the difficult and complex issues around their self-harm. He describes how the staff wrestled with issues about their own need to control at the same time as trying to work alongside young people, and the importance of young people making changes through the group.

Wood *et al.* (2001) compared routine care and group CBT with routine care alone and found that young people receiving CBT were significantly less likely to self-harm. Burns *et al.* (2005) reported a randomised study of group therapy and aftercare versus usual aftercare for 12–16 years olds who had self-harmed at least once in the previous year. The group therapy involved techniques from DBT, CBT and problem-solving approaches. The young people who received the group therapy had significantly fewer occurrences of self-harm at follow-up.

 Activity

Mairi is a 16-year-old girl who has been suffering from depression for the last 2 years. Her depression has remitted for 2 or 3 months at a time but keeps recurring. She acknowledges that her mood has improved but still feels quite low.

Mairi started to hurt herself about 6 months ago, the intensity and frequency increasing over the months until she is now hitting her arms with a hammer almost daily. She says she gets great relief from it. She has no social life, where previously she was an outgoing person. She wants to stop hurting herself but nothing relieves her feelings in the same way. Describe the things you would consider when thinking about working alongside Mairi?

4.14 The personal impact of working alongside children and young people who self-harm

Working with children and young people who are distressed and in emotional pain is difficult; it is therefore understandable that we may wish to distance ourselves from our reactions and feelings about this hurt. It can be an emotionally painful experience when someone we work alongside self-harms; unpleasant or uncomfortable feelings such as shock, disappointment, anger or being let down may be invoked. How could someone we are trying to help do this to themselves? Why couldn't they speak to us? As Spandler (1996: 117) highlights, this search for truth and reasons may not in itself be helpful. Processing, understanding and making sense of our feelings are essential if we are to avoid becoming indifferent and uncaring. We need to work alongside young people, understanding their accounts and work together to find a different path.

 Activity

Consider how you process your work with young people – do you receive supervision? If you are not being supervised, how do you bring a different perspective to you work?

In 1996, 42nd Street published a report on young people, self-harm and suicide; one of the chapters titled 'Not a Clue' reported young people's views of service provision, views which were critical and uncomfortable to read (Spandler 1996). There are positive signs that attitudes and values are changing. The NICE Guidelines on self-harm clearly state that the treatment of people who self-harmed has been 'often been unacceptable' (NICE 2004b: 7) and that people should be treated with dignity and respect. The Ten Essential Shared Capabilities in the UK and the Recovery Approach in Scotland have agendas focused on values, rights, relationships, respect and a collaborative approach to mental health practice (Department of Health 2004, Scottish Executive 2006). Translating such laudable policy and guidelines into practice will be a challenge, but it is a challenge to the prevailing culture, which is both refreshing and inspiring. Bosma and van Meijeil (2008) reviewed the literature on self-injury in psychiatry examining service user and nurse perspectives. None of the studies looked at children or young people's views but service users reported helpful interventions as one's which 'nurture hope, self confidence and self esteem' (Bosman and van Meijeil 2008: 183). This is a message which we must incorporate in our work with children, young people and their families/carers. Focusing on communication and relationships which promote such positive change may therefore be more important than focusing on a particular treatment or intervention.

4.15 Conclusion

This chapter has presented core issues about self-harm. The public perception is that self-harm is increasing and such perceptions seem to be supported by the evidence. The studies around prevalence appear to challenge the conventional view that self-harm is a predominantly female problem and research is ongoing in this area. Understanding and connecting with children and young people who self-harm must be a focus for all adults who work alongside children and young people. Establishing a consensus on what self-harm actually is would contribute to the understanding of issues around self-harm. It may be that we have to see self-harm and self-injury as separate entities as there may different motivations for different acts. Finally, the focus on relationships and the shift in mental health policy, particularly in Scotland, towards a recovery focus is a welcome move, the benefits of which are yet to be assessed.

Recommended reading

Hawton, K., Bergen, H., Casey, D., *et al.* (2007). Self-harm in England: a tale of three cities. Multicentre study of self-harm. *Social Psychiatry and Psychiatric Epidemiology* 42 (7), 513–521.

Scottish Government (2009). *Towards a Mentally Flourishing Scotland: Policy and Action Plan 2009–2011*. Edinburgh: Scottish Government.
Solomon, Y. and Farrand, J. (1996). Why don't you do it properly? Young women who self-injure. *Journal of Adolescence* 19 (2), 111–120.
Sourander, A., Aromaa, M., Pihlakosk, L., *et al.* (2006). Early predictors of deliberate self-harm among adolescents. A prospective follow-up study from age 3 to age 15. *Journal of Affective Disorders* 93 (1–3), 87–96.
Spandler, H. and Warner, S. (2007). *Beyond Fear and Control: Working with Young People Who Self-harm*. Ross on Wye: PCCS Books.
Stanley, N. (2007). Young people's and carers' perspectives on the mental health needs of looked-after adolescents. *Child and Family Social Work* 12 (3), 258–267.
The Mental Health Foundation (2006). *Truth Hurts – Report of the National Inquiry into Self-harm Among Young People*. London: Mental Health Foundation.
Wadman, S. (2007). Scratching the surface. *Mental Health Practice* 10 (8), 18–19.

Resources

The National Children's Bureau
http://www.selfharm.org.uk/default.aspa
http://www.bebo.com/Profile.jsp?MemberId=4253888538

The Basement Project
The Basement Project provides support groups for those who have been abused as children and people who self-harm. These are free to individuals. They also provide training, consultation and supervision for workers in community and mental health services. They publish a number of publications which offer advice to workers.
http://www.basementproject.co.uk/

Young People and Self-Harm
http://www.selfharm.org.uk/
Information resource for young people who self-harm and their carers.

National Self-Harm Network
PO Box 16190
London
NW1 3WW
Campaigns for the rights and understanding for people who self-harm and provides information and leaflets.
http://www.nshn.co.uk/

Bristol Crisis Service for Women
PO Box 654
Bristol BS99 1XH
Information, publications and training about self-harm
Tel.: Office/Admin 0117 927 9600
Email: bcsw@btconnect.com
Helpline 0117 925 1119 Friday and Saturday Nights 9.00 p.m. to 12.30 a.m.
http://www.users.zetnet.co.uk/BCSW/youngwomen.htm

SIARI – Self Injury and Related Issues
Extensive information on self-harm:
http://www.siari.co.uk/

Chapter 5

DEPRESSION

Martin Gaughan

School of Nursing, Midwifery and Social Care, Edinburgh Napier University, Edinburgh, Scotland

5.1 Introduction

In the age group 15–44 years, depression is currently the second highest cause of life lost due to an early death or a productive life lost to disability (World Health Organization (WHO) 2008b). In high-income countries in 2004, depression was the main cause of disability. The WHO has predicted that, by 2020, major depression will be the second leading cause of disability across all ages (WHO 2010). Depression in children and young people is perceived as an increasing health problem. A survey of the mental health of children and young people in the UK found prevalence rates for depression of 0.2% in children between 5 and 10 years old and 1.2% for young people aged 11–16 years (Green *et al.* 2005). In the USA, 1.3 million young people between 15 and 19 years of age are reported as experiencing depression (Angold *et al.* 1998). Estimated rates of major depression in children between the ages of 9–17 years is thought to be 5% (Shaffer *et al.* 1996a) and the point prevalence rate for young people is estimated to be between 4% and 6% (Kessler *et al.* 2001). A study in Spain of preschool children aged 3–6 years old found a prevalence of 1.12% for major depression (Doménech-Llaberia *et al.* 2009). Depression is seen as a serious problem, a problem which is often undetected, and a problem in need of treatment. This chapter will explore the prevalence of depression in children and young people and consider why depression has become an issue of such concern. We will discuss issues relating to the diagnosis of depression and reflect on the proposition that rather than being under-diagnosed, depression may be over-diagnosed because it is being confused with sadness. We will examine factors which make young people vulnerable to

Understanding Children and Young People's Mental Health, first edition. Edited by Anne Claveirole and Martin Gaughan. Published 2011 by John Wiley & Sons Ltd. © 2011 John Wiley & Sons Ltd.

depression and conclude with a review of current strategies for helping young people who are depressed.

Learning outcomes

After reading this chapter, you should be able to:

1. Discuss why depression is more prevalent in young people than children.
2. Describe the features of childhood depression.
3. Describe the difference in the presentation of depression between boys and girls.
4. Compare two different intervention methods for depression in children and young people.
5. Consider the evidence for the effectiveness of medication in treatment of depression.

5.2 Defining depression

Depression is a serious mental health problem which can significantly affect a child or young person's development. Experiencing depression at such an important developmental phase can be difficult to cope with for the child and their family. Depression is widely recognised as a common problem in children and young people, in contrast to the earlier view that children in particular could not become depressed because of lack of maturation in their personalities (Harrington 2005). However, this perspective is not shared by all clinicians: Timimi (2004) argues that there is no convincing evidence to reliably distinguish between depression and sadness in children. Because non-specific symptoms are often used to diagnose depression in children, there is uncertainty about the true frequency of depression before puberty. The symptoms associated with depression will be outlined later in this chapter.

Diagnosing depression in children is complex. Children may have difficulty in distinguishing between feelings such as sadness and anger (Bamberg 2001) and in recognising the duration of problems, so they may not good at describing how long they have experienced particular feelings. In using adult definitions with children, depression was previously diagnosed without the presence of a majority of adult symptoms. It has been argued that symptoms of depression are difficult to detect in children as they can be masked by other phenomena such as phobias, delinquencies, eneuresis and somatic symptoms (Glaser 1967, Bschor 2002). Abdominal pain is regarded as a potential or coexisting symptom of depression (Dowrick *et al.* 2005). However, as Goodman and Scott (2005) argue, depression should not be diagnosed unless affective symptoms are present. Deciding whether a young person has a depressive disorder or is simply experiencing depressive symptoms is challenging.

The *Diagnostic and Statistical Manual of Mental Disorders* (DSM) (American Psychiatric Association (APA) 2000) makes minor distinctions between childhood and adult criteria, while the *International Classification of Diseases* (ICD) (WHO 1992) makes no mention of differences in the diagnosis of children or adults. Using diagnostic criteria for depression in children which bear little relationship to those of adult depression is problematic and of concern to a number of commentators.

Activity

Consider the signs and symptoms of depression in children and young people and outline how you would distinguish these from everyday feelings of sadness experienced by children and young people.

A difficulty of diagnosing depression in children and young people is that everyday feelings, behaviours and emotions can be interpreted as signs of 'disease or illness'. The medicalisation of children's behaviour and emotions has been widely discussed elsewhere (Blum 2007, Conrad 2007, Timimi 2007) and we will not repeat the debate. However, it is essential that at the very least we are aware of differing views about the definition and diagnosis of depression in children and young people.

Previously depression was seen as either endogenous (occurring from within, having a biological cause) or reactive (a combination of stressful external events and a vulnerability to depression). The advent of DSM-III changed this perspective and depression was categorised along a continuum of minor to major depression. This has significantly influenced our view of depression and what was previously a rare illness has become commonplace. This medicalisation of everyday emotions has created a new set of challenges for young people not experienced by previous generations. However, there is minimal engagement with this debate in the Child and Adolescent Mental Health Services (CAMHS) literature. Depression is seen as under-recognised in primary care and children's symptoms of depression are overlooked (Weller and Weller 2000). If, however, depression is over-diagnosed, the development of these children and young people may be adversely affected, particularly their resilience.

Horwitz and Wakefield (2007) analysed the rise in the diagnosis of depression across the lifespan and proposed that normal sadness had become confused with depression; that normal experiences of loss and unhappiness were being reinterpreted as illness. They argued that due to the increasing influence (it could be argued dominance) of DSM-IV criteria, depression had become over-diagnosed. Horwitz and Wakefield (2007) saw a number of factors influencing our view of depression from what was a relatively rare illness 30 years ago to one that is now commonplace. The context of people's sadness is often ignored when considering whether someone is depressed. The context is important because without context, other factors affecting people's mood, such as loss, are ignored. Horwitz and Wakefield (2007) argue that DSM-IV criteria, while useful in clinical practice, are used as a framework to diagnose depression in the community – this leads to an over-recognition or over-estimation of depression in both children and young people. This argument is important because children and young people end up receiving medical treatment for a perceived illness, which may in fact be an existential problem – a problem of being human. Rather than medicalising such problems, young people need to be given an opportunity to overcome and manage their distress.

5.3 Prevalence

Concern has been expressed about an epidemic of depression in children and young people. Costello et al. (2006) reviewed the evidence and suggested that while clinicians increasingly recognised depression, the actual rate had remained the same for the last 30 years or more. The British Child and Adolescent Mental Health Survey 1999 (Ford et al. 2004) found prevalence rates of around 0.9% for all depression and 0.6% for major depression in children aged 5–15 years. A number of studies have reported prevalence rates of around 1–2%, others report 3% of major depression in 9–12 year olds and 4–6% in young people (Kessler et al. 2001), while a study of secondary school pupils in Edinburgh found prevalence rates of 8.4% (Moor et al. 2007). Children with learning disability are at higher risk of depression than children without (Emerson and Hatton 2007, Tonge and Einfeld 2003, Tonge 2007), although some studies show little difference in clinical depression between children who have a learning disability and those who do not (Stevenson and Romney 1984). The ability of ICD-10 and DSM-IV criteria to identify psychological difficulties in children and young people has been called into question given the over-reliance on verbal communication; this is particularly true of children and young people with learning disabilities.

There are gender differences in rates of depression; in pre-pubertal children, depression is just as common in boys as it is in girls, with some studies suggesting a greater preponderance of depression in boys (Anderson *et al.* 1987, Weller *et al.* 2006a). By adulthood, women have higher rates of depression than men. Salokangas *et al.* (2002) argue that differences in prevalence rates for males and females may be due to gender-biased items in the screening instruments. A study of 5- to 8-year-old girls in Pittsburgh found that less than 1% of the girls studied had depressive symptoms and that in 7 year olds it was more common than not to have a symptom of depression (Keenan *et al.* 2004). This study reflects Horwitz and Wakefield's (2007) concerns, as existential issues such as *I felt lonely, thought nobody loved me, was very restless* were categorised as symptoms of depression. The measure used in this study was the Short Moods and Feelings questionnaire (Angold *et al.* 1995), a measure commonly used in assessing depression in young people.

 Activity

Consider what factors might contribute to the difference in prevalence rates of depression for males and females both before and after puberty.

5.4 Vulnerability

A combination of environmental and biological factors has been strongly implicated in vulnerability to depression, examples of these are outlined in Table 5.1. The development and maintenance of depression depend on a complex interplay between these factors and will be different for each individual.

These vulnerability factors are not direct causes of depression, it is the interaction between these vulnerabilities which may lead to depression. Factors may combine to produce depression; however, the development of depression is complex and experiencing a number of vulnerabilities may not result in a young person becoming depressed.

There may be a genetic component to depression as there are high rates of mental health problems amongst relatives, particularly parents of children who have depression (Klein *et al.* 2001). There is a strong association between depression and young people who have problems forming peer relationships. However, it is not clear whether peer problems are a cause or

Table 5.1 Vulnerability Factors for Depression

Early Experiences	Individual Disposition	Family and Social Disposition	Current Adversities	Maintenance Factors
Attachment	Genetics	Poverty	Bereavement	Severity of depression
Lack of parental/ guardian care	Difficulty in forming relationships	Social class	Loss	Family stress
Physical abuse	Negative styles of thinking	Adverse family environment	Rejection	Temperament
Emotional abuse	Low self-esteem	Parents who are/have been depressed	Abuse	Difficult social relationships
Sexual abuse	Temperament	Divorce	Being bullied	Isolation
Neglect	Attributional style	Parental educational attainment	Adverse life events	Poor academic and school experiences
Domestic violence	Control	Parental substance misuse	Disasters	Hopelessness/helplessness

a result of depression, or whether both are influenced by a third factor. Goodyer and Altham (1991) have suggested that either depressed children act in a way which has a negative impact on their friends, or the negative thinking in depression reduces the types of behaviour necessary to maintain or develop friendships. Other studies have shown that having the qualities which bring out positive social responses in others are protective against depression (Radke-Yarrow and Sherman 1990).

The onset of depression in children has been associated with undesirable life events and maternal distress (Goodyer 1990, Tamplin *et al.* 1998); however, there are no specific life events particularly associated with depression in young people. In a study of the effect of stressful life events on the development of depressive symptoms, the impact of life events disappeared when the study controlled for previous depressive symptoms, and the authors' caution against a simplistic approach of correlating stressful life events and depression (Waaktaar *et al.* 2004). Adverse childhood experiences (ACEs) such as emotional or sexual abuse are known to have an influence on the development of depression and may continue to do so decades after the traumatic event/s (Chapman *et al.* 2004).

 Activity

Is depression inherited? Read Hansson *et al.*'s (2008) paper. Consider arguments for and against the proposition of a direct or indirect genetic link to depression.

5.5 Assessment

When assessing a young person, it is important to consider information from different sources, as children usually behave differently depending on the setting. Parents are an obvious source of information: they can explain why they believe there is a problem and why now. When interviewing the child, an understanding of child development, particularly of language, emotional and cognitive development, is essential because children have different understandings and different ways of describing things depending on their age. It is important to consider alternative influences or explanations, and take a holistic approach. If enquiries are made in the context of specific environmental events, children can differentiate basic emotions such as sadness or irritability. However, in the absence of a context, children may confuse basic emotions such as sadness and anger (Bamberg 2001, Martin *et al.* 2010). While parental perspectives should be noted, parents may have a limited knowledge of their children's inner world (or even if they are aware may not act on their knowledge). A study by Puura *et al.* (1998) suggested that while parents and teachers readily saw symptoms of depression in children, they were on the whole unlikely to seek help for the child. A study in four secondary schools in Edinburgh found that teachers were unlikely to recognise depression in young people prior to receiving specific training in the recognition of depression (Moor *et al.* 2007).

Interviews are usually used in assessments and can be structured, semi-structured or unstructured. Other methods of assessment include questionnaires, such as the Beck Depression Inventory (Beck *et al.* 1961) or the Birleson Depression Inventory (Birleson 1981), and schedules for semi-structured interviews, such as the Kiddie-SADS (Puig-Antich and Chambers 1978), which has been revised by Ambrosini *et al.* (1989), and the Child Assessment Scale (Hodges *et al.* 1982). Rating scales have been developed to assess depression in people with learning disabilities, although they tend to be used with adults. Meins (1993) modified the Children's Depression Inventory to diagnose depression for adults with learning disabilities and Marston *et al.* (1997) developed a checklist of 30 items from ICD-10 criteria to assess depression in people with a learning disability. The Glasgow Depression Scale was developed to specifically assess depression in people with a learning disability and is written in easily understandable language (Lunsky and Palucka 2004). The level of care and support someone with a learning disability receives may mask symptoms. Whether someone is taking physical care of themselves may be hidden by the fact they are receiving personal care from someone else.

Questionnaires and inventories while useful should never be the sole method of assessment – the child or young person should always be interviewed or observed. Play therapy approaches are important techniques when working with younger children. Creative approaches in assessment, using techniques such as externalising the problem or giving the depression a name can be helpful. Nylund and Ceske (1997) describe a narrative approach to understanding depression in young women – some children and young people respond quite well to the use of such an approach in the assessment.

Multiple areas of a child or young person's functioning need to be considered. Some symptoms of depression such as low mood, withdrawal or loss of appetite are more immediately accessible. Changes in the way a child or young person speaks or behaves should be investigated. However, there are many events and experiences that result in a child or young person feeling sad. It is important that adults do not jump to the conclusion of a medical explanation for life events which bring sadness to a young person's life.

The assessment of emotional problems with a child or young person who has a learning disability can be particularly challenging. Helping young people with a learning disability to describe their feelings can be difficult as communication is often impaired and it may be hard for the child to describe how they feel. The more severe the level of learning disability, the more difficult it can be for the child to communicate their feelings. Information from other sources such as parents and school teachers is therefore important. Observing the child or young person and recognising changes in behaviour such as sleep, appetite and level of activity can be helpful (Bouras and Holt 2007) as well as taking into account the developmental stage the child is at – not the stage they 'should' be at.

The risk of suicide or attempted suicide increases as children grow older. There is a clear connection between depression and suicide, with one review finding between 49% and 64% of young people who completed suicide also had depression (Gould *et al.* 2003). There is the concern that the problem of suicide in children under age 12 years is increasing (Tishler *et al.* 2007). Even though suicide is more common in young people, it should not be dismissed in children as some children have suicidal thoughts and act on these. It is unclear at which age a child is able to understand the consequences of their actions, i.e. that their actions may result in their death and what death is. Chapter 6 discusses the assessment of suicide in children and young people and should be consulted if you are concerned about suicide risk.

5.6   Symptoms of depression in children and young people

Before discussing some of the symptoms of depression in children and young people, we will outline the symptoms of depression as defined in DSM-IV-TR (APA 2000). For a diagnosis of an episode of major depression to be made, at least five of the criteria outlined in Box 5.1 should have been present for at least 2 weeks, and one of the criteria must be depressed mood or loss of interest or pleasure. The symptoms must also cause significant distress, affect the person's social and vocational functioning, not have a physical cause such as substance misuse or hypothyroidism, and not be due to bereavement. There are two exceptions in the diagnosis of depression in children and young people; the depressed mood may be an irritable mood and the weight loss may be a failure of a child to gain weight expected in their physical development. ICD-10 and DSM-IV-TR categorise the range of depressive disorders differently and you should consult both guidelines to familiarise yourself with the differences.

Box 5.1 Symptoms of Depression

- Diminished ability to think or concentrate
- Depressed mood nearly all or most of the day
- Thoughts of death – suicidal thoughts
- Sleep disturbance, either lack of sleep or markedly increased sleep nearly every day
- Psychomotor retardation or agitation
- Feelings of worthlessness or excessive or inappropriate guilt
- Fatigue or loss of energy
- Marked changes in appetite or weight
- Loss of interest or pleasure in most or all activities

Young people can present with some or most of these signs and symptoms of depression, but may also show differences from adult depression. In young people, irritability and social withdrawal are more marked, loss of pleasure in activities is less common, physical pain as an indicator of depression is more frequent as are suicidal thoughts (Dowrick *et al.* 2005, Weller *et al.* 2006). Self-harm may be a way of managing feelings of depression for some young people.

There are differences in the signs of depression between pre- and post-pubertal children. Children may express more somatic complaints, irritability, separation anxiety, crying, school refusal and abdominal pain (Goodman and Scott 2005, Weller *et al.* 2006). Young people experience greater hopelessness and helplessness, guilt, anhedonia (absence of enjoyment of anything), hypersomnia (too much sleep) and use of alcohol and drugs to manage their depressed feelings (Goodman and Scott 2005, Weller *et al.* 2006b, Wu *et al.* 2006). Hallucinations may also be present in severe depression (Cepeda 2000). For children and young people who have learning disabilities, careful consideration of assessment of depression should be undertaken. Box 5.2 outlines some of the areas to consider, or symptoms to look for. It should be clear that a multiple perspectives of a young person's life should be taken, rather than simplistically relying on straightforward explanations.

An episode of major depression is a serious problem for a child or young person and if recurrent can have significant effects on a young person's development. Young people who become depressed may continue to experience depressive episodes throughout their adult life. Depression is associated with increased rates of substance misuse and affects interpersonal, social, vocational and academic functioning (Fergusson and Woodward 2002). Depression in young people is usually preceded by a

Box 5.2 Areas to Consider for Symptoms of Depression

- Low mood
- Feelings of worthlessness
- Thoughts of suicide
- Loss of enjoyment and interest in activities which were previously enjoyable
- Motor agitation
- Hallucinations
- Infrequent attendance at work or school
- Alcohol or substance misuse
- Helplessness
- Unexplained pain
- Changes in the young person's appetite
- Loss of weight or significant weight gain
- Delusional thoughts
- The child and family's understanding of what is happening
- Cognitive abilities
- Irritability
- Coherence, speed of thinking and concentration
- Relationships
- Change in the young person's social functioning – social withdrawal
- Sadness
- Thyroid functioning (to exclude hypothyroidism)
- Negative thinking
- Self-esteem
- Psychomotor retardation
- Significant life events
- Diet and nutrition
- Changes in sleep pattern are also common – often an inability to get to sleep or early morning wakening, but also over-sleeping
- Self-blame
- Weight loss
- Feeling defeated
- Medication

childhood history of generalised anxiety disorder, or dysthymia (Chavira 2004, Weissman *et al.* 2005). Dysthymia is a mood characterised by depressed feelings, loss of interests and pleasure, which has persisted for more than 2 years but is not serious enough to meet the criteria for major depressive disorder. Feelings of worthlessness can appear from middle-childhood, guilt is usually seen later in the child's development (Goodman and Scott 2005). Thoughts and acts of self-harm tend to occur from around 12 to 14 years old (see Yates 2004 for review), but may be seen earlier, particularly in children who have lived in an environment where they have seen self-harm in others. Ollendick *et al.* (2005) argue that symptoms of depression are normal for children but actual depression occurs much less often.

5.7 Protective factors and promoting resilience

If children at risk of depression can be identified, it may be possible to reduce depression through mental health promotion and prevention. It is everyone's responsibility to promote the mental health of children and young people, and a move away from mental health being the domain of professionals to mental health being everyone's business is key to this process (Scottish Needs Assessment Programme (SNAP) 2000). There are a number of everyday things which can be done to promote mental health. Parents and schools, particularly Health Promoting Schools, can play a major part in promoting healthy eating and good nutrition. Schools which have clear anti-bullying policies and pupil-led strategies to tackle bullying have proven to be successful (Mukoma and Flisher 2004, Rowe *et al.* 2007). Children are incredibly creative and intuitive when it comes to solving problems within the playground or classroom, so we should tap into their emotional intelligence and provide structures to support them. Parents can provide opportunities for children by encouraging them to become involved in after-school activities which promote mental health. The SNAP (2000) cite a meta-analysis by Durlak and Wells (1997) of mental health promotion activities with young people which found the majority of the activities analysed produced significant positive effects. Clarke *et al.* (1995) found that depression could be successfully prevented in at-risk groups of young people using a cognitive group prevention intervention.

 Activity

Hansson *et al.* (2008) discuss the concepts of shared and non-shared environment – how might such concepts be useful in the assessment of depression? Can you identify both shared and non-shared environmental factors which are resilience factors and others which are vulnerability factors?

Interpersonal therapy–adolescent skills training (IP-AST) has been used as a preventative intervention with groups of school pupils (Young *et al.* 2006) as have cognitive–behavioural group approaches such as the Penn Prevention Program (PPP) although results have been mixed (Freres *et al.* 2002, Roberts *et al.* 2003, 2004). Single gender groups for females may be a more effective way of delivering the Penn Prevention Program (Chaplin *et al.* 2006) although the evidence for this needs to be more firmly established. The Positive Thinking Program (Rooney *et al.* 2000) for 8–9 year olds uses cognitive and behavioural approaches. The programme employs a sessional approach, looking at such issues as connecting thoughts to feelings, positive thinking styles, challenging negative thoughts and decatastrophising. In a pilot study of the programme, Rooney *et al.* (2006) reported that symptoms of depression were reduced and more optimistic styles of thinking were apparent directly after the intervention; however, these reductions were not maintained over time. Collins and Dozois (2008) reviewed prevention of depression programmes and found the elements in the programmes that made a difference were the improvement of cognitive skills, interpersonal approaches and the inclusion of parents in the programme.

5.8 Interventions

Treatment of depression in children and young people is contested – particularly the use of medication. Clinical practice is often at odds with research evidence. This may be because clinical practice is ahead of research findings or because it is difficult to establish the effectiveness of some psychotherapeutic interventions. A related factor is that children and young people who access CAMHS often have complex needs which do not fit neatly into particular research categories or diagnoses. Young people with a learning disability have problems in accessing appropriate mental health services and often have unmet mental health needs (Foundation for People with Learning Disabilities 2002).

5.9 Cognitive–behaviour therapy

Cognitive–behaviour therapy (CBT) has developed as a first-line intervention for depression with growing evidence that it is an effective treatment in both individual and group formats (Wood *et al.* 1996, Lewinsohn and Clarke 1999, Pfeffer *et al.* 2002, Nelson *et al.* 2003, Dudley *et al.* 2005, David-Ferdon and Kaslow 2008). While the evidence is growing, there are relatively few extensive follow-up studies.

The core beliefs, assumptions and negative automatic thoughts (NATS) we hold about ourselves are examined during the process of CBT where the child or young person is helped to challenge and modify their thoughts to help them think differently and feel better about themselves.

The age at which a child is able to engage with CBT is debatable, although Stallard (2002) argues this should be possible by the time a child reaches the concrete operational stage of cognitive development (around 7–12 years of age). CBT should be adapted for use with children, employing the use of visual stimuli such as thought balloons, emotional dictionaries,

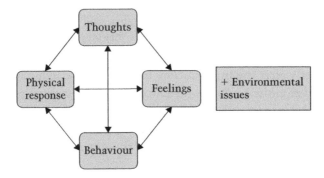

Figure 5.1 Hot cross bun model.

feelings worksheets, as well as creative approaches such as positive self-talk, games, puppets and storytelling. Younger children may have difficulty distinguishing whether feelings derive from external events or internal thoughts, and need plain and straightforward instructions if they are to engage with CBT. There is very little evidence of psychological interventions with children and young people with learning disabilities and depression, although there are case study reports of interventions with adults which reported some level of effectiveness (Lindsay *et al.* 1993, Dagnan and Chadwick 1997, Lindsay 1999). For CBT to be effective, the child needs to be ready and parents usually need to be involved (Stallard 2005). CBT can be delivered by a trained therapist or through self-help manuals. Curry and Reinecke (2003) use a modular therapy approach for young people. Dummett and Williams (2008) outline a five-areas approach to overcoming teenage depression; the five areas are shown in the 'Hot Cross Bun' model in Figure 5.1.

5.10 Interpersonal psychotherapy for depressed adolescents

Interpersonal psychotherapy (IPT) (Weissman *et al.* 1979) has been adapted for use with adolescents (IPT-A). It is a brief, structured, time-limited intervention. In IPT-A, young people identify and target interpersonal problems that maintain depression. Part of the contract of treatment is that the young person accepts they are sick and seeks help as they would with a physical illness. During the initial phase, the young person creates a review of their current social functioning and relationships (interpersonal inventory). The therapist develops an interpersonal formulation – linking the depression to one of four interpersonal problem areas: grief, interpersonal role disputes, role transitions and interpersonal deficits. IPT-A addresses the *here and now*; problems occurring in the present. In IPT-A an effort is made to consolidate the therapeutic gains which have been made by the young person (Frombone 1998, Weissman *et al.* 2000, Mufson *et al.* 2004a, b, Coleman 2006).

 Activity

Choose one of the psychological therapies for depression and research the approach. How might this intervention be used with a child or young person you know?

5.11 Medication

The use of medication with children is contested – in this section we will look at the evidence. The main approaches to the medical treatment of depression in children and young people are tricyclic antidepressants (TCAs), selective serotonin reuptake inhibitors (SSRIs) or serotonin reuptake inhibitors (SRIs). There is general agreement that TCAs should not be prescribed as they are no more effective than placebo in the treatment of depression in children and young people (Hazell *et al.* 1995, 2002, Kutcher 1997, Geller *et al.* 1999). Not only are they ineffective, they also cause some unpleasant side effects such as dry mouth, sweating and constipation, as well as potentially fatal cardiovascular toxic effects (Birmaher *et al.* 1998). Similarly, monoamine oxidase inhibitors (MAOIs) are not proven to be effective for children and young people and there is little evidence to support their use (Heyman and Santosh 2005).

 Activity

Tricyclic antidepressants were still being prescribed for children and young people after research indicated they were ineffective in this age group. Consider the issues which may have affected a decision to continue to prescribe, despite this evidence.

The use of antidepressants with children and young people has been increasing (Zito *et al.* 2003, Mitchell *et al.* 2008). Murray *et al.* (2004) reviewed the prescription of TCAs and SSRIs in the UK between 1992 and 2001. Overall 93,091 prescriptions were given to 24,976 individuals, 51,869 TCAs (55.7%) and 33,429 (41.3%) SSRIs. Prescriptions increased by 1.7-fold over the period studied, with a 30% reduction in TCAs and a 10-fold increase in SSRIs, 50% of children and young people had discontinued treatment after 2 months. In 2007, it was estimated that 50,000 children in the UK were prescribed antidepressants and that prescriptions were increasing (Hansard 2007). At the time of writing, a Scottish Government target is to halt the increase in prescription of antidepressants.

There has been concern expressed about the effectiveness and safety of SSRIs (Jureidini *et al.* 2004a and b). In a meta-analysis of studies involving 2,318 patients receiving either antidepressant medication or placebo, Kirsch and Sapirstein (1998) argued that virtually all the variation in the effect of the drug was due to the placebo. They reported the inactive placebo produced improvement equal to 75% of the drug. They suggested that a quarter of the drug response was due to the administration of an active medication; half was placebo effect and a quarter due to non-specific factors. The Committee on the Safety of Medicines in the USA recommended the withdrawal of all SSRIs (with the exception of fluoxetine) because of the increased risk of suicide in children and young people connected with their use, although this is not supported by all studies (Isacsson *et al.* 2005).

Initial reports of the effectiveness of SSRIs were favourable (Emslie *et al.* 1995, Geller *et al.* 1999) and SSRIs were seen and continue to be seen by many as an effective treatment for depression in children and young people because of reduced cardiotoxicity in overdose and fewer side effects. The evidence for the use of SSRIs with children and young people however is equivocal. The main evidence for the effectiveness of SSRIs relies on the Treatment of Adolescent Depression Study (TADS) (March *et al.* 2004, 2006, 2007, TADS Team 2004), a study looking at the effectiveness of commonly used treatments for depression in young people in the USA costing $17 million over 6 years. TADS reported a combination of CBT and fluoxetine was most effective in treating depression.

Overall, the evidence for the effectiveness of SSRIs with children and young people is weak, with the only positive evidence being for fluoxetine (Whittington *et al.* 2004, Goodyer *et al.* 2007). In a meta-analysis of 30 randomised-controlled trials of antidepressants prescribed to children and young people, Tsapakis *et al.* (2008) found only modest evidence for the effectiveness of antidepressants and found limited difference in outcomes between SRIs and TCAs. Tsapakis *et al.* (2008) argue that fluoxetine might be more effective in young people, but SRIs and antidepressants did not show effectiveness in children. They call for more research particularly on more severely depressed and suicidal children and young people.

A review by Usala *et al.* (2008: 70) largely favourable to the use of SSRIs with children and young people concluded:

> This systematic review and meta-analysis shows that SSRI treatment (fluoxetine in particular) in children and adolescents may be more effective on the symptoms of depression than placebo.

The finding that SSRIs may be more effective than placebo needs to be considered alongside concerns raised about SSRIs and increased suicidal behaviour in children and young people, and the influence placebo may have in the treatment of depression. In a study comparing routine care and SSRI adding or omitting CBT, Goodyer *et al.* (2007) argued that a placebo trial was not used as it would be unethical in young people who were so unwell; this has been criticised by Jureidini (2007) who argues that placebo has been found to be at least as effective as SSRIs in a number of studies. Further evidence of the role of placebo in treating depression can be found in Cohen *et al.* (2008) who reviewed 23 trials between 1972 and 2007 of mainly non-TCAs and found that the average placebo response rate was 49.6% for major depression, ranging from 17% to 90%.

Following criticism that only positive research results had been published, there have been calls for the publication of all results by drug companies, which has increased the concern that SSRIs may not be as effective as previously thought. The Food and Drug Administration (FDA) Center for Drug Evaluation and Research in the USA reviewed the effectiveness of the data and approved only one SSRI – fluoxetine (FDA 2004). The evidence for the efficacy of SSRIs is limited; however, their use remains commonplace. This is worrying given we know there is a greater risk of suicidal behaviour in children and young people than in adults taking SSRIs (Stone *et al.* 2009). Shearer and Bermingham (2008) argue that there are ethical problems in the prescription of SSRI medication with children and young people – such as whether the antidepressant medication is more effective than placebo, and the short- and long-term effects on the physical and psychological development of those receiving the medication. Jureidini (2009) argues that an approach which involves 'watchful waiting' and attention to the emotional and physical needs of children can be used as an alternative to medication. The effects of neural imprinting – the continued effect of the drug after discontinuation (Andersen and Navalta 2004) – are under-researched. Various claims are made for the effectiveness of antidepressant medication, given the concerns about efficacy and safety SSRIs should be prescribed with caution; there should be careful and rigorous monitoring and psychological interventions should be tried first.

5.12 Psychodynamics

With the advent of CBT and manual-based therapies, there has been a move away from psychodynamic-based therapies, as they are regarded as too expensive, labour intensive and time consuming. However, it is important to recognise that young people diagnosed with depression may have complex problems which it may only be possible to address with long-term therapy. The cognitive approaches may suit a majority of mild to moderate problems; however, the long-term effects of depression may themselves require a long-term solution. In a meta-analysis of cognitive and non-cognitive (including psychodynamic treatments), Weisz *et al.* (2006) found no difference between cognitive and non-cognitive psychotherapies in that both produced modest effects in the treatment of depression. Trowell *et al.* (2007) found that psychodynamic psychotherapy was effective at treating childhood depression and dysthymia with 74.3% young people recovering, and young people continued to improve with 100% showing no symptoms of depression at follow-up. Working in the context of a long-term therapeutic relationship can be of benefit for children and young people – particularly children who have suffered trauma. NICE (2005) guidelines recommend that individual child psychotherapy be considered when previous combined treatments have been unsuccessful. Group psychodynamic approaches are used with young people and the context of a psychodynamically oriented day programme may be of benefit to some young people. There are very few studies of psychodynamic psychotherapies, e.g. in Watanabe *et al.*'s (2007) study of the 27 studies reported only one used a psychodynamic approach.

5.13 What else helps?

Other interventions include social skills interventions, academic help and supporting the child or young person at school. Focusing on peer relationships can be helpful as they can be used to help in the young person's recovery. Some young people may also require inpatient or day-patient treatment. Inpatient treatment is helpful, particularly if the young person is suicidal, while day-patient treatment can help a young person deal with issues of social isolation. Group-based interventions may help the young person make sense of their difficulties, reduce their sense of aloneness and promote effective and supportive social networks.

Narrative therapies can be helpful with children and young people who are depressed – proponents argue narrative therapies are *therapies of curiosity* in comparison to traditional therapies which are seen by some as *therapies of certainty* (Amundson *et al.* 1993). Narrative therapy uses storytelling, playing out familiar stories and using the children's own stories and often employs drama techniques. Solution focused therapy is increasingly used in practice and is seen by practitioners as a helpful approach, although the evidence base of effectiveness with children and young people has yet to be established. Music therapy has been used to treat depression in young people (Hendricks and Bradley 2005). Other important areas to consider are diet, routine and physical exercise which all have a helpful role in helping young people to recover from depression.

5.14   The family

Having a child who is depressed can be worrying for family members. Families may blame themselves and look for explanations in their own behaviour and functioning. To help families understand, they need to be informed about depression and what it means. Education about signs and symptoms can help the family to understand depression in relation to their child; this will involve discussion and making sense of a child or young person's behaviour, e.g. is lying in bed until 2 p.m. a sign of depression or is it normal adolescent behaviour? Does a child who continually worries about their performance at school have depression? Discussing these and other issues with parents can help provide some clarity and help parents to have ordinary expectations of their child. Some families will benefit from education, some from family support and for others family therapy will be helpful. NICE (2005) guidelines recommend that individual systemic family therapy be considered when previous combined treatments have been unsuccessful (see Chapter 2). While the vast majority of families are supportive to young people, some families can be detrimental to a child's development, supports for the parents/carers and the family as a whole should of course be the first consideration; however, there will be occasions when child protection measures have to be taken to protect a child. Assessment of the family's views of treatment such as a discussion of medication or the role psychotherapy might play is important. Answering questions at an early stage and entering into a collaborative dialogue with parents can help engagement.

5.15   Conclusion

Depression is a serious mental health issue which can have long-term negative effects on children and young people's development. Early recognition of depression has been the focus of health promotion and prevention campaigns. Alongside a greater recognition of depression has been the concern that there is an over-medicalisation of children and young people's mental health. This tension is particularly apparent when we consider drug treatment in children and young people. Of course we should be concerned that we may be affecting young people's development by the prescription of antidepressants at an early age. Recognising when children and young people are depressed is difficult, because as we have seen a number of 'symptoms' of depression can be easily confused with other behaviours in children and young people. Developing appropriate interventions which are effective and encourage young people to develop their own solutions to emotional problems will help them later in life. Taking a thoughtful, watchful, waiting approach and understanding the whole context of children and young people's lives may be a helpful starting point. Some of the solutions to young people's depression may lay in political and societal responses rather than be located in the individual.

Recommended reading

Andersen, S. L. and Navalta, C. P. (2004). Altering the course of neurodevelopment: a framework for understanding the enduring effects of psychotropic drugs. *International Journal of Developmental Neuroscience* 22 (5–6), 423–440.

Emslie, G. J., Wagner, K. D., Kutcher, S., et al. (2006). Paroxetine treatment in children and adolescents with major depressive disorder: a randomized multicenter, double-blind, placebo-controlled trial. *Journal of the American Academy of Child and Adolescent Psychiatry* 45 (6), 709–719.

Goodyer, I. (ed) (2001). *The Depressed Child and Adolescent*, 2nd edition. New York: Cambridge University Press.

Hansson, K., Cederblad, M., Lichtenstein, P., et al. (2008). Individual resiliency factors from a genetic perspective: results from a twin study. *Family Process* 47 (4), 537–551.

Horwitz, A. V. and Wakefield, J. C. (2007). *The Loss of Sadness: How Psychiatry Transformed Normal Sadness into Depressive Disorder*. New York: Oxford University Press.

Jureidini J., Tonkin, A. and Mansfield, P. R. (2004b). TADS study raises concerns. *British Medical Journal* 329, 1343–1344.

Leo, J. (2006). The SSRI trials in children: disturbing implications for academic medicine. *Ethical Human Psychology and Psychiatry* 8, 29–41.

March, J. S., Silva, S., Petrycki, S. (2007). The Treatment for Adolescents with Depression Study (TADS): long-term effectiveness and safety outcomes. *Archives of General Psychiatry* 64 (10), 1132–1143.

Shireman, T. I., Olson, B. M. and Dewan, N. A. (2002). Patterns of antidepressant use among children and adolescents. *Psychiatric Services* 53 (11), 1444–1450.

Simpson, D. and Miller, L. (eds) (2004). *Unexpected Gains: Psychotherapy with People with Learning Disabilities*. London: Karnac Books.

Thapar, A. and McGuffin, D. (1994). A twin study of depressive symptoms in childhood. *British Journal of Psychiatry* 165, 259–226.

Timimi, S. (2004). Rethinking childhood depression. *British Medical Journal* 329, 1394–1396.

Websites

Learning disability
The Royal College of Psychiatrists leaflet for people with learning disabilities who may have depression can be found at:
http://www.rcpsych.ac.uk/mentalhealthinfoforall/problems/depression/learningdisability.aspx

The surgeon general and depression
A chapter on depression from the USA's surgeon general can be found at:
http://www.surgeongeneral.gov/library/mentalhealth/chapter3/sec5.html

NIMH
The National Institute for Mental Health have information about depression in children and adolescents which can be accessed at:
http://www.nimh.nih.gov/health/topics/depression/depression-in-children-and-adolescents.shtml

Treatment effectiveness
This website by the *BMJ* looks at the evidence for the effectiveness of various treatments of depression in children and young people – updated April 2009.
http://www.clinicalevidence.com/ceweb/conditions/chd/1008/1008.jsp

Australian optimism
The Aussie optimism website run by the School of Psychology at Curtin University of Technology has useful information about programmes for the prevention of depression.
http://psych.curtin.edu.au/research/aussieoptimism/pt_program.cfm

Mood juice
Is a website run by the NHS in Scotland which aims to help people think about emotional problems and resolve them.
http://www.moodjuice.scot.nhs.uk/index.html

Chapter 6
SUICIDE

Martin Gaughan

School of Nursing, Midwifery and Social Care, Edinburgh Napier University, Edinburgh, Scotland

6.1 Introduction

Suicide is of worldwide public concern, and one of the main causes of death in young people (Patton *et al.* 2009). While uncommon in children, in the teenage years the rate of completed suicide starts to rise steeply (WHO 2004a). Suicide is a major problem from the early teenage years throughout the lifespan, with estimates that a million people commit suicide worldwide each year (WHO 2009b). This chapter will consider issues relating to suicide in young people, starting with a discussion of how suicide is defined, how common suicide is, what makes young people more vulnerable to suicidal behaviour and how to promote resilience to suicide. In this chapter, we will examine assessment of suicide and discuss particular models of assessment and intervention. Prevention of suicide has been an area of focus for the WHO's Suicide Prevention Programme (SUPRE) (WHO 2010); we will consider particular suicide prevention programmes and conclude with a discussion of postvention, i.e. the after-effects of attempted and completed suicide.

Learning outcomes

After completing your study of this unit, you should be able to:

1. Outline factors which make children and young people vulnerable to suicide.

Understanding Children and Young People's Mental Health, first edition. Edited by Anne Claveirole and Martin Gaughan. Published 2011 by John Wiley & Sons Ltd. © 2011 John Wiley & Sons Ltd.

2. Develop an awareness of gender differences in the rates of suicide in children and young people, and discuss factors which contribute to these differences.
3. Discuss the strengths and weaknesses of a suicide prevention programme.
4. Consider reasons for the different suicide rates across Europe.
5. Outline an assessment method for a young person with suicidal ideation, and suggest a programme of intervention.

6.2   What is suicide?

At first glance agreeing a definition of suicide may seem relatively simple; on further examination it becomes a little more complex. Issues such as the meaning of suicidal behaviour, intent, suicidal acts and parasuicide have meant that researchers have struggled to find an agreed definition of suicide and associated behaviours. In fact consensus on a single definition has yet to be agreed (O'Connor and Sheehy 2000). Researchers often ask young people if they have ever made a suicide attempt and young people's responses to this question are used to estimate the prevalence of suicidal behaviour. However, what is seen as suicidal behaviour can range from a relatively superficial attempt with no intention of dying, to the use of lethal methods with the expressed intent of death (Kidd 2004).

O'Carroll *et al.* (1996) developed a classification for suicidal and self-harming behaviours using two broad headings: (1) 'risk-taking thoughts and behaviors' and (2) 'suicide-related thoughts and behaviors'; these were subdivided into the immediacy of the risk and the level and persistence of suicidal intent. These classifications have been refined and developed further by Silverman *et al.* (2007) and reflect an ongoing debate within the suicidology research community on establishing a shared definition of suicidal behaviour. In this chapter, we will use the definition of suicide employed in the UK by Choose Life, the National Strategy and Action Plan to Prevent Suicide in Scotland which states:

Suicide: an act of deliberate self-harm which results in death (Scottish Executive 2002b: 12).

6.3   How common is suicide?

Suicide accounts for over 20% of all deaths of young men aged between 15 and 24 in England and Wales (Biddle *et al.* 2008). The overall rates of suicide in the UK and Ireland have fallen over the past 20 years (Palmer 2008). Over this period, rates of suicide in Scotland have been consistently higher than in England, Wales, Northern Ireland and Ireland, and the rates of suicide in the most deprived areas of Scotland are double the Scottish average (National Statistics 2006, Choose Life 2010). During the 1980s, there was a large increase of suicide in males in the 15–24 age group which since 1991, despite a peak in 1998, has declined in England and Wales (Centre for Suicide Research 2010). In Scotland, the suicide rate for this age group was on an upward trend from the 1980s to 2001 since then the trend has been downward (General Register Offices for Scotland 2009).

It is quite common for young people to have suicidal thoughts with some studies reporting 20–45% of young people having suicidal thoughts at some point in their adolescence (Hawton and James 2005) and some research suggesting that suicidal thoughts are normative (Marcenko et al. 1999). In a systematic review of population-based studies, Evans et al. (2005) found 10% of young people had made a suicide attempt and 30% had thought about suicide at some point in their lives. The reporting of suicide can be problematic for a number of reasons; car accidents may actually be suicides but be reported as accidents; coroners may be reluctant to categorise a death as suicide unless there is clear and unequivocal evidence (Langer et al. 2008). It is generally accepted that suicide is underreported, with estimates of underreporting being up two or three times current practice (Gosney and Hawton 2007).

The reduction in the number of suicides has been a concern of a number of governments worldwide. The Scottish Choose Life Campaign was introduced in Scotland in 2002 (Scottish Executive 2002b); there was a 10% reduction in overall suicides between 2000–02 and 2006–08 (Choose Life 2010). Similar results have been found from other national campaigns in the UK and Australia (NIMHE 2006, Morrell et al. 2007).

More males commit suicide at all ages across the lifespan; in fact males are two to four times more likely to commit suicide than females (WHO 2002). Females are more likely to engage in suicidal behaviour but are less likely to die (Hunt et al. 2006). In 2007 in the 15–24 age group, 379 young people (309 males and 70 females) committed suicide in the UK and Northern Ireland; in the 5–14 age group 10 boys and 4 girls committed suicide during this period (WHO 2009a). While the differences between children and young people are marked, these figures challenge the perception that children do not commit suicide.

There are considerable differences in worldwide suicide rates of 15–19 year olds as reported by WHO (2004a), with some countries such as Kuwait, Philippines and Egypt reporting an absence or very low suicide rates (0.00–0.02 per 100,000 population). In the USA, suicide is the second most common cause of death in young people, accounting for 10 deaths per 100,000 population. In Eastern Europe, generally the rates are significantly higher; e.g. Lithuania (38.4 males and 8.8 females, per 100,000 population), Poland (14.1 males and 2.4 females, per 100,000 population) and the Russian Federation (36.5 males and 9.6 females, per 100,000 population). There may be a number of factors which affect these figures, such as how suicide is viewed in a particular country, religion may also play a role, as may alcohol consumption, poverty and other socio-economic issues. It is difficult to establish worldwide trends as the year of reporting ranges from 1986 to 2001 depending on the country. However, when comparing the same year (1995) of collection, four out of five of the highest suicide rates for 15–19 year olds were in countries in Eastern Europe, the exception being New Zealand. Worldwide rates are also difficult to establish as there is an absence of data from the African continent, parts of Asia and Alaska. There are, however, some generalisations which can be drawn; suicide is much higher in males than in females, the only exception being China (selected rural and urban areas); and the rates of suicide are generally higher in the Northern Hemisphere than in the Southern Hemisphere (WHO 2004a).

 Activity

Read the statistics on the WHO website on the suicide rates in different countries – consider why there are different suicide rates in different countries.

6.4 Vulnerability

The reasons children and young people commit suicide are complex and often involve an interconnection of different factors and events. A difficulty in relationships, either with a partner or family member, is a commonly cited reason (Stoep *et al.* 2009). Parental conflict and rigid family systems can be factors influencing suicidal behaviour (Wise and Spengler 1997). In young people, events that have an impact on the young person's identity, autonomy and independence can play a part. Depression, hopelessness and a history of sexual abuse can also be factors (Mazza and Reynolds 1998, Fleischmann *et al.* 2005, Brent *et al.* 2009) and are seen to be more present in young people who make more serious suicidal attempts (Grøholt *et al.* 2000). Substance misuse, aggression, risky sexual behaviour and health problems have been found to be related to suicidality (Epstein and Spirito 2009). A negative perception of body image and lack of attention to their own physical needs is seen as a risk for suicidal behaviour in some young people (Orbach 2006). Fleming *et al.* (2007) found that knowing someone who had attempted suicide, having symptoms of depression, alcohol misuse, violence and Lesbian, Gay, Bisexual and Transgender (LBGT) relationships were associated with an increased risk of suicide. A number of studies have looked at factors that make people more vulnerable to repeating a suicide attempt; these include low self-esteem, early puberty, relationship difficulties, being physically impaired due to illness or injury, substance/alcohol misuse, hopelessness, a previous suicide attempt and a recent suicide attempt by a friend (Wichstrøm 2000, Fergusson *et al.* 2005). Studies of homeless young people found that they reported feeling trapped by their experiences and factors which made them vulnerable to suicide were drug use, experiencing familial abuse as a child, having low self-esteem and feeling lonely (Kidd 2004, 2006, Kidd and Carroll 2007).

Box 6.1 outlines some of the reasons young people give for contemplating suicide, and factors which make a young person vulnerable to suicide.

Family functioning is more important than family structure; the way a family functions in particular relationships with parents can be both a protective and vulnerability factor (Fotti *et al.* 2006). The effect of the media is open to question with some studies reporting that young people and young adults were less likely to have 'copycat' effect, although it is thought that reports of suicide in teenagers may be an influence on imitative behaviour (Schmidtke and Schaller 2000, Stack 2005). The death of a family member can make the possibility of suicide four to six times more likely (Rubenstein *et al.* 1989). Feeling connected to others is a protective factor and when these connections are broken, suicide risk may increase. Multiple stressors may be a problem and having depression and being victimised at school has been found to increase vulnerability (Brunstein 2005). Abuse as a child is a predictor of suicide attempts later in life; the more often a child is abused the stronger the association is with a suicide attempt. The relationship the abuser has to the child is also important; the closer the relationship (e.g. immediate family member) the stronger the association with suicide (Brezo *et al.* 2008).

Shaffer *et al.* (1996b) found that 21% of young people who committed suicide had seen a mental health professional within 3 months of their death. Suominen *et al.* (2004) found that two-thirds of young people did not have treatment contact 1 month before their attempt. Wannan and Fombonne (1998) found 11% of around 5,500 Child and Adolescent Mental Health Services (CAMHS) outpatients showed some type of suicidal behaviour.

It is thought that between a fifth and half of young people with early onset psychosis consider suicide at some point in their lives (Petersen *et al.* 2005,

Box 6.1 Some Vulnerability Factors for Suicide in Children and Young People

- Emotional abuse
- Attention deficit hyperactivity disorder
- Unemployment
- Depression
- Knowing someone who has died by suicide
- Psychosis
- Sexual abuse
- Anorexia
- Poverty
- Impulsivity
- Reporting of suicides in the media
- Self-harm
- Physical abuse
- Bulimia
- Deprivation
- Bullying
- Parental mental illness
- Chronic illness
- Family difficulties
- Low problem-solving
- Menstrual cycle
- Rejection
- Parental substance misuse
- Being recently disciplined
- Lack of parental support
- Genetic predisposition
- Lower social class
- Lack of social connectedness
- Death of a family member
- Substance misuse

Bertelsen *et al.* 2007) and that 5.65% will commit suicide (Palmer *et al.* 2005). Early psychosis intervention programmes have lower rates of suicide than generic services (Harris *et al.* 2008). The risk of suicide has been found to be higher in the first month of treatment (Fedyszyn *et al.* 2010). In a follow-up study of 282 young people/adults with psychosis, 61 people made a suicide attempt during the follow-up period, including 12 completed suicides (Robinson *et al.* 2010). Some of these factors which make young people with a psychosis more vulnerable to suicide are outlined in Box 6.2.

Box 6.2 Vulnerability Factors for Young People with Psychosis

- Male
- Severe onset of illness in previous 5 years
- Poor attachment
- Single
- Previous suicide attempts
- Depression
- Unemployed
- Good premorbid personality
- Substance misuse
- Long-term illness
- High expectations of self
- Insight
- High IQ
- Feelings of paranoia
- Frequent relapses
- Depression
- Negative attitudes towards treatment
- Impulsive behaviour

Children commit suicide less frequently than young people – a number of factors may play a part. Children on the whole suffer from less severe depression. Their lack of cognitive maturity may make them less able to feel hopelessness or plan a successful suicide. Relationships and structures in school and the community may be more supportive for children than for young people, e.g. children at primary school are usually taught by one teacher and may therefore have the opportunity to develop closer and more supportive relationships. However, despite children being less vulnerable, children do commit suicide, and childhood suicide may be on the increase; therefore, any concern that a child might be suicidal must be taken seriously.

An increase in alcohol consumption is related to an increase in suicide rates (Nemtsov 2003, Bye 2008). Being intoxicated can affect thinking and reasoning, and may promote disinhibition. Alcohol and substance misuse have been shown to be significant predictors of adolescent suicide (Waldrop et al. 2007). Students aged 16–19 are more likely to attempt suicide if misusing substances, and substance use has been found to have a significant correlation with suicidal ideation (Dunn et al. 2008).

There are particular groupings of young people who are vulnerable to suicide. One of these groups is young Asian women and a number of hypothesis have been posited, including cultural differences, the emphasis on success in both education and work, and the expectation of obedience and compliance in younger females as possible reasons (Thompson and Bhugra 2000). LBGT young people are another vulnerable group. Eisenberg *et al.* (2006) reported that of 2,555 students who reported a same sex experience 37.4% reported that they had made a suicide attempt. However, if protective factors were in place, such as a supportive family, school safety and feeling connected to an adult, then they argue the level of risk would be considerably reduced. Scourfield *et al.* (2008) found a link between the experience and prevalence of homophobia and self-harming behaviours in LBGT young people. Looked after and accommodated children have increased risk factors for suicide which make them a particularly vulnerable group (Scott and Hill 2006).

Eckersely (1993) argued that modern Western societies are harmful to the psychological and social well-being of young people – citing examples of problems in interpersonal relationships, poverty, family conflict and breakdown, unemployment, hopelessness and educational pressures as indicators of harm. Lester (1998) argued that suicidal behaviour in affluent societies increases because young people cannot blame their shortcomings or hopeless feelings on external sources, i.e. if a lot of other people are successful there are fewer excuses for not being successful. Young people therefore blame themselves for their failures and become depressed. Lester (1998) argues that comparing themselves to successful role models compounds these feelings in young people.

Activity

Consider five factors which may make children or young people more vulnerable to suicide and reflect on how you might be able to promote resilience in a child or young person.

6.5 Resilience

There is a paucity of evidence for factors which make children and young people resilient to suicide; this is particularly true of children who are looked after and accommodated. McLean *et al.* (2008) conducted a systematic international literature review of factors across the lifespan which protect against suicide. We have identified those of particular relevance to children and young people as well as factors identified in other studies (see Box 6.3).

If we are to increase resilience in children and young people, we need to enhance these factors in children and young people. Reflecting on how you

Box 6.3 Protective Factors Against Suicide

- Perception of positive health
- Access to treatment by a health professional
- Exposure to suicidal behaviour
- Good social skills
- Participation in sporting activities
- Employment (for the older adolescent)
- Traditional social values (for girls)
- Engagement and enjoyment at school
- Good problem-solving
- Access to health professionals at school
- Individualistic values (for boys)
- Internal locus of control
- Playing sports
- Hopefulness, optimism and reasons for living
- The presence of multiple protective factors
- Supportive school environments
- Positive family relationships
- Self-control of thoughts, behaviour and emotions
- Religious faith and spirituality
- Supportive peer relationships

would promote some of the factors outlined in Box 6.3 with a young person you know may help you to think about the issue of resilience.

Canetto (1997) examined the meaning of suicidal behaviour in high school students in the USA and found gender differences in the perception and construction of suicide. Non-fatal suicidal behaviour was perceived as more feminine, particularly when attempted suicide was in response to relationship problems. Suicide attempts prompted by achievement failure were perceived as masculine. Males were more critical of people who attempted suicide, and avoided suicidal people, particularly other males. Surviving a suicide attempt was seen as culturally unacceptable by men and they tended to structure suicidal acts in such a way as to reduce the likelihood of survival. Canetto and her colleagues (Canetto 1997, 1998, Dahlen and Canetto 2002) suggests that intervention should involve the assessment of the young person's beliefs about gender and suicidal behaviour. Intervention should focus on male meanings of the right to kill oneself, while reducing the stigma of surviving a suicidal act. Scourfield et al. (2008) examined young people's interpretations of suicidal behaviour in males and females in the UK. Male suicide was associated with strength, courage, honour, impulse and decisiveness. Female suicide was associated with love and relationships, manipulation and revenge and a cry for help. Understanding how males and females perceive and view suicide in others may offer insights into developing interventions which take account of gender perspectives.

6.6 Risk assessment

Children and young people face multiple and significant stressors unique to these phases of life which may make assessment difficult. When assessing a child or young person for suicidal intent, a number of factors need to be taken into account. The context of the assessment is important, such as whether the assessment is taking place before or after a suicide attempt. If after, there will be more information on which to base the assessment. The following guidelines relate to post-attempt assessment, but can easily be modified to assess whether a child or young person is at risk of suicide. It is important to establish the level of lethality of the attempt or intended act. To help do this, the following areas should be enquired into:

- Was the attempt timed so that intervention was unlikely, e.g. did the child or young person take an overdose while everyone else was in bed?
- Were precautions taken to avoid discovery, e.g. did the child or young person hide from others so that they were unlikely to be found in time?
- Were there preparations for death, such as giving away treasured possessions prior to the act?
- Had the child or young person told someone they were going to commit suicide?
- How premeditated was the act?
- Was a suicide note left?
- Has the child or young person told someone after the attempt?
- What was the child or young person's intent – did they want to die?

Answers to these and similar questions will help uncover the risk level for further suicide attempts. With children words may be less important and it may be through other media such as drawings, paintings or play that suicidal thoughts may become accessible.

There is some evidence from the literature on adult suicide that people who make multiple suicide attempts are no different in their risk of suicide than those who make single attempts (Tuckman 2007). There is also a view that young people who make numerous low lethality suicide attempts are not trying to kill themselves. At the other end of the spectrum, there are young people who take numerous potentially fatal overdoses without intent to die. There is no quick or simple way to understand a child or young person's reason/s for attempting suicide. Getting to know the particular young person, understanding their emotional pain and their reason for suicide at that particular time is key in offering assistance.

 Activity

Cameron is a 15-year-old boy with no history of depression, anxiety or relationship difficulties. He commits suicide by hanging in his bedroom following a family argument. There is no suicide note. Cameron lived with his mum and dad, and his 14-year-old sister. Consider what the parents might be feeling and how Cameron's sister might be affected? Discuss with your colleagues resources which may be of help to the family.

6.7 Models of assessment and intervention

There are numerous methods employed to assess suicidal behaviour in children and young people such as structured and semi-structured diagnostic interviews, e.g. the Child and Adolescent Psychiatric Assessment (CAPA) (Angold and Costello 2000), self-report inventories and behaviour checklists, e.g. the Beck Scale for Suicidal Ideation (Beck *et al.* 1979), scales which attempt to predict future suicidal behaviours such as the Child–Adolescent Suicidal Potential Index (CASPI) (Pfeffer *et al.* 2000), multi-tiered survey assessments to identify high-risk populations of children and young people, e.g. the Columbia Teen Screen and Diagnostic Interview Schedule for Children (Shaffer and Craft 1999), instruments to assess the level of intent and lethality of suicidal behaviour, e.g. the Pierce Suicide Intent Scale (Pierce 1977).

The array of instruments to measure current and future suicidal behaviour can be bewildering, and while useful for research, evaluation or audit purposes may not be of direct utility in practice. The following section outlines three different approaches to working alongside and assessing someone at risk of suicide.

A process model for assessing adolescent risk for suicide

Stoelb and Chiriboga's (1998) model is used to build a picture of the risk of suicide for the young person. This assessment is usually achieved by interviewing the child or young person. In the model, risk factors for suicide are categorised as primary, secondary and situational. Primary factors are having an affective disorder, having made a previous suicide attempt and hopelessness. Secondary risk factors are substance misuse and having difficulty with emotional regulation. Situational risk factors are issues such as a family history of substance misuse, being exposed to violence, child sexual abuse, exposure to suicide, life stressors, rejection and humiliation. We have made two changes to the wording of the model: 'personality disorder' has been changed to young people 'having difficulty with regulation of emotions' and 'homosexual' has been changed to LBGT young people. The model has four stages:

- *Stage 1* Involves assessing primary risk factors, if present, the young person is seen as being at 'severe' risk of suicide. If the interviewer is not concerned, a hypothesis of 'low' or 'moderate' risk is made. Even in the absence of a primary risk factor, a hypothesis of 'severe risk' can be made if the interviewer is concerned the young person might be suicidal.
- *Stage 2* Involves the assessment of suicidal ideation, intent and plan. Suicidal ideation is defined as thoughts and ideas concerning death, suicide and self-harming behaviour. The frequency and intensity of these thoughts and ideas are important – as are underlying reasons, such as to escape or get revenge, to evoke guilt or a cry for help. The interviewer establishes whether the child or young person has a plan and the method to be used. Whether a date has been set and the availability of implements are very important – the more specific these are, the more dangerous it is for the young person (Bonner 1990, Nock *et al.* 2008). From this assessment of the level of ideation, intent and plan, the young person is categorised as at 'severe', 'moderate' or 'low' risk of suicide.
- *Stage 3* Is the assessment of secondary risk factors: substance misuse and emotional dysregulation. These two factors are seen as adding impulsivity to the young person's risk, as these two factors are seen as being related to impulsivity. In turn, impulsivity is seen as being connected to increased risk of suicide. If there are no secondary risk factors, the category is not changed. If secondary risk factors are present, 'with impulsivity' is added to the model, or the model is upgraded to 'severe' risk.
- *Stage 4* Is the assessment of situational risk factors – one factor adds the specification 'with situational factors' to the model. By interviewing the child and family, the impact of situational risk factors can be seen, and the influence these situational risk factors may have on a young person's suicidal behaviour can be established.

The more factors the young person has, i.e. the more primary, secondary and situational factors present, and the more clear the young person is about their plan or intent, the more at risk of suicide the young person is considered to be. Once the level of suicidal ideation has been established, a plan of help can be put in place which will focus on the safety of the young person.

 Activity

Read Stoelb and Chiriboga's (1998) paper on assessment of adolescent risk for suicide. Think about a child or young person you know who was suicidal and apply the model. Where does the child or young person fit on the model?

6.8 Applied suicide and intervention skills training

Applied suicide and intervention skills training (ASIST) aims to develop suicide safer communities where suicide is recognised, discussed and where people are 'willing, ready and able' to help people at risk of suicide. Over a period of 2 days, ASIST participants:

- explore their own attitudes to suicide
- review vulnerability to suicide
- examine professional and lay people's attitudes to suicide
- develop an understanding of a suicide intervention model (SIM)
- through a series of simulations use the model to help people at risk of suicide.

The course is interactive and skills-based and requires active engagement by the course participants. ASIST can be seen as both intervention and prevention, in that course participants are taught how to intervene with a SIM to help someone at risk of suicide, coupled with a philosophy of prevention through building suicide safer communities. ASIST has been implemented in numerous countries throughout the world and was reviewed in the Choose Life evaluation in Scotland. Griesbach et al. (2008) reported that over 10,000 people had been trained in ASIST in Scotland and that ASIST had an effect on participant knowledge and skills in suicide intervention. They also reported that there has been little research on the effectiveness of ASIST. ASIST is only suitable for young people aged 14 years and older.

6.9 Skills-based training on risk management

Skills-based Training On Risk Management (STORM) is a suicide intervention programme developed by the University of Manchester (Gask *et al.*
2006, Hayes *et al.* 2008). While ASIST is aimed at the whole population,
STORM is aimed at frontline staff working in areas such as health care, the
criminal justice system and voluntary agencies. The training uses a modular structure, with two compulsory modules: Assessment (of the risk of
suicide) and Crisis Management (keeping the person at risk safe); two
optional modules: Problem Solving (the person at risk-taking control of
problems) and Crisis Prevention (how to manage should the person feel
suicidal again). There is a focus on the development of clinical skills in
working with people at risk of suicide, using role-play and video feedback.
The programme is flexible and designed to meet the needs and the level of
training and experience of individual participants (Morriss *et al.* 2005).
While STORM was originally designed for adults, a training package for
frontline staff working in children and young adults services has been
developed – STORM Children and Young Adults (CYA).

There are numerous other methods for intervening and helping children
and young people at risk of suicide such as Coping and Support Training
(CAST) (Thompson *et al.* 2001) found to be useful in reducing hopelessness
in young people at risk of suicide, The ZUNI Life Skills Development curriculum which is aimed at teaching young people at risk of suicide and also
addresses hopelessness (LaFromboise and Howard-Pitney 1995, LaFromboise
2006), The Collaborative Assessment and Management of Suicidality
(CAMS) (Jobes 2000) which uses a manualised, collaborative approach to
assess and treat people at risk of suicide. These and other approaches should
be examined and further knowledge obtained about these approaches. There
are however key principles which should underpin all interventions/pre-
ventions and a number of myths which need to be addressed. The key
principles can be summarised as the 3E's:

1. Engaging with the child or young person
2. Establishing whether the child or young person is at risk of suicide
3. Ensuring that the child or young person is safe

Engaging with the child or young person involves noticing that changes
have occurred. When children feel suicidal their behaviour changes. This
may show itself by changes in their pattern of sleeping or eating, they may
become withdrawn, they may not look after themselves as well as they used
to. They may look preoccupied or distracted. Their school work may be

affected; they may shun friends and lose interest in previously enjoyed activities. The changes in the child or young person's behaviour may be quite subtle and prior knowledge of them is often helpful. The child may look troubled or worried, or say something in an off-hand way, such as 'it's not worth it anymore', or 'I just can't be bothered'.

At surface level, changes in behaviour and statements do not indicate whether a child or young person is suicidal. It is only after engaging with the young person and noticing change that questions about suicide can be asked. Asking someone straight away if they are suicidal is probably not a helpful strategy, but it is a question which ultimately has to be asked if risk of suicide is to be established. Direct questioning is important – the meaning of vague questions such as 'are you thinking of ending it all?' may be clear to the questioner, but may mean something different to the child or young person. Barker and Buchanan-Barker (2005: 69) provide a succinct but powerful example of a simple but often effective assessment by asking 'have you ever thought about killing yourself?' – if the answer is yes enquiring further, if the answer is no, asking 'why not?' This is not only an effective way of establishing whether a child or young person is at risk of suicide, but it also links into reasons for living. There is a myth that asking about suicide you might encourage people to think about suicide when they previously had not thought about it. There is no evidence that you can put the idea of suicide into someone's thoughts, but there is evidence that people who are feeling suicidal feel relieved when someone asks them if they feel suicidal. Exploring young people's reasons for dying and living will help the child and young person feel engaged and understood.

6.10 Intervention

Suicide has been described as a long-term solution to a short-term problem. Helping a child or young person recognise that suicide is not the only option is key to intervening. Establishing reasons for living and having the young person engage with those reasons may be helpful. It is only through engagement and connecting with the children and young person's reasons for living and dying that we can really connect with their pain. What drives a child or young person to attempt suicide will vary from individual to individual. Intervention should therefore take account of difference and involve an approach which is tailored to the young person's particular needs. Little is known from research on intervention with children and young people about which therapeutic techniques work, in particular which methods work with whom and how change is maintained over time. This section will examine different approaches to intervention with children and young people. Linehan (2008) has argued that the effectiveness of interventions for people with suicide remains poorly researched and the suicide intervention is an area in need of much more focused and robust research.

Rudd and Joiner (1998) have developed a three-phase intervention approach which focuses on crisis intervention, short-term treatment and long-term treatment. Each specific intervention period targets a particular area using a specific therapeutic focus and intervention techniques. More time is spent in the early stages on examining stress in the young person's life. As the intervention progresses, the focus shifts to addressing skill deficits, then self-image and interpersonal functioning. The intervention is not time-limited, but achievement focused. The approach recognises that achievement of goals of therapy will be different for each child or young person.

Admission to hospital of a young person intent on suicide is often seen as essential, although the effectiveness of this strategy is contested (Katz et al. 2004, Steele and Doey 2007). For young people with moderate suicidal intent, outpatient intervention can work. Admission of a young person, however, needs to be balanced with the lack of emergency psychiatric beds for young people in the UK. For most young people, particularly those past their sixteenth birthday, admission to hospital may mean admission to an adult ward. Admission of children and young people to adult wards can expose them to patterns of behaviour which are at best unhelpful and at worst damaging to their identity. On occasions, admission to hospital may be unavoidable; however, consideration should be given to planning care so that the admission is brief, and supported by outpatient and day-treatment as constructively as possible.

Box 6.4 outlines the factors which Rudd and Joiner (1998) identify as requirements if outpatient treatment is to be successful.

Research with adults shows that longer-term care and lengthier interventions are more effective in reducing suicidal ideation. Psycho-education, problem-solving and psychosocial approaches have been useful in reducing suicidal ideation and suicide attempts, as well as reducing depression, anxiety, hopelessness and the need for emergency services (Linehan 1993, Rudd et al. 1996).

Working alongside the family may reduce hostility between family members, create a more supportive environment and improve the communication skills of the child or young person. Social skills training may help the young person to be able to elicit support from peers, which can be an important factor in preventing further attempts.

There has been an increasing interest in the use of cognitive–behavioural based interventions to help reduce suicidal behaviour. Katz et al. (2004)

Box 6.4 Factors Needed to Support Successful Outpatient Treatment (from Rudd and Joiner 1998)

- Ongoing evaluation of the need for hospitalisation
- Active involvement of the family or carers
- A 24-hour crisis line for the young person and family/carers
- Medication is reviewed regularly
- An assessment of risk indicators is obtained from the young person and their family/carers
- Increased frequency if outpatient visits
- Ongoing evaluation of treatment goals
- Telephone consultation is available for the young person and their family/ carers
- Suicide risk is frequently re-evaluated
- Professional consultation for staff

report on the use of dialectical behavior therapy (DBT) with young people comparing it with treatment as usual (TAU) with a group of young people who were inpatients. They report that both TAU and DBT showed a highly significant reduction in parasuicidal behaviour, depressive symptoms and suicidal ideation. DBT in the Katz (2004) study also showed a significant reduction in behavioural incidents compared to TAU. Woodberry and Popenoe (2008) found DBT to be helpful in an outpatient setting in reducing self-harming and suicidal behaviour in young people.

Tarrier *et al.* (2008) performed a systematic review and meta-analysis of the effect of cognitive–behavioural interventions on suicidal behaviour and found that while cognitive–behaviour therapy (CBT) appeared to be effective in modifying suicidal thoughts with adults, the effect was not significant with adolescents. However, they acknowledged that the number of studies with young people was poor compared with the adult studies. March *et al.*'s (2008) study found that CBT was effective in reducing suicidal thoughts in young people. Steele and Doey (2007) argue that most research has been carried out on young people with depression rather than suicidal behaviour, and that more research is needed on the effectiveness of psychological interventions.

 Activity

Jane is a 14-year-old girl who until recently was doing well at school. Since splitting up with her boyfriend after a 6-month relationship she has been truanting from school. She looks withdrawn in class and teachers have noticed she is more irritable.

There is a family history of anxiety and an uncle committed suicide 5 years ago. Jane has been writing gloomy essays in her English class and seems preoccupied with thoughts of death. Her teacher has suggested her to see her GP and the GP has subsequently referred her to your outpatient department.

What risk factors for suicide can you identify for Jane?

What might help Jane?

What further information would you need to assist your assessment?

6.11   Prevention

Suicide prevention is an area where government interventions have been implemented worldwide (WHO 2000, 2008a, c, Department of Health 2002, Scottish Executive 2002b, Mann et al. 2005), and while there are signs that such strategies are having an effect in reducing suicide the evidence is not conclusive (Palmer 2008). As well as national strategies, there are also local and school-based approaches. In a study of suicide prevention programmes in the USA, it was found that there was no relationship between the programmes and suicide rates (Metha et al. 1998). The authors made a number of recommendations to reduce suicide attempts, such as controlling firearms, family support, the identification treatment of at-risk youth and education of the media about the dangers of social imitation.

Aseltine et al. (2007) evaluated the effectiveness of the signs of suicide (SOS) in reducing suicidal behaviour in school children. The SOS programme has been adopted by hundreds of schools in the USA. The programme involves the use of a video 'Friends for Life' which illustrates issues relating to depression/suicide, how to respond to someone who is feeling depressed or suicidal, and accounts from people who have been touched by suicide. Students are also screened for suicidal behaviour using the Brief Screen for Adolescent Depression (BSAD). Students who scored above 16 on the BSAD are seen as clinically depressed and encouraged to seek help from a counsellor or teacher. The programme centres on two factors associated with suicide in young people: mental illness (in particular depression) and alcohol misuse. Young people are taught to recognise signs of depression and to respond to these by using ACT – *acknowledge* (the person's feelings), *care* (ensure that the student knows they are cared about) and *tell* (let a responsible adult know about the situation). At 3-month follow-up, those students taking the SOS programme reported 40% less suicide attempts than the control group. The SOS group had an increased knowledge of depression and suicide, but the programme did not have a statistically significant effect on suicidal ideation and help-seeking behaviour. Encouraging help-seeking is of importance for males as we know they are less likely to seek help than females. It should be noted that previous evaluations of psycho-educational groups to prevent suicide have found those not aimed at specific groups may at best have no effect and at worst have a negative effect on suicidal thinking (Shaffer and Gould 2000).

There is a suggestion that males may dismiss educational programmes aimed at suicide prevention and that participation in them may increase their rejection of suicidal peers. Males also report feeling depressed when attending these programmes, although this may be a sign they are beginning to confront some difficult issues concerning suicidal behaviour and masculinity (Canetto 1998). Katz et al. (2004) examined young people's style of coping – i.e. young people with 'maladaptive' coping strategies and young people with help-seeking strategies. Boys were more likely to display 'maladaptive' styles – and the authors suggest that concentrating strategies on young people with 'maladaptive' styles may increase help-seeking and potentially reduce suicide.

While there is debate whether prevention programmes are helpful, a combination of prevention and treatment programmes may reduce the rate of suicide and therefore be preventative. A prevention/intervention programme introduced into a school system in 1989–90 saw a 62.79% reduction in suicides in the period 1989–94 compared to the period 1980–88 (Zenere and Lazarus 1997). In the Zenere and Lazarus study, the mean number of completed suicides fell from just under 11 per year in the 5 years before the start of the programme to just fewer than 7 per year during the 5 years of the programme. The number of suicide attempts progressively fell from 243 in 1990 to 95 attempted suicides in 1989–94. Using what they perceived to be the successful factors in the programme, the authors made a number of recommendations including providing teachers with knowledge of the early warning SOS and introducing preventative programmes from the age of 5 years, which should be rigorously evaluated. The development of problem-solving skills, positive coping behaviours and improving self-esteem in children and young people were also seen as strategies to reduce suicidal behaviours.

Thompson et al. (2000) looked at the factors which produced change in the prevention of suicide – they found that the skills and experience of the group leader were central to the group's effectiveness. They also found that selecting teachers who wanted to work with this often 'unpopular' group of young people, providing them with training and videotaping their evaluations were also helpful. The support provided by the young person's peer group could increase their sense of personal control and reduce suicide risk behaviours.

6.12 Postvention

Postvention is concerned with help offered after a suicide attempt and can involve helping the bereaved come to terms with the loss of a loved one, or helping those who have attempted suicide negotiate the effects of their suicide attempt. We have discussed earlier assessment following a suicide attempt. During the assessment, issues of loss should be considered. Young people may have suffered physical damage as a result of their suicide attempt and may also be feeling psychological or emotional loss in terms of their identity and relationships.

The events associated with a suicide attempt ripple outwards and touch many other people's lives. These ripples can feel like overwhelming waves of emotions for those close to the child or young person and may feel unmanageable or overpowering. Loss through bereavement can be difficult to cope with, but loss through suicide can involve other issues such as shame, guilt, isolation, feelings of rejection and stigma (Beautrais 2004). Helping survivors work through the bereavement is an important task following a suicide. The ripples may extend well beyond family and friends, to the community, school and other social links the child or young person may have. Parents and family members may review what they could have done, looking for missed warning signs and missed opportunities to ask. Their grief may be further complicated as friends and relatives may be unsure what to say, and may even avoid the immediate family – this is difficult enough when a child dies but is complicated by the shame and stigma which can be attached to suicide. This silence is further compounded as there may be no public acknowledgement of the suicide and obituaries may not mention the suicide. In Norway, there has been an attempt to face up to this issue and newspaper obituaries now mention that someone has died by suicide rather than covering it up – this may be helpful in addressing the stigma and secrecy surrounding death by suicide.

Blame is a common emotion during the early period of bereavement. We want someone to take responsibility for what has happened and be called to account. Health and social care professionals may share in this guilt and blame. Like the parents they may feel responsible, and think they should have prevented the suicide. It is important that like parents and families, professionals are able to work though their own grief – suicide reviews can be helpful, as long as they focus on understanding and making sense, rather than looking for someone to blame. The effective use of supervision can be invaluable in making sense of our own feelings and role.

Parrish and Tunkle (2005) provide a useful overview of issues to be addressed following the suicide of a young person, which includes addressing the needs of family, friends, school pupils and professionals. The period following the death of a son or daughter is a tremendously sad and difficult time and may involve using support groups and professionals, but will inevitably be best supported by caring and understanding family and friends. As Owens *et al.* (2008) found in their study of parents understanding of their sons' suicides, it is by attempting to make sense of what happened and who played which part that parents can negotiate the past and be prepared to face the future.

> The parents all resist drawing on an available medical discourse in order to account for the disintegration of their sons' lives, employing instead a moral discourse that relies heavily on notions of agency and accountability. As they struggle to work through their intense pain and question whether they were in any way to blame for what happened, their stories focus not just on what took place but on who played the decisive role. There is an overwhelming concern with the moral integrity of key players. (Owens *et al.* 2008: 250).

6.13 Conclusion

The loss of a child or young person through suicide can have a devastating effect on family and friends, and can be one of the most difficult experiences to overcome. In this chapter, we have looked at factors which make children and young people more vulnerable to, or at risk of suicide and how these vulnerabilities and risks can be assessed. Vulnerability to suicide is complex and a simple correlation does not exist between factors of vulnerability and suicide. Being aware that children and young people may be vulnerable to suicide can help us to be open to the distress and hurt young people are experiencing. By reflecting on the various approaches to risk, assessment and intervention, we may be able to reach out to young people who are at risk of suicide. Involving the family and friends in postvention can be a painful but essential part of the work with children and young people who are suicidal. Those in the helping professions may have to be containers of powerful and primal emotions as parents and families work through their loss. This can be particularly difficult when those trying to help may share in the same loss. This chapter has outlined different approaches to prevention, intervention and postvention. The approaches discussed in this chapter are not definitive, and will not address everyone's needs. Continuing to search for effective and acceptable interventions should continue to be the task of all those who work with children and young people at risk of suicide.

Recommended reading

Anderson, M. and Standen, M. J. (2007). Attitudes towards suicide among nurses and doctors working with children and young people who self-harm. *Journal of Psychiatric and Mental Health Nursing* 14 (5), 470–477.

Barrero Pérez, S. A. (2008). Preventing suicide: a resource for the family. *Annals of General Psychiatry* 7, 1.

Fortune, S. and Clarkson, H. (2006). The role of child and adolescent mental health services in suicide prevention in New Zealand. *Australasian Psychiatry* 14 (4), 369–373.

Gunnell, D. and Ashby, D. (2004). Antidepressants and suicide: what is the balance of benefit and harm. *British Medical Journal* 329, 34–38.

Platt, S., Boyle, P., Crombie, I., Feng, Z. and Exeter, D. (2007). *The Epidemiology of Suicide in Scotland 1989–2004: An Examination of Temporal Trends and Risk Factors at National and Local Levels*. Edinburgh: Scottish Executive.

Scottish Executive (2002). *Choose Life: A National Strategy and Action Plan to Prevent Suicide in Scotland*. Edinburgh: The Stationery Office.

Websites

Choose Life – a National Strategy and Action Plan to Prevent Suicide in Scotland

The Choose Life site contains information about suicide, local action plans for Scotland, statistics about suicide evidence about different interventions, and suicide prevention training opportunites. There is also a resource database in which some resources are downloadable.
http://www.chooselife.net/home/Home.asp

PAPYRUS

PAPYRUS is a UK voluntary organisation founded in 1997 by a group of parents who had lost children through suicide. PAPYRUS supports people who work with children and young people at risk of suicide. They produce resources for families and professionals as well as disseminating expertise, good practice and commissioning research.
http://www.papyrus-uk.org/

Compassionate Friends

This is a charity which supports bereaved parents and their families; their home page can be found at http://www.tcf.org.uk/index.htm

They produce a leaflet specifically for parents who are bereaved by a child suicide, which can be accessed at: http://www.tcf.org.uk/leaflets/lesuicide. html

Cruse Bereavement Care
The aim of Cruse is to promote understanding about bereavement and promote the well-being of people who have been bereaved.
http://www.crusebereavementcare.org.uk/index.html
Cruse have a leaflet about support for people bereaved by suicide.
http://www.crusebereavementcare.org.uk/pdf%20files/suicide_factsheet. pdf
Cruse also has a website written by young people for young people called the 'Road for you', RD4U, which aims to support young people after the death of someone close to them: www.rd4u.org.uk

National Registry of Evidence-based Programs and Practices
National Registry of Evidence-based Programs and Practices (NREPP) is a service of the Substance Abuse and Mental Health Services Administration (SAMHSA). NREPP is a searchable database of interventions for the prevention and treatment of mental and substance use disorders. SAMHSA has developed this resource to help people, agencies and organisations. Type your search subject in 'find interventions' and you will be able to search by subject and age group.
http://www.nrepp.samhsa.gov/index.asp

Promising Strategies. Aboriginal Youth: A Manual of Promising Suicide Intervention Strategies
Written by Jennifer White and Nadine Jodoin. This manual reviews the literature around Aboriginal suicide prevention, examines preventative factors and provides an overview of prevention strategies. The focus is on using the manual to develop culturally relevant programmes.
http://www.chooselife.net/web/FILES/Tool_Kit/aboriginal_youth_manual_ of_promising_suicide_prevention_strat.pdf

Preventing Suicide: a Toolkit for Mental Health Services
An audit toolkit to measure services against existing standards from recommendations made by National Confidential Inquiry into Suicide and Homicide by People with Mental Illness. The toolkit has a list of resources to help develop practice.
http://www.chooselife.net/web/FILES/Tool_Kit/preventing_suicide_toolkit_ mental_health_services.pdf

Suicide Prevention Resource Center
The Suicide Prevention Resource Center (SPRC) provides a number of resources such as the Best Practice Registry – which reviews and disseminates information about suicide prevention, support from suicide prevention specialists as well as training, a library and prevention news.
http://www.sprc.org/featured_resources/index.asp

The Aeschi Working Group
Discusses therapeutic approaches to working with people who are suicidal and provides an overview of CAMS model.
http://www.aeschiconference.unibe.ch/cams1.htm

The National Centre for Suicide Research and Prevention
The University of Oslo have established a research and suicide prevention unit whose aim is to support research and disseminate knowledge about research and counselling.
http://www.med.uio.no/ipsy/ssff/english/index_english.html

WHO – Preventing Suicide How to Start a Survivors' Group
This is part of SUPRE, the WHO worldwide initiative for the prevention of suicide and a useful resource in developing survival groups in localities.
http://www.chooselife.net/web/FILES/Tool_Kit/preventing_suicide_start_survivors_group.pdf

Chapter 7

CHILD ABUSE AND CHILD PROTECTION

Julie Hendry[1] and Marlene Macinnes[2]

[1] *Child Sexual Abuse Team, NHS Lothian Child and Adolescent Mental Health Services, Edinburgh, Scotland*
[2] *Child and Adolescent Mental Health Team, Edinburgh, Scotland*

7.1 Introduction

Child abuse has occurred over centuries and across cultures, but it was perhaps the founding of children's charities such as the National Society for the Prevention of Cruelty to Children (NSPCC) at the end of the nineteenth century that first brought it to the public's attention in the UK. At that time the main focus was on abandoned or neglected children.

Awareness of child abuse grew slowly: in 1962 the paediatrician Henry Kempe wrote about 'battered baby syndrome' and suggested that physical abuse was occurring on a wider scale than previously thought (Kempe *et al.* 1962). Sexual abuse has gained increasing recognition since the mid-1980s.

In 1973, the enquiry into the death of Maria Colwell (DHSS 1974) led to child protection procedures being created in the UK. Despite this, subsequent public enquiries on the deaths of children such as Jasmine Beckford (London Borough of Brent 1985) and Tyra Hendry (London Borough of Lambeth 1987) criticised professionals for failing to protect them, whereas the Cleveland Inquiry (Butler-Sloss 1988) and the Orkney Inquiry (Clyde 1992) raised serious concerns about the removal of children without evidence of abuse.

Many child protection procedures and much of the legislation introduced over the last 30 years have been influenced by similar events. The Victoria Climbie Inquiry (Laming 2003) and recent concerns over 'Baby Peter' have demonstrated that we are still struggling to find the right balance between too much intervention and too little.

Understanding Children and Young People's Mental Health, first edition. Edited by Anne Claveirole and Martin Gaughan. Published 2011 by John Wiley & Sons Ltd. © 2011 John Wiley & Sons Ltd.

Learning outcomes

After studying this chapter, you should be able to:

1. Outline categories of child abuse.
2. Demonstrate knowledge of incidence and prevalence in child abuse.
3. Understand the possible impact of child abuse.
4. Describe what child protection assessments may involve.
5. Discuss the legislation used to protect children in the UK.
6. Outline a range of interventions used in child protection.

7.2 Definitions of child abuse

Child abuse can involve physical, emotional or sexual maltreatment and neglect, all of which may harm a child's health and development. It can be perpetrated by parents, carers and other adults known to a child or by strangers. There are degrees of overlap between different types of child abuse, because a number of risk factors are associated with all types of abuse.

Physical abuse

Physical abuse can involve causing physical harm to a child, such as hitting, shaking, burning or suffocating. In some cases particularly for children under the age of 5, it can result in death. In the UK, some forms of physical chastisement are deemed reasonable in law, but an observable injury and hitting or shaking a child under the age of 3, a blow to the head, or the use of an implement are defined as abuse in Scotland.

Fictitious or induced illness

Fictitious or induced illness, sometimes referred to as Münchausen syndrome by proxy (Bass and Adshead 2007), occurs when parents or carers repeatedly bring their children for medical intervention, for conditions they have induced or fabricated which may cause physical and emotional harm or be life-threatening. Examples of induced illness include the manufacturing of symptoms, altering laboratory samples – e.g. adding blood to urine samples. The main conditions which are produced in children affect the gastrointestinal, central nervous, respiratory and genitourinary systems (Sheridan 2003). The prevalence of induced illness is contested and the use of objective measures to test induced illness has been brought into question (Lawrence 2004).

Emotional abuse

Emotional abuse is the persistent psychological maltreatment of a child that is likely to impair their development. It can involve recurrent criticism, humiliation, threats, negative attributions, isolation, frequent rejection and emotional unavailability. It can occur when a parent or carer has inappropriate developmental expectations, which may be beyond a child's capabilities. Alternatively, parents may be overprotective and prevent a child from exploring their environment or engaging in social interaction (Glaser and Prior 2002).

Emotional abuse can involve a parent or carer using a child to meet their own emotional needs, failing to recognise the child's individuality and boundaries, encouraging prejudice or exposing them to domestic abuse or other criminal activity. It may lead to children feeling in a persistent state of fear or danger. Some form of emotional maltreatment exists in all types of child abuse, but it can occur on its own.

Sexual abuse

Child sexual abuse is the exploitation of children for the sexual gratification of adults. It can involve forcing or persuading children to view or take part in sexual activities, including penetrative (e.g. rape) and non-penetrative acts. Sexual abuse can include forcing the child into prostitution, to look at or be involved in the production of pornography (Browne and Hamilton-Giachritsis 2007). The organisation of child sexual abuse and the distribution of child pornography have greatly increased as a result of the Internet. A distinction is made between intra-familial (within the family) and extra-familial (outside the family) sexual abuse.

Neglect

Neglect is the failure to meet a child's basic physical or emotional needs, and it is likely to impair a child's health or development. Neglect during pregnancy may occur as a result of maternal substance misuse. It can involve a parent or carer not providing adequate food, clothing or accommodation, not protecting a child from harm or ensuring access to appropriate medical attention. It can involve a parent or carer being unresponsive to a child's need for stimulation and social interaction. Neglect is often seen as having the most adverse outcomes in terms of psychological problems and educational difficulties in later life (De Bellis 2005). In some cases neglect can also result in death (Horwath 2007).

Non-organic failure to thrive

Non-organic failure to thrive was first recognised by Spitz (1945) in a study of babies raised in institutions who failed to grow despite reasonable calorific intake. It is not caused by any hereditary or medical condition. It results in a child failing to meet weight and height norms or developmental milestones, and traditionally is diagnosed when a child is below the third centile for height and weight (Batchelor and Kerslake 1990). If a child is on the third centile for height, it means that for every 100 children of the same age 97 are taller and 3 shorter.

Non-organic failure to thrive is of course not limited to children raised in institutions and is a problem across society. More recently there has been little agreement on the criteria used to describe failure to thrive children, with identification methods being seen as over or under inclusive (Olsen 2006, Olsen *et al.* 2007).

Historical abuse

Historical abuse involves allegations of child abuse that are usually made by adults, about events that occurred in their childhood. In a large number of cases, allegations have been made about abuse where a group of adults have acted together in a school or residential institution.

Child abuse can lead to physical injuries, developmental delay, relationship difficulties and mental health problems. Not all children and young people who have experienced child abuse go on to develop long-term difficulties. Resilience factors can be a protection, but the frequency and severity of the abuse, and the co-occurrence of more than one type of abuse, puts them at greater risk (Carr and O'Reilly 2004).

 Activity

Rosie (6) and Beth (8) are regularly absent from school. They have problems with recurring head lice, poor dental hygiene and are often dressed unsuitably for the weather. There are concerns about Rosie's learning and aggressive behaviour, while Beth is described as very withdrawn. Both girls have had a number of accidents and injuries in the home resulting in cuts and bruises.

What types of child abuse may be occurring in this case?
What are your reasons for thinking this?

7.3 Incidence and prevalence

Despite an increased awareness of child abuse, and many millions of pounds being spent on child protection each year in the UK, research indicates that child abuse and neglect are under-reported. Incidence studies look at the number of reported cases of child abuse, and prevalence studies try to identify all cases whether they were reported or not, by asking a sample of adults if they were abused in their childhood. Most prevalence studies have been conducted in Western countries, but it is important to be careful about making comparisons between them because of differing definitions of child abuse and methods used (Wekerle and Wolfe 2003).

Creighton reviewed research studies from 1998 to 2003 in England, North America and Australia and reported on the incidence of child maltreatment found in these studies. Neglect was found to be the most frequent form of child abuse across countries, and emotional abuse the least commonly reported, although in Australia emotional abuse and neglect are substantiated or registered in equal numbers. The rates of child maltreatment ranged from 2.7 per 1,000 children in England to 12.4 per 100,000 in the USA. In England, nearly 20 times more cases were reported or referred than were substantiated or registered (Creighton 2004).

Cawson et al.'s (2000) prevalence study of young adults in the UK found that 7% reported serious physical abuse, 6% reported serious neglect, 6% had experienced emotional abuse and 1% said they had been sexually abused by their parents or carers, predominantly their fathers or stepfathers. This study did not include people who were homeless or living in hospitals or prisons who are thought to have experienced higher rates of child abuse.

Finkelhor (1994) looked at surveys of child sexual abuse in 21 countries and found it was not possible to make comparisons across countries because of the different definitions used. Creighton's (2004) overview of self-reported studies of child sexual abuse in Europe, the USA and New Zealand from the 1980s to the present day found the overall prevalence to be 8–42% for females and 3–25% for males. Prevalence for contact child sexual abuse was 6–20% of females and 1–16% of males. However, the annual incidence of child sexual abuse reported in the UK, North America and Australia was between 0.02% and 0.12%.

 Activity

What is the difference between incidence and prevalence?
  List some reasons why studies report such a wide range of prevalence?

7.4 Risk factors

While there are a range of risk factors associated with all types of child abuse and neglect, it is important to state that the existence of risk factors in itself does not mean a child will be abused. Neither will all parents who were abused or neglected as children harm their own children. Many risk factors have been established from research on recorded abuse, but there may be other unidentified risk factors for unreported abuse.

When assessing risk it is not possible to say that the greater the number of risk factors, the larger the risk of abuse and neglect. Gelles (1991) argued that while some abuse developed along a continuum from mild to severe, this is not always the case. Some parents and carers are qualitatively more harmful to children than others.

The child

A number of risk factors are present in a child and some relate more to the relationship they have with their parent/s. A premature or ill child or a child with a developmental delay or learning disability may be more vulnerable because of the additional demands they place on their parent or carer. Similarly a child thought to have a 'difficult' temperament such as being fractious or continually crying is thought to be more at risk of abuse.

The parent or carer

There are many risk factors that place parents or carers at risk of abusing their children. Glaser and Prior (1997) found that 69% of children who were abused or neglected came from families with parents who had a mental illness, misused substances or where there was domestic violence.

Other risk factors include parents or carers with a disability or chronic illness, parents with poor emotional regulation, young or single parents, step-parents and those who struggle to have a positive parent-child attachment. Parents or carers may also have experienced abuse or neglect in their childhood, have poor knowledge of child development and inappropriate expectations of their child or have an authoritarian style of parenting.

The environment

Risk factors coming from the environment tend to relate to poverty, poor housing and overcrowding, and antisocial neighbourhoods. If neighbourhoods are not constructed to support parents, vulnerable families are more at risk of abuse. There is also an increasing awareness of the poorer outcomes experienced by children who have been looked after and accommodated and the more difficult challenges they face in life (Barber and Delfabbro 2004).

Resilience factors

It should be no surprise that resilience factors are often the direct opposite of those factors that make children vulnerable to abuse. Promoting resilience in children, families and their environment is an obvious area of focus and one which is receiving increasing attention (Gilligan 2005, 2008).

The child

Resilient children place fewer demands on their parents and they may have an easy temperament or be physically healthy. This can be a protective factor particularly if parents have a low threshold for tolerating difficult behaviour. Other factors which provide what might be regarded as constitutional resilience include high intelligence quotient (IQ), the ability to make and sustain friendships (Lynskey and Fergusson 1997), to feel good about oneself, to develop self-efficacy (Hauser and Allen 2006) and to be assertive. A strong attachment to a non-abusing parent or carer can also be a protective factor against abuse or neglect (Graham-Bermann *et al.* 2006).

The parent or carer

Resilience in a parent is affected by inherent qualities, such as high IQ, and also by environmental factors, such as being able to access social support when needed (Ghate and Hazell 2002). Having a positive relationship with a partner, accurate knowledge of child development, an authoritative parenting style and a secure parent-child attachment are all resilience factors.

The environment

Coming from a high socioeconomic group and living in an environment where there is good housing and infrastructure, where people can feel safe, valued and have social and educational opportunities are protective to children (Daniel and Wassell 2002).

 Activity

Connor (4) lives with his teenage mother Lisa, who has a history of postnatal depression. Connor is physically healthy and is making good progress at nursery where he has friends. Lisa has been attending a parenting course and has regular contact with a community psychiatric nurse. She has recently been reconciled with Connor's father who has just been released from prison.

What makes Connor vulnerable to abuse?

What might help Connor to be resilient?

In what way do you think that Connor is at risk of abuse and neglect?

7.5 Policy

'Every Child Matters' (HM Government 2003) introduced in England and Wales following the Victoria Climbie Inquiry (Laming 2003), 'It's everyone's job to make sure I'm alright' (Scottish Executive 2002a) in Scotland and 'Our Children, Our Young People, Our Pledge' (Northern Ireland Government 2006) in Northern Ireland emphasise that we all have a part to play in the detection and prevention of child abuse and neglect. Professionals involved in childcare have mandatory training in child protection and procedures are in place for reporting concerns about children and young people without delay. Sharing information where there is cause to believe a child may be at risk of harm overrides an agency's confidentiality requirements.

There has been increased recognition of the particular needs of children and young people in foster care and residential settings. For example, the Scottish Government commissioned a systemic review of residential schools and children's homes between 1950 and 1995; the recommendations made include focusing on children's rights, staff training and regular reviews (Shaw 2007).

Emphasis on identifying and monitoring adults who are considered to pose a risk to children in the community led to national guidance on Multi-Agency Public Protection Arrangements (MAPPA) in 2001, which were most recently updated in 2009 (National MAPPA Team 2009). This guidance provides agencies with the mechanisms to work together to manage individuals thought to pose a high risk of harm to children.

7.6 Assessment

Initial assessment

Following a child protection referral, assessment of abuse is multi-agency involving social services, police and health professionals. The initial assessment is concerned with establishing if abuse has occurred, and a risk assessment should involve a systematic collection of information to ascertain the likelihood of a child being abused or neglected in the future.

Assessment should be seen as a continuing process throughout the investigation and should consider the child's health, education and social circumstances rather than simply focusing on a specific allegation. It may reveal no cause for concern, or that parenting is 'good enough' (Adcock and White 1985) by reaching a set of standards of care seen as necessary for healthy child development. In some cases, it may be decided that a child is 'in need' and additional support or services required, but in others there may be evidence emerging that the child is at risk of 'significant harm', as stated in relevant legislation.

Agencies have been accused of ignoring race, culture or ethnicity during the assessment period, and making subjective judgements on the basis of white middle-class norms, which have led to black and mixed raced children being over-represented in the care system. Workers need to be culturally competent to be able to work with families, meaning that they need broad cultural knowledge and 'variability both within and between cultures' (Korbin 2007: 134). Similarly concerns exist that disabled children may be more negatively valued, and that child protection services are not set up to meet their needs during investigations.

Interviewing the child

The primary aim of any interview is to establish the child's account of any alleged abuse, by using non-leading questions. The main role of the police is the detection of crime, while social services need to assess the levels of risk and protective factors within the child's family. To prevent the need for children to undergo multiple interviews, it is common for police and social services to question children together. Interviewing siblings or other children in the household may be necessary to assess if they have also been abused, or to gather more information about the family's circumstances.

With extra-familial abuse where the alleged abuser lives outwith the child's home, it may be possible for police and social services to gather information by interviewing the child with the family's knowledge without placing them at risk of further abuse. This would not be possible, however, if parents had a close relationship to the alleged abuser or they were likely to disbelieve the child.

In cases of intra-familial abuse, there is a need to assess the child so that they do not feel intimidated by their parents or carers to retract any disclosure. In some cases where severe abuse is suspected, it may be necessary for a child to be accommodated under emergency protection legislation to allow this to occur.

Medical examination

If physical abuse, neglect or child sexual abuse is suspected, a full forensic medical assessment needs to be arranged. Consent is required from parents or carers, unless this is seen as placing the child at greater risk. If parents refuse to give consent to a medical examination in conjunction with other concerns, it may be grounds for emergency child protection procedures. Children and young people may also provide consent if a medical practitioner deems them to be capable of understanding the nature of the examination.

Child Protection Case Conference

In a non-emergency situation where there is concern that a child may be at risk of abuse, it is the responsibility of social services to arrange a Child Protection Case Conference. The meeting is attended by relevant professionals, parents or carers and the child or young person where appropriate, to enable a comprehensive risk assessment of the needs of the child, the parents' capacity to care for them and the family's circumstances.

The Child Protection Case Conference may decide that the child is not at risk of abuse and the case may be closed or family support and services may be provided. When a child is assessed by the Child Protection Case Conference to be at risk of abuse, their name is placed on the Child Protection Register. Professionals involved then formulate a child protection plan to consider supports and services to reduce the risks of abuse.

A child's registration must be reviewed within 6 months to consider the progress of the child protection plan, and whether the risks have decreased sufficiently to remove their name from the Child Protection Register.

A referral to the family courts or the Scottish Children's Reporters Administration may occur concurrently to consider compulsory measures of supervision or care.

 Activity

Zoe (14) tells a teacher at school that she has been sexually abused by her stepfather over the past 2 years. He has told her that no one will believe her and that he will abuse her younger sister Stacy (8) if she goes to stay with her father.

How would you plan the assessment?

Can Zoe give consent to a medical examination?

Can Stacy? What would you do if Zoe's mother did not believe abuse had occurred?

The United Nations Convention on the Rights of the Child

The United Nations Convention on the Rights of the Child 1989 was ratified by the UK in 1992. Some of its general principles include:

■ The welfare of the child is paramount.
■ Children have the right to be protected from abuse neglect and exploitation.
■ Each child who can form a view has the right to express those views.
■ Parents should normally be responsible for the upbringing of their children.
■ Public authorities should promote the upbringing of children by their families.
■ Any intervention by public authorities must be properly justified.

Child Protection Legislation in the UK

The UK, Scotland, England and Wales, and Northern Ireland have separate legal systems. The United Nations Convention on the Rights of the Child influence on child law led to the Children Act (1989) in England and Wales, the Children (Scotland) Act 1995 and the Children (Northern Ireland) Order 1995, which all embody its general principles.

Despite this there is no single piece of legislation that covers child protection in each jurisdiction, and laws are regularly amended, e.g. the Children Act (2004) updated the law in England and Wales on physical punishment, and information sharing between professionals. Laws are changed through Acts of Parliament but it is left to the courts to interpret the legislation.

Child Protection Legislation is civil law, and for legal proceedings to go ahead there must be sufficient evidence in the balance of probabilities that child abuse has occurred. The level of proof for criminal legal proceedings is higher, and it must be shown beyond reasonable doubt that abuse has occurred. It is not uncommon therefore to have a situation where a child may be removed from their home as a result of abuse, but the alleged abuser is not prosecuted, or if prosecuted found not guilty.

Legal definition of a child

The classification of a child in law is a person under the age of 16 in Scotland and under the age of 18 in England, Wales and Northern Ireland.

Partnership and the no order principle

Legislation refers to the importance of working in partnership with families, which suggests power sharing. In the case of child protection, however, there can be a conflict of interests between parents and children. The law also requires that no court order should be made, unless it is thought that doing so would be better for the child. This is sometimes referred to as the 'positive advantage principle' (Lyon 2007: 225).

This has led to the belief by some social workers that work has to be undertaken with families on a voluntary basis, unless relationships have completely broken down. This was never the intention of the law however, and it is still possible to have some form of partnership with families where there is compulsory supervision or care.

Recent child deaths have also raised concerns about the interpretation of these laws with local authorities being seen to place too much emphasis on the principle of keeping families together, rather than the protection and welfare of the child being the paramount consideration.

Statutory intervention

Child law in the UK recognises that local authorities have a duty to 'safe-guard and promote the welfare of children in need' by providing services to children and families. This can include resources such as day care, parenting programmes or respite. In cases where it is thought that voluntary support may not be sufficient, there are various statutory interventions available.

Child Assessment Orders

Where there is concern as stated in the legislation that 'a child is suffering or is likely to suffer significant harm' and an assessment of a child's health or development is required, which parents or carers do not consent to, a Child Assessment Order can be sought through the courts. This should be used for planned assessments when all efforts to persuade families to co-operate have been made, and not for emergencies.

Emergency and Child Protection Orders

In cases where there is concern that 'a child is suffering or is likely to suffer significant harm if they are not moved to a place of safety', an Emergency Protection Order or a Child Protection Order in Scotland can be obtained through the courts. In an absolute emergency, where there is no time to apply for an order, a police officer may remove a child to a place of safety if they believe the grounds for an Emergency or Child Protection Order would be satisfied. These are short-term measures for the immediate protection of children, and the child would be referred to family courts or the Scottish Children's Reporters Administration following this action.

Exclusion orders

Legislation exists in the UK to exclude the alleged abuser from the home rather than removing the child, where appropriate.

Supervision and care orders

A supervision order or supervision requirement in Scotland places a child under the supervision of the local authority, and can have various conditions attached, such as regulating contact with any person or accessing medical treatment. A child who is subject to supervision is referred to as being 'looked after' in law.

In Scotland a supervision requirement can also have a condition of residence outwith a child's home with a relative (where possible), foster carer, residential unit or secure accommodation. In England, Wales and Northern Ireland, a Care Order would be sought for this purpose. If a court decides a child is to live away from home, they are 'looked after and accommodated' under law. These orders and requirements are regularly reviewed, and can be varied or terminated. There is also a right of appeal for children and their families.

 Activity

Outline the steps you would take to address the following scenarios:

1. A mother who is experiencing depression and is struggling to set limits for her three children.
2. A family of six children who are not brought to routine health checks.
3. A teenage boy who has been bruised by his father when trying to protect his mother from domestic abuse.
4. A baby who has head injuries which medical staff believe are a result of shaking.

7.7 Prevention

Social policy and legislation emphasise the need for agencies to prevent as far as possible abuse from occurring. Knowledge of risk factors for abuse should enable families where children are seen to be in need, to access the support and resources they require. Preventive work is primarily provided by voluntary agencies, but short-term funding, limited resources and a lack of a strategic overview often mean that the majority of children's services remain reactive.

7.8   Interventions

Initial intervention

The principal consideration following a disclosure of abuse is to ensure the child is safe, with the minimum disruption to their lives. In a number of cases of emotional abuse, neglect or physical abuse, a range of supports can be provided to the child and his family in the home. In some cases of extra-familial sexual abuse, when parents believe their children, arrangements can be put in place to prevent them from having further contact with the alleged abuser. In some cases of intra-familial sexual abuse or physical abuse, where non-abusing parents believe their children, the perpetrator can be excluded from the household using legislation.

In some cases, it is not possible to protect children from further episodes of abuse by leaving them at home, and there is a need for them to be looked after and accommodated. In such circumstances, steps should be taken to keep children in their schools, and maintain links with their family and communities.

Multi-agency interventions

Multi-agency interventions are thought to be more effective, and form the basis of a child protection plan. They can include the following.

For the child

Specialist day care or nursery
Befriending service
Respite
Individual therapy
Group therapy
Family therapy
Prosecution of the alleged abuser

For the parent or carer

Treatment for mental illness
Treatment for substance misuse

Family therapy
Group therapy for non-abusing parents or carers
Parenting classes and information on child development
Advice on debt and benefits
Help with a housing transfer
Home care
Respite
Mobilising the extended family to provide support where possible

Culturally sensitive treatment

In all cases it is important to be culturally sensitive to a family's beliefs and values, and that this will also help with engagement and build good working relationships between the family and the professionals involved. All communication must be appropriate to the child and family's level of understanding; interpretation and translation services must be used where required.

Problems in helping children who have been abused

While there has been an increase of awareness about child abuse in society, and more procedures put in place to investigate and identify it, there is concern that there are fewer resources left to monitor and treat children and families. More research is also needed about what interventions work best for children who have been abused and neglected.

It may also be difficult to help children who have been abused when:

- parents or carers deny the abuse
- parents or carers refuse to co-operate with the child protection plan
- co-ordination and co-operation between professionals is lacking
- resources are limited
- legal proceedings are protracted
- short-term care placements are of poor quality
- interventions are not culturally sensitive.

All these are considered risk factors for further abuse and long-term adjustment to the abuse.

    Activity

Mark (12), Louise (6) and twins Declan and Jamie (1) live with their mother Lauren, and the twins' father John. Both Lauren and John have a history of opiate misuse. The children's names have been recently put on the Child Protection Register following an incident where Louise took some of her parents' methadone to school.

What interventions would you include in a child protection plan?

What would be your reasons for this?

What would you do if Lauren and John did not allow the social worker to see the children?

7.9 Conclusion

In the UK, there has been an increase in the awareness of child abuse over the last 30 years, with policies, procedures and legislation put in place. Much of this has been in response to public enquiries where there have been professional failings, and the emphasis has moved from demands for high levels of state intervention to low levels, and back again. Child protection is a complex field, and it may not be possible to completely eliminate child abuse from our society. This chapter has demonstrated that there are systems in place in the UK, which work to protect thousands of children each year, but more research is needed on effective interventions, and more government funding and commitment is required to resource them for real change to be achieved.

Recommended reading

Batchelor, J. (2008). 'Failure to thrive' revisited. *Child Abuse Review* 17, 147–159.

Becker, F. and French, L. (2004). Making the links: child abuse, animal cruelty and domestic violence. *Child Abuse Review* 13, 399–414.

Creighton, S. J. (2002). Recognising changes in incidence and prevalence. In: Browne, K. D., Hanks, H. H., Stratton, P. and Hamilton, C. (eds). *Early Prediction and Prevention of Child Abuse: A Handbook*. Chichester: Wiley.

Department for Education and Skills (2006). *Working Together to Safeguard Children*. London: Department for Education and Skills.

Earnshaw, S. (2005). Disorders of parenting and child abuse. In: Gowers, S. (ed). *Seminars in Child and Adolescent Psychiatry*, 2nd edition. London: Gaskell.

Edinburgh and Lothians Child Protection Committee (2003). *Report of the Caleb Ness Inquiry*. Edinburgh: Edinburgh and Lothians Child Protection Committee.

Finkelhor, D., Ormrod, R. K., Turner, H. A. and Hamby, S. L. (2005). The victimization of children and youth: a comprehensive, national survey. *Child Maltreatment* 10 (1), 5–25.

Horwath, J. and Tidbury, W. (2009). Training the workforce following a serious case review: lessons learnt from a death by fabricated and induced illness. *Child Abuse Review* 18 (3), 181–194.

Sawyer, M. G., Carbone, J. A., Searle, A. K. and Robinson, P. (2007). The mental health and wellbeing of children and adolescents in home-based foster care. *The Medical Journal of Australia* 186 (4), 181–184.

Scottish Executive (2007). *Getting It Right for Every Child – Guidance on the Child or Young Person's Plan*. Edinburgh: Scottish Executive.

The Royal Society for the Prevention of Cruelty to Children (2006). *The Child Protection Companion*. London: RSPCC.

Wilson, K. and James, A. (2007). *The Child Protection Handbook*, 3rd edition. London: Balliere Tindall Elsevier.

Web resources

Barnardos:
www.barnardos.org.uk
Children 1st:
www.Children1st.org.uk
National Society for the Prevention of Cruelty to Children:
www.nspcc.org.uk
Royal College of Paediatrics and Child Health:
www.rcpch.ac.uk

Chapter 8

EATING DISORDERS

Gavin Cullen

NHS Lothian Child and Adolescent Mental Health Services, Royal Edinburgh Hospital, Edinburgh, Scotland

8.1 Introduction

We have all seen pictures of emaciated models, celebrities and sometimes ordinary people with anorexia, and we are constantly exposed to media reports celebrating this star's latest diet or supposedly expressing concern about that diet's effects on their health. Such mixed messages may lead us to believe that eating disorders are a self-indulgent fad for rich and famous people, albeit an occasionally dangerous one, or just diets gone wrong. But if we have a relative or a friend with an eating disorder, we know that such ideas are very far from the mark: eating disorders such as anorexia are complex, long-term conditions that may deliver enormous suffering to the person concerned and those who love them, irrespective of social status, and they can result in death. There is a continuum of eating disorders with less severe eating problems at onc cnd to the more severe and enduring problems at the other. It is the more severe and enduring problems which will be discussed in this chapter.

Where eating disorders in children and young people are concerned, we may hold a range of views, from underestimating their significance to seeing their causes and effects everywhere and an epidemic on our hands. In this chapter, we will examine the main types of eating disorder seen in a Child and Adolescent Mental Health Services (CAMHS) setting and outline some of their potential risks. We will also consider how common eating disorders are and examine key theories of vulnerability, including known risk and resilience factors. Next, we will consider assessment and the evidence for treatment for eating disorders in CAMHS. Along the way we will question some of the myths about eating disorders and there will be the opportunity to

Understanding Children and Young People's Mental Health, first edition. Edited by Anne Claveirole and Martin Gaughan. Published 2011 by John Wiley & Sons Ltd. © 2011 John Wiley & Sons Ltd.

reflect on issues raised in the chapter in reflective exercises. We would encourage you to work through these, and access the resources recommended, as the topic can be distressing and sometimes perplexing.

Strictly speaking, in CAMHS children can present with either an *eating* disorder or a *feeding* disorder. In eating disorders food intake is restricted, avoided or expunged due to its perceived fattening effects, while in feeding disorders food is restricted or avoided for other reasons. For example, a child with *functional dysphagia* may avoid eating due to fear of swallowing or being sick, making the dysphagia a feeding disorder. This chapter will focus on eating disorders in general and *anorexia* and *bulimia* in particular given the concern, suffering and controversy that surround them.

Learning outcomes

After reading this chapter, you should be able to:

1. Outline the main eating disorders seen in a CAMHS setting.
2. Identify the main explanatory models for eating disorders.
3. Identify key vulnerability and resilience factors for eating disorders.
4. Reflect on how a child or young person with an eating disorder might be helped.

8.2 What are eating disorders?

There are four main terms used by psychiatrists to classify eating disorders: anorexia and bulimia, which most people have heard of; eating disorder not otherwise specified (EDNOS); and binge eating disorder (BED) (American Psychiatric Association 1994, Fairbairn 2008). People with anorexia and bulimia share beliefs that they are overweight and are preoccupied with their weight and body shape, take extreme measures to control those things and often mostly or wholly base their self-esteem on their ability to do so (Bryant-Waugh and Lask 2007, Fairbairn 2008). To receive a diagnosis of anorexia, a person will have a significantly lower body mass index (BMI; see Box 8.1) than expected for their height and age and will be taking steps to keep their weight down. People with bulimia tend to have relatively healthy BMI scores, regardless of their perception of their weight, but will engage in *bingeing* several times a week (Freeman 2002). Binges involve eating an objectively large amount of food (e.g. 2,000 calories worth) in one sitting, often of foods the person has otherwise denied themselves, perhaps as part of dieting. Binges are accompanied by a sense of being out of control, and induce

Box 8.1 Body Mass Index

BMI is calculated by taking a person's weight in kilograms and dividing it by their height in metres squared. For example, the author's own weight is about 84 kg and his height is 1.76 m; this gives a BMI score of 27.1.

There are numerous Internet sites which will calculate BMI for you, but it is important to remember that most of these are for adults (aged 18 plus). For children and teenagers, you need specific age-adjusted charts/calculators to take account of expected growth rates, often referred to as percentiles.

Nonetheless it is interesting to note the following general guidance commonly referred to in relation to BMI scores:

■ A BMI score of 17.5 or less is considered significantly underweight (17.5 is the cut-off point for anorexia).
■ A score of 19.9 or less is considered underweight.
■ A score of 20–24.9 is within a healthy range.
■ A score of between 25 and 29.9 is considered overweight.
■ A score of 30 or above is defined as obese.

guilt, which leads to *purging* behaviour – getting rid of the extra calories by vomiting, exercising or taking laxatives. People with EDNOS are those who have an eating disorder but do not meet *all* official criteria for anorexia or bulimia, and those with BED are people who engage in the bingeing but not the purging behaviour seen in bulimia.

There are striking similarities between anorexia, bulimia and EDNOS, and the same person, in diagnostic terms, can often 'move' between the three (Fairbairn 2008). Anorexia and bulimia both involve diets, rules about food, avoiding eating, binges and intense exercising. People with anorexia can develop bulimic symptoms on the path to recovery (up to about 50% do), and people with bulimia can develop anorexic symptoms (Carr 2006). EDNOS, almost by definition, includes elements of and movement between anorexic and bulimic problems.

Fairbairn (2008) helpfully suggests that clinicians are in effect seeing one eating disorder with different phases or aspects over time. His stance has important implications, chief among them is validation of the service user and their carers' experience. There are also treatment implications, which are outlined below, and the need to be aware of different risks at different times for the young person. For a summary of the main risks associated with eating disorders, see Box 8.2.

You may have noticed that obesity is not included here as an eating disorder. There is no doubt that obesity is a significant health risk; it

Box 8.2 Risks and Physical Consequences of Eating Disorders*

Anorexia

General: weight loss; emaciation/skeletal appearance; dehydration; hypothermia; delayed growth/short stature; mood fluctuations, and anger or flat affect.

Dermatological: pale and/or dry skin; dry, cracked lips; lanugo hair (fine, downy hair also seen on babies); thinning hair; and brittle nails.

Muscular: atrophy of the muscles.

Abdominal: constipation.

Brain changes: reduced reflexes; impaired concentration and memory; and peripheral neuropathy.

Cardiac: irregular heartbeat; heart rate and blood pressure changes; low blood pressure; cold extremities; delayed capillary refill; oedema; and heart failure.

Bulimia

General: weight fluctuations; dehydration and mood changes.

Dermatological and oral: dry lips and tongue; erosion of teeth enamel; tooth decay and inflammation of the gums.

Abdominal: tenderness.

Brain changes: impaired concentration and memory.

Cardiac: irregular heartbeat; low blood pressure and oedema.

*Note that this is by no means a full list of possible medical consequences. Readers interested in learning more are directed to the resources noted at the end of the chapter and to consult with medical colleagues about these issues.

---

brings increased potential for developing high blood pressure, diabetes and coronary heart disease, and is on the increase in the UK (Scottish Public Health Observatory 2007). Obesity is also a significant health problem facing people with BED (Zipfel *et al*. 2005). However, obesity is also more often considered a consequence of modern, sedentary lifestyles, where nutritional supply and consumption often exceed energy expenditure, rather than a mental health problem per se (van Hoeken *et al*. 2005, Scottish Public Health Observatory 2007). Psychological support could help some people with obesity, and people with eating disorders sometimes need and request help for both (Scottish Health Observatory 2007, Fairbairn 2008). What is being questioned here is the assumption that obesity is in general and automatically a *mental health disorder* – for further discussion about these and wider issues consult Fairbairn and Brownwell (2005) and Gilman (2008).

8.3 How common are eating disorders?

Methodological problems abound in epidemiological eating disorders research. These include different age ranges being used in different studies, e.g. adolescents sometimes being included in adult studies. Also, people with eating disorders can take a long time to agree they have a problem, making it less likely they will participate in research at certain times (Treasure *et al.* 2007). Nonetheless, we can note that:

- Most people with an eating disorder are thought to be between 15 and 35, and in this age range incidence is estimated to be increasing (van Hoeken *et al.* 2005).
- Approximately 0.3–0.5% of the population up to age 18 develop anorexia and 1% bulimia (Gowers and Bryant-Waugh 2004, Carr 2006).
- Bulimia is rare under 12 years, with a mean age of onset of between 15 and 18 – compared to 15 for anorexia.
- The female:male ratio for eating disorders is about 4:1 for under 12 and 9:1 for 13–18 year olds (Carr 2006).
- In the West it is not only the rich, famous or privileged individuals who develop eating disorders (Freeman 2002). Anorexia and bulimia are known to affect people from any social or cultural background (Freeman 2002, Muise *et al.* 2003, van Hoeken *et al.* 2005). Much less is known or documented about the prevalence of eating disorders in the rest of the world. The most common theme in the literature is that there is increasing recognition of problems in different countries around the world and that eating disorders are more likely in countries experiencing rapid economic change – with a consequent change in the roles women have in those countries (Gordon 2001).

We can also note that eating disorders are by no means a new phenomenon, having been recognised in children from the 1600s onwards, and that available objective evidence does not support the view that there is a dramatic increase in eating disorders in children and adolescents. Nor is there any agreed explanation(s) for the apparently disproportionately high numbers of females with eating disorders compared to males. What is certain, however, is that children as young as 6 can be acutely aware of body image issues, including the perceived link between being slim and being attractive (Faulkner 2007). We will return to these ideas when we discuss the social climate surrounding eating disorders.

Activity

1. BMI calculations are not the only way to measure a person's healthy weight range. Using the Internet can you find an alternative and consider the relative advantages and disadvantages of the different methods?
2. Why do you think that more females are recognised as having an eating disorder than males?

8.4 What causes eating disorders?

A biopsychosocial approach

Surprisingly, given the high personal and literal costs eating disorders involve, no single unifying explanatory model has been established. Also, many experts contend that no one risk factor is ever likely to explain disorders so inherently complex (Nicholls 2007). Instead, eating disorders research examines a number of key causative theories and associated risk and resilience factors. Unsurprisingly, some of this research is contentious and intermittently contradictory.

The solution to these problems lies with a pragmatic approach that eating disorders arise as a combination of biological, psychological and social forces (Lucas 2008). The precise interaction involved is unique to each person, as is the trigger to their illness beginning, and often their paths to recovery (Lucas 2008). It is only at certain points, e.g. when people are starving as a result of anorexic behaviour that eating disorders appear similar (Lucas 2008).

We will now examine the main biological, psychological and social themes in turn.

Biological Factors

Genetic vulnerability

Most psychiatrists are confident that eating disorders run in families, although researchers are unsure exactly how that risk is realised, including the extent of inherited traits, such as perfectionism, versus environmental influences (Goodman and Scott 2005, Nicholls 2007, Treasure 2007). The number of genes involved and the precise extent to which they influence the development of a disorder are also unknown and vary in the literature. Lucas (2008), for example, states that genes account for up to 70% of a disorder developing, with the remaining 30% arising from a person's environment.

Neurological vulnerability

Neuroscientific research proposes that specific deficits in brain structures and functions are involved in eating disorders, and that the neurological, physical and social changes puberty brings influence their development (Southgate *et al.* 2005). Neuroscientific suggestions, mainly for people with anorexia, include:

- disruptions to the brain structures related to appetite and food-as-pleasure
- being less adaptable to change
- tendencies to become so absorbed in details they stop seeing the bigger picture
- difficulties identifying and describing their own feelings, and, in a few cases, being able to tell what others are feeling.

Southgate *et al.* (2005), Treasure (2007)

Unfortunately, existing neuroscientific research findings are inconsistent and unable to explain fully which things are related to cause and which to effect (Treasure 2007). Future research may clarify these issues and help shape clinical interventions. However it is also prudent to wait and see how a person functions once they have more fully recovered their weight and health, given the well-known effects of starvation on brain functioning and structure.

Starvation effects

Denying the body and brain the essential nutrients food and water provide will lead to a person being unable to think clearly or make decisions and a reduction in brain chemicals which stimulate hunger and delayed gastric emptying (Freeman 2002, Pinhas *et al.* 2007). Delayed gastric emptying itself will cause a person to feel like they are full when they have eaten little, to feel bloated when eating, or to be constipated – which will put them off further eating (Pinhas *et al.* 2007). Starvation during puberty is also believed to leave people's brains underdeveloped psychologically. Thus it is clear that starvation itself carries significant risks for maintaining an eating disorder once it has begun. (Treasure *et al.* 2007). These starvation effects are universal, i.e. they are not specific to anorexic behaviour and happen to anyone who starves. Amongst other known universal starvation effects are an intense preoccupation with food and eating, and an understandable depressed-like lethargy and inactivity in some or a more physically active, restless response in others (Freeman 2002).

Psychological Factors

Function(s) of eating disorders

Some experts have constructed hypotheses related to the purposes eating disorders, or the behaviours associated with them, might serve. Treasure *et al.* (2007) describe a situation in which eating disorders allow people with them to manage difficult feelings. For example, starvation effects may dampen strong emotional pain, binges may offer temporary distraction from it, and purges may get rid of 'too many' difficult thoughts and feelings (Treasure *et al.* 2007). Goss and Gilbert (2002) also describe disordered eating behaviour as helping people manage potent negative feelings. These range from feelings of low self-worth, inadequacy, feeling like a failure, to feelings related to loss (Goss and Gilbert 2002). For Goss and Gilbert (2002), these feelings are themselves part of people with eating disorders experiencing an ongoing sense of shame, shame that is tied to body image and fear of being overweight.

It seems logical, then, to identify things which cause those feelings noted above to find more specific psychological risk factors. Painful or traumatic life events, such as the death of significant people, parental divorce or sexual abuse, have been linked with eating disorders. Having to negotiate significant transition points in life, such as adolescence, in combination with stressful life events, is also thought to play a role (Freeman 2002, Carr 2006). However, these risk factors, in terms of objective research evidence, are linked more with developing psychological problems generally than with eating disorders specifically (Freeman 2002). But stating that does not minimise two essential points here:

1. People with eating disorders are psychologically vulnerable and often in great distress.
2. Every person with an eating disorder has their own life story, aspects of which will have a significant bearing on the development of it.

Coexisting mental health problems

People with anorexia and bulimia often experience other mental health problems, including:

■ depression, which is associated with anorexic or bulimic difficulties;
■ substance and alcohol abuse, which is associated more with bulimic problems;

- anxiety disorders and phobias;
- obsessive–compulsive disorder (OCD). OCD, unfortunately, is also associated with poorer outcomes for people with anorexia and therefore must be highlighted as a risk factor in its own right. The precise relationship(s) between coexisting psychological problems and eating disorders is not yet fully understood.

Particular activities, hobbies or occupations

Athletics, ballet dancing and fashion modelling have all been associated with developing eating disorders, with ballet dancers particularly being described as a high-risk group (van Hoeken *et al.* 2005, Ringham *et al.* 2006, Model Health Inquiry 2007). However, it is not really known if those highly competitive, perfectionist worlds attract people with those tendencies or create (or worsen) those attributes in them (van Hoeken *et al.* 2005). Certainly, all three areas focus intently on body shape, image and performance, and at least one of those areas, the fashion industry, is very defensive about being linked with eating disorders or perpetuating an ideology of thinness being equated with attractiveness (Model Health Inquiry 2007).

Meanwhile, clinicians tend not to believe that activities *cause* eating disorders, but they sometimes see evidence of perfectionism, competitiveness, over-exercising and other eating disordered behaviours being displayed in pursuits like swimming, ballet or other dancing forms, aerobics, or indeed any sport. Simultaneously, these activities are highly valued by people with eating disorders and their families as contributing to positive self-esteem and maintaining friendships.

Social factors

These factors are probably the most controversial and experts are not in agreement about their role. On the one hand, many commentators note the pressures within Western society and in places aspiring to Western values on females to be slim to be attractive (and males to be a particular shape), which arise from a variety of sources, including the media, an interest in celebrity and diet fads (Faulkner 2007, Model Health Inquiry 2007, O'Hara and Smith 2007). Others, on the other hand, question the extent of social influences by reminding us that eating disorders have existed for centuries and different values in different times have apparently led to the same ultimate problem (Lucas 2008).

We cannot ignore the social context within which any mental health problem exists; society provides the backdrop for an individual's roles within it, their choices and self-esteem. We have already noted that children as young as 6 are aware of the perceived relationship between slimness and attractiveness (Faulkner 2007). Children are also acutely sensitive to remarks made by their parents and significant others about their weight (Nicholls 2007).

Dieting is one of the main means by which attractiveness, or a more desirable weight, can be achieved and can be seen as a contributory factor in developing an eating disorder. Orbach (2006) points to a widespread profit-making industry surrounding dieting to evidence just some of the pressure to diet. She would also argue that the need for women to diet to be slimmer is a socially constructed falsehood. Interestingly, recent American evidence suggests that diets do not work to keep weight down long term, with some adults and young people gaining more weight than they began with, and dieting sometimes contributing to the development of binge eating habits (Mann *et al.* 2007).

Dieting features as a clear precursor to developing bulimia, and therefore is a risk factor for it, especially in those who had previously been overweight or where being overweight runs in the family (Nicholls 2007). The evidence to support a link between dieting and anorexia is more tenuous, perhaps because the spirit and purpose of dieting in people with anorexia is so different (Freeman 2002, Nicholls 2007). People with anorexia are often secretive about dieting and perceive themselves as becoming more and more overweight, even though they are actually getting thinner (Freeman 2002).

8.5   Resilience factors

In the person with the eating disorder

A high IQ, relatively good self-esteem, an optimistic but mature outlook and good problem-solving abilities are all considered important factors that can influence recovery from eating disorders. The ability to make and keep friends is also helpful (Carr 2006).

In the family

Families do not cause eating disorders, and good practice views the family as a central resource in helping young people recover (Carr 2006, Treasure *et al.* 2007). Families in which there are good parent–child bonds, where the parents have a happy marriage and where they share child care can all do better. Familial resilience is also linked with the capacity of the parents to be *authoritative* with their children. This is the ability to be in charge of situations firmly but with compassion, as opposed to being distant or being authoritarian and harsh. Parents also need to have compassion for themselves, and everyone in the family, in order to maintain the energy needed to support the person with the eating disorder and to look after their own health (Treasure *et al.* 2007). This might mean asking extended family members or friends to help out, and having time off.

Families also have a crucial role in helping young people accept that they have an eating disorder (Treasure *et al.* 2007). This is not an easy task, given the understandably strong feelings the situation provokes. Parents often feel guilty, and facing up to an eating disorder can make everyone feel worse in the short term. Simultaneously, the person with the eating disorder might be very reluctant to hear what even loved ones have to say. Nonetheless, acceptance is a vital foundation for all future interventions, and one that good staff teams will support families carefully with.

 Activity

Young people are or can be as resilient and resourceful as adults. What strengths do you think young people have to help each other and themselves cope with eating disorders?

8.6   Assessment

There is no room here to explain fully the physiological complications associated with anorexia and bulimia. The following is a summary only, and for more information interested readers are directed to the risks noted in Box 8.2 and the resources suggested at the end of the chapter.

In primary care

GPs are often the first point of contact for people with eating disorders, who might present to them for other health concerns including low mood, anxiety, stomach or bowel problems and problems with menstruation (NHS QIS 2006). Primary care staff therefore have a significant role in beginning the assessment process and knowing when to refer a person on to specialist services (NHS QIS 2006). They will also need to exclude alternative medical explanations (Pinhas *et al.* 2007).

Referral to specialist services

Specialist services are mental health services with expertise in managing eating disorders or services exclusively for eating disorders. The lower a person's weight is, e.g. where their BMI is 16 or less and they are losing weight continually, the more advisable their referral to specialist services is (NHS QIS 2006). If a person's BMI is 13 or less, and they are losing 1 kg or more per week, the referral is urgently required. For bulimic problems, referral to specialist services is needed if the person's symptoms are severe, continue for more than 6 months and do not respond to advice or self-help methods. In both cases, referral on to mental health agencies is also indicated where the person is experiencing very low mood, other coexisting mental health problems or engages in self-harm (NHS QIS 2006). People with eating disorders may also need treatment in general hospitals to ameliorate physiological emergencies, such as dehydration, prior to beginning treatment in a mental health service.

Assessment in specialist services

Around the UK, there are a variety of NHS and private health care services for people with eating disorders (NHS QIS 2006). It is outwith the scope of this chapter to comment on the regional, organisational and philosophical differences between them. Here, we will focus on services provided by CAMHS to describe assessment (and, later, interventions).

Most people with eating disorders can be seen as outpatients, but CAMHS sometimes have day- or inpatient units, and each of these settings could be used to assist initial assessment and engagement (Gowers and Bryant-Waugh 2004). This involves building trust and rapport with the young person, and their family, from the outset, and includes taking account of:

■ a person's diet, weight and physical health from birth to present date
■ important life events for the person and the family
■ any history of mental health problems in the person or the family
■ peer relationships and important friendships
■ relationships within the family
■ the person's attitude to eating, their body shape and the prospect of treatment.

Assessment ideally involves psychiatrists who have experience of managing physiological as well as psychological aspects of eating disorders, dieticians, nurses, occupational therapists and psychologists who are in a position to offer individual psychological support to the person and/or family support (Pinhas et al. 2007).

8.7 Interventions

Motivation to change

Provided it is physiologically safe to do so, clinicians must work with a person's variable readiness to engage with help. To avoid doing this increases the likelihood that people with eating disorders will resist changing their behaviour, and may also contribute to staff or carers becoming frustrated or stressed themselves – and thus less likely to be offering the right kind of support at the right time.

Clinicians can formally train in *motivational interviewing*. This balances counselling skills such as warmth, empathy and active listening, with reflecting back to people their current motivational stance. Thus, people retain a sense of responsibility for change themselves.

Physical care

All physical health complications must be addressed in turn, beginning with the most urgent, such as heart problems. Simultaneously, an overall treatment goal is to establish healthy, stable eating and exercise patterns, which necessitates an agreed diet plan, the setting of *target weights* and regular weight and BMI monitoring to review progress (Gowers and Bryant-Waugh 2004).

Where anorexic behaviour is concerned, the effects of starvation need to be stopped then reversed, which takes time, and involves a gradual re-introduction to healthy eating and developing a healthy appetite (Treasure *et al*. 2007). This process needs to be carefully monitored to avoid *re-feeding syndrome* (Pinhas *et al*. 2007). This is a very dangerous possibility in which a person's stomach and body cannot cope with suddenly being asked to take on too much food after a period of starvation, resulting in cardiovascular, neurological and/or blood chemistry complications. The person could, therefore, in extremis, die, and at the very least experience considerable distress and discomfort, and perhaps a loss of confidence in eating and in those caring for them.

Long-term, re-establishing healthy eating gives the person's body and brain the best chance of recovering fully (Freeman 2002, Treasure *et al*. 2007). In the short term, it can also help a person recover enough so that they can then use formal psychological supports.

8.8 Psychological support

Individual

Cognitive–behavioural therapy (CBT) focuses on understanding and positively challenging the possible links between a person's thoughts, actions and how they feel. It is a logical choice for eating disorders given that key maintaining factors in them revolve around people's dissatisfactions with themselves and beliefs they are overweight. CBT is indeed recommended for treatment of anorexia, and has a reasonable evidence base to support the treatment of bulimic symptoms (NICE 2004a, NHS QIS 2006).

Interpersonal therapy (IPT) is a good alternative to CBT for people with bulimia, although the treatment takes longer (NICE 2004a). Dialectical behaviour therapy (DBT) is an adapted version of CBT. It has recently begun to be used to treat people with eating disorders and has a small amount of evidence to support it (Gowers and Bryant-Waugh 2004).

Two important points are worth noting here. First, psychotherapies like CBT are typically developed for adults then adapted for younger populations. This means that all clinicians using them must adapt them according to the specific developmental needs of the young person (Gowers and Bryant-Waugh 2004). Second, therapists must be prepared to offer long-term, stable commitments to children and young people, and forge therapeutic, non-judgemental alliances as a platform for reducing the control eating disorders have over them (Gowers and Bryant-Waugh 2004, Lask and Bryant-Waugh 2007).

Family

In CAMHS, family work is highly recommended in the treatment of eating disorders, and anorexic problems particularly. Families can understandably adapt to eating disorders in ways that then maintain them, and the type of family work showing most promise aims to address this by offering skills training, education and emotional support (Carr 2006, Treasure *et al.* 2007). For example, families can be shown how staff support a young person to manage mealtimes. In this, staff and, later, parents support young people in their fight against a shared enemy – anorexia, an approach called *externalisation* (Lask and Bryant-Waugh 2007).

Medicine

Psychiatric medication is not the first treatment of choice for young people (Gowers and Bryant-Waugh 2004). There is little evidence to support the use of medication for anorexic problems, and much caution needs to be exercised here anyway, as some psychological problems may recover with weight restoration and medication side effects may be intolerable at lower body weights (NICE 2004a). Where bulimic problems are concerned, antidepressants can be used to augment treatment for adults (NHS QIS 2006). However, few studies have examined specific effects on adolescents, and there are ongoing concerns about the potential of anti-depressants to increase suicidal thinking in young people (Le Grange and Schmidt 2005).

Inpatient care

In emergencies, e.g. where a person has very low mood, dangerous self-harming behaviour and/or their weight is very low, inpatient treatment may be needed (NICE 2004a, NHS QIS 2006). When a person's BMI has reached 13.5 or lower, there is a potentially life-threatening emergency (NHS QIS 2006, Treasure *et al.* 2007). Inpatient services may be able to arrest weight decline, restore weight or both. They can also allow families to rest, pause and gather the necessary energy and resources to help their child.

Unfortunately, available evidence is mixed where inpatient treatment is concerned. Qualitative studies have shown that inpatient staff, if they become too strict or controlling, can reinforce young people's negative self-beliefs (Offord *et al.* 2006). Some quantitative studies have also shown that people often do not sustain the weight gains made in inpatient units (Offord *et al.* 2006, Gowers *et al.* 2007). In one very recent study, no advantage was found in the long run in a person having an inpatient admission compared to outpatient treatment (Gowers *et al.* 2007). More research is needed in this important area, and the above is not presented as conclusive evidence. Perhaps the most pertinent comment here is the recommendation that inpatient admissions are only made to units with ongoing experience and expertise in helping people with eating disorders (NHS QIS 2006). Where that is the case, an inpatient admission can be a vital first step in the person's recovery – and indeed often a very necessary one.

 Activity

Motivational interviewing was mentioned above. At the beginning of treatment, it often seems like a young person with an eating disorder has the opposite motivation or readiness to change (i.e. they might not be ready or want to) compared to staff or the person's family. How do you think the young person might show that they are not ready and how do you think other people should manage that? (You may need to read up on this or ask a colleague who has been involved in this sort of work.)

8.9 Conclusion

Anorexia and bulimia are complex and dangerous disorders which affect children, young people and their families. Considerably, more research is needed to satisfactorily explain their causes and how to prevent and treat them at a personal and societal level. In the meantime, there are a number of biological, psychological and social factors which combine in ways particular to the person to influence the onset and outcome of an eating disorder.

Working with a young person's motivation, engaging well with their family (and utilising their strengths), teamwork and careful management of any physiological consequences of eating disorders are all fundamental to recovery. And most young people with eating disorders do get better. However, some will go on to have long-term problems and some risk death as a consequence of their eating disorder. It is literally vital, therefore, that continued efforts are made to expand on the existing evidence base and identify the most effective interventions; that the evidence is followed wherever it leads – including into the sociological and economic spheres; and that clinicians and service users work together to alleviate the suffering eating disorders bring.

Resources

On the Internet
Beat/beating eating disorders: A UK website for people with eating disorders and their families:
www.beat.co.uk
The Scottish Eating Disorders Interest Group, SEDIG:
www.sedig.co.uk
NHS Quality Improvement Scotland (QIS):
www.nhshealthquality.org
National Institute for Clinical Excellence:
www.nice.org.uk

Books

Clinical
Fairbairn, C. and Brownwell, K. (2005). *Eating Disorders and Obesity: A Comprehensive Handbook*. New York: Guilford Press.
Gilman, S. (2008). *Fat: A Cultural History of Obesity*. Oxford: Polity Press.
Lucas, A. (2008). *Demystifying Anorexia Nervosa: An Optimistic Guide to Understanding and Healing*. USA: Oxford University Press.
Morris, J. (2008). *ABC of Eating Disorders*. Oxford: Wiley Blackwell.

Sociological
Orbach, S. (2006). *Fat Is a Feminist Issue*. London: Arrow Books.
Orbach, S. (2009). *Bodies*. London: Profile Books.

For people with eating disorders and their parents or carers
Treasure, J., Smith, G. and Crane, A. (2007). *Skills-Based Learning for Caring for a Loved One with an Eating Disorder: The New Maudsley Method*. Abingdon, Oxford: Routledge.

Chapter 9

EARLY ONSET PSYCHOSIS

Martin Gaughan

School of Nursing, Midwifery and Social Care, Edinburgh Napier University, Edinburgh, Scotland

9.1 Introduction

Over the last few decades, our understanding of psychosis has increased and interventions have improved. Early detection has been the focus of increased research; early intervention services have grown considerably and are viewed positively from service users' perspectives. The introduction of 'atypical' antipsychotic medication has been heralded as an important step forward in the medical treatment of psychosis. However, the experience of psychosis for a child or young person can be bewildering, perplexing and is often lived through without a shared framework to help the child make sense of their experiences. In Western societies, stigma is associated with psychosis; consequently, a child may feel as though they have no one to turn to, and may worry that even their family does not understand.

In this chapter, we will provide an overview of psychosis in children and young people. The chapter will begin with a discussion of terminology particularly around the use of the term 'schizophrenia'. We will discuss the prevalence of and vulnerability to psychosis, and briefly outline a stress-vulnerability model. We will examine some of the experiences associated with psychosis and conclude with a discussion of current interventions, particularly around medication, psychosocial approaches and methods of early intervention.

Understanding Children and Young People's Mental Health, first edition. Edited by Anne Claveirole and Martin Gaughan. Published 2011 by John Wiley & Sons Ltd. © 2011 John Wiley & Sons Ltd.

Learning outcomes

After studying this chapter, you should be able to:

1. Consider the impact experiencing an episode of psychosis may have on a child or young person.
2. Outline the main components of psychological interventions for children and young people.
3. Discuss the prodromal phase.
4. Describe the importance of family work with children and young people who have experienced or are experiencing a psychosis.
5. Consider approaches to early intervention for children and young people.

 Activity

Consider the terms 'psychosis' and 'schizophrenia' – what do these terms mean to you? How do you think they are viewed and understood by society?

9.2 Time to change?

Throughout the chapter, we will use the term psychosis to outline the experiences described. In the main we will avoid specific diagnostic labels such as 'bipolar disorder', 'schizo-affective disorder' and 'schizophrenia'. We regard the label 'schizophrenia' as unreliable, harmful and think it should be changed. We are not convinced that any single diagnosis will reflect the multitude of difficulties and experiences currently covered by this umbrella term and think that people's individual experiences should be taken account of.

The validity and reliability of the term 'schizophrenia' have been challenged (Bentall 2003, Read 2004, Romme and Morrison 2007), it is seen by some as a diagnosis which is scientifically meaningless because it brings together a range of disparate problems under a particular label, is heterogeneous in nature and is difficult to verify (Fink and Taylor 2008). The criteria for 'schizophrenia', 'schizo-affective disorder' and psychosis in 'bipolar disorder' have been criticised as they overlap (Lake and Hurwitz 2007). Different practitioners may use the terms 'psychosis' and 'schizophrenia' interchangeably to mean the same thing.

People diagnosed with 'schizophrenia' are subjected to stigma and expect to experience stigma (World Psychiatric Association 2002, Thornicroft *et al.* 2009). The World Health Organization (WHO) (2002) recognises that stigma associated with 'schizophrenia' should be challenged – some organisations have addressed this challenge. The Japanese Psychiatric Federation change of name from *Seishin Bunretsu Byo* (mind-split-disease) to *Togo Shitcho Sho* (integration disorder) has been received in a largely positive light by carers and clinicians (Sato 2006). Prior to the name change, only 36.7% of people diagnosed with *Seishin Bunretsu Byo* were informed of their diagnosis, this increased to 69.7% following the change. In the UK, the Royal College of Psychiatrists acknowledge that people feel stigmatised because of their diagnosis of 'schizophrenia'.

There are inherent difficulties in making an accurate diagnosis, when a child or young person first experiences an episode of psychosis, and making a diagnosis to match DSM-IV-R or ICD10 criteria can be problematic. The young person's presentation may change over time leading to diagnostic instability, particularly between 'schizo-affective disorders' and 'schizophrenia'. Early Psychosis, Prevention and Intervention Center (EPPIC) (McGorry and Edwards 1997) suggest two possible approaches: – (1) use current classifications such as 'schizophrenia' and 'bipolar disorder', and make changes to the diagnosis in light of new evidence; (2) the preferred alternative is to have a simple, clear and general diagnosis such as 'acute psychotic episode'.

There are of course challenges in presenting research using the approach we have taken, and where necessary we have reported research in terms used by the research authors. However, we believe research approaches need to take account of each individual's lived experience, and interventions should be geared towards the individual needs of a child and family. Using categorical terms such as 'schizophrenia' to report on such broad and different experiences does little to enhance an inclusive approach.

 Activity

Outline the pros and cons for changing the name of 'schizophrenia'. What other ways of describing people's experiences might be more helpful or acceptable?

9.3 Prevalence

Psychosis occurs more often than is generally thought – around 3.4% of the population across the lifespan will experience a psychosis (Perälä *et al.* 2007).

Hallucinations, a common symptom of psychosis, are thought to occur in around 10–15% of the population (Tien 1991) and about 15% of the population are thought to experience psychotic-like symptoms (PLIKS) in their lifetime (Zammit *et al.* 2008). In a study of young people in Scotland, Boeing *et al.* (2007) found that a 3-year prevalence for psychosis of 5.9 per 100,000 of the general population, 20% of who were not in contact with mental health services; and approximately 50 per 100,000 adolescents were seen to be at risk of developing a psychosis. Around 20% of young people who have a learning disability are thought to have a psychosis (McClellan and McCurry 1998) although this may not be the true picture as research studies may have learning disability as an exclusion criterion.

9.4   Vulnerability to psychosis

Given the breadth of research and different theories proposed for causes of psychosis, we are at a relatively early stage in our understanding. There are competing views on the causes of psychosis, with a number of fields offering different although interrelated perspectives including genetic, environmental, neurodevelopmental, neurodeteriorative and multi-factorial. There is however no single cause and it is unlikely that one will be identified, because an interaction of multiple factors is probably what leads to the development of a psychosis (Keshavan *et al.* 2005, 2008).

The environment in which a young person has grown is thought to have some influence, with young people from urban environments being more vulnerable (Sundquist *et al.* 2004). Migration may also play a part (Veling *et al.* 2008). Children who develop a psychosis often experience developmental delays, have cognitive impairments and may be anxious or socially isolated (Cannon *et al.* 2002, Muratori *et al.* 2005). Other important risk factors include a family history of psychosis, eccentric behaviour and anomalies of thinking (Jones *et al.* 1994) as well as psychosocial issues including hostility in families, racism and poverty (Janssen *et al.* 2003, Read *et al.* 2005). There is some agreement that being exposed to bacterial or viral infections in the womb and other obstetric complications such as bleeding during pregnancy, diabetes, pre-eclampsia, difficulties in the growth of the foetus, asphyxia or caesarean delivery may increase vulnerability to psychosis (Koenig *et al.* 2002). There is an association between winter births and the development of psychosis (Torrey *et al.* 1997) although this may be less influential with early onset psychosis (Fouskakis *et al.* 2004).

Trauma experienced during childhood can significantly affect a child's development and there is growing evidence that it may influence the development of psychosis (Morrison *et al.* 2003, Bebbington *et al.* 2004, Janssen *et al.* 2004, Rosenberg *et al.* 2007, Shevlin *et al.* 2007). Trauma can be experienced in many different ways including abuse, neglect, bullying, domestic violence, divorce, parental problems of substance misuse, parental mental health problems or parents who have been incarcerated. Schreier *et al.* (2009) found that the risk of psychosis increased twofold if the young person had been bullied, particularly if the bullying was long standing or severe in nature. Trauma has a 'dose' influence – if the trauma is repeated and/or severe, it increases vulnerability. Whitfield *et al.* (2005) found a significant relationship between childhood trauma and hallucinations. In the past, trauma had been overlooked, or even dismissed as a possible cause of psychosis. Connections were not made between the content of people's delusions and hallucinations and their previous traumatic experiences. It is now generally accepted that helping young people talk about their hallucinations and delusions can help them manage and gain control over these experiences.

Research into the genetic origin of psychosis has been carried out for more than a century. Numerous studies and reviews have examined the influence of genetics in the development of psychosis, amongst twins (Gottesman *et al.* 1987, Gottesman 1991) and in adopted children of birth mothers with 'schizophrenia' (Tienari *et al.* 2003). Kendler *et al.* (1993, 1995, 1996) and Straub *et al.* (1997) argue genetic factors constitute the most important known risk factor for 'schizophrenia'. Werry (1992) has argued that genetic links are higher when the onset occurs in childhood. Tandon *et al.* (2008) reviewed the literature relating to genetics, outlining that 'schizophrenia' is known to run in families and that the closer the relative is to the child, the more likely they are to develop 'schizophrenia'. In monozygotic twins, the risk is 40–50% while in dizygotic twins the risk is 10–15%. The influence of genetics is hypothesised to be the interaction of the small effect of multiple genes which influence the development of 'schizophrenia' (Harrison and Weinberger 2005). Despite scientific advances, the understanding of the specific role of genetics in psychosis has developed relatively slowly.

Research into gene–environment interactions as a vulnerability to psychosis is growing (Van Os and Poulton 2008). The study of gene–environment interactions is complex; it can be difficult to unpick which elements are implicated. In what way do day-to-day experiences (micro elements) play a part in comparison with wider influences, such as the child's community or school environments (macro elements)? The

European Network of Schizophrenia Networks for the Study of Gene–Environment Interactions (EU-GEI) (2008) argue that despite the difficulty in unravelling these complex interactions, the study of gene–environment influences should play a major part in understanding vulnerability.

Psychosis may be induced or influenced by misusing drugs. Amphetamines (Tucker 2009), cocaine or crystal methamphetamine (crystal meth) are believed to cause psychosis. The relationship between cannabis use and psychosis has been subject to intense scrutiny, as the use of cannabis amongst young people is considered to be growing worldwide. Young people are thought to be particularly vulnerable to developing cannabis influenced psychosis because of their developmental stage (Stefanis *et al.* 2004) with reports of a twofold increased risk of psychosis for those using cannabis (Arseneault *et al.* 2004). In the general population, very few people using cannabis will develop a psychosis. Sewell *et al.* (2009) argue that cannabis use on its own is unlikely to cause psychosis but may combine with other factors to increase risk.

It is also important to understand how people make sense of the development of their own psychosis. Dudley *et al.* (2009) examined how people understand their own psychosis. From 48 different explanations they found four major categories: (a) drug misuse, (b) trauma in adulthood, (c) personal sensitivity and (d) developmental vulnerabilities. Perhaps unsurprisingly, these categories are the subject of increased research attention.

The stress-vulnerability model

The stress-vulnerability model, which has become widely accepted, suggests a process by which psychosis may develop. The model proposes we are all vulnerable to psychosis, with some more vulnerable than others. There are many factors which may be involved in the development of psychosis; a traumatic life event may be a precipitant of psychosis in some people but not in others. While vulnerability can be seen as something innate, people can also acquire vulnerability, e.g. through trauma or family experiences.

The stress-vulnerability model initially developed by Zubin and Spring (1977) has been incorporated by others. Zubin and Spring's (1977) model is a two-factor theory, with vulnerability and precipitating factors. Velleman (2001) proposed extending the model by adding perpetuating factors, therefore becoming predisposing, precipitating and perpetuating (the three Ps). There has been criticism that the original model was too mechanistic; therefore, how people cope and manage stress and trauma has been incorporated into modifications of the model (Davidson and Strauss 1995).

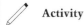

Activity

Think about a child or young person you know who has developed a psychosis – what do you think are stress and vulnerability factors for this child or young person?

9.5 Early and very early onset psychosis

Psychosis in children and young people usually develops slowly, and can be difficult to identify because early signs of psychosis may be mistaken for normal difficult behaviour, particularly in teenagers. Yet we know that earlier recognition is likely to produce more positive long-term outcomes. Early onset occurs between 13 and 18 years and very early onset occurs before this age (Asarnow *et al.* 1994). Around 5% of young people who develop psychosis do so before their 15th year, and 20% develop a psychosis before 20 years of age (Asarnow and Asarnow 1994).

Positive and negative symptoms

Symptoms of psychosis are often categorised as positive and negative. Negative symptoms are those such as apathy, lack of motivation and social withdrawal, which affect the young person's ability to socialise and be a part of their peer group. They are referred to as negative because they are seen as taking something away from the person. Positive symptoms include hallucinations, delusions, thought disorder, excitement and suspiciousness. They are called positive because they are seen as being active parts of the experience of psychosis. While both positive and negative symptoms are generally recognised as core symptom categories, a third one, 'disorganisation' has been proposed, which because of its effect on development may be particularly relevant to early onset psychosis (Dollfus *et al.* 1991).

Recognition of psychosis will be influenced by the child's communication skills and cognitive ability. Younger children may find it more difficult to give an accurate account of their experiences and may confuse hallucinations with fantasy and sleep-related illusions. The onset in younger children is often accompanied by increased disorganisation, particularly of thoughts and sense of self, and a reduction in social and cognitive skills. Delusions and hallucinations are less complex and there may be a theme of monsters. Delusions may be fleeting or half-formed. Hallucinations are generally auditory, involving commands, and there may very occasionally be visual hallucinations.

In older children hallucinations, delusions and thought disorder occur more often. Hallucinations are the most consistently reported experiences, yet they are not in themselves a definite indicator that the young person is developing a psychosis (Werry 1992). Hallucinations are usually auditory and often paranoid in nature, but may be visual, tactile, olfactory or somatic. There may also be persecutory delusions, or ideas of reference. Other possible symptoms include illogical thinking and loose associations, flattened or inappropriate affect, and depressive symptoms. Less common is catatonic behaviour which can also be experienced with other mental health problems (Cohen *et al.* 2005). The main negative symptoms are social withdrawal, poor rapport and lack of spontaneity (Russell 1992).

9.6 Phases of psychosis

Werry and Taylor (1994) identified five phases: prodromal, active, recuperative, residual and chronic. Miller and Mason (2006) talk about the acute, healing and maintenance phases. McGorry and Edwards (1997) list three phases: prodromal (or early warning), acute and recovery. We will follow the latter categorisation as it is more commonly used. The prodromal phase occurs prior to the acute onset, although prodromal also refers to the period preceding a relapse of acute psychosis (Birchwood *et al.* 1989). During the prodromal phase, there is a change in the young person's behaviour and their subjective experience of the world. Their concentration and attention may be reduced, they may lack drive and motivation, experience low mood, sleep disturbance and withdraw socially. The young person may become suspicious, irritable and there may be an overall reduction in their functioning. The length of this phase can vary from days to years, with the average phase lasting between 1 and 2 years (Sheitman *et al.* 1997). If the young person is experiencing mania or hypomania, the prodrome is likely to be very brief.

In the acute phase, experiences such as hallucinations, delusions and thought disorder are present. This period can last from 1 month to several years. Interventions in this phase include medication, psychoeducation, family work, psychological and psychosocial interventions.

In the recovery phase, the child or young person may be completely recovered or still experience difficulties such as inattention, lack of energy or depression.

Recovery focused services which are engaging to young people can be helpful (Edwards *et al.* 2005). The meaning of the word *recovery* has changed. Recovery used to mean becoming well and being free of symptoms. It has now taken on a more subtle meaning involving a process and taking into account individual lived experience and service users journeys. Frak (2005) defines recovery as:

.... a personal process of tackling the adverse impacts of experiencing mental health problems, despite their continuing or long-term presence. It involves personal development and change, including acceptance. There are problems to face, a sense of involvement and control over one's life, the cultivation of hope and using the support from others, including direct collaboration in joint problem-solving between people using services, workers and professionals. Recovery starts with the individual and works from the inside out. For this reason it is personalised and challenges traditional service approaches. (Frak 2005: 1).

Recovery is an individual experience, unique to the young person, it is not something imposed or decided on by a service and of course it applies to children and young people experiencing any kind of mental health problem. It is important that the process of recovery be considered at an early stage, as the psychosis may be enduring and affect the young person's life in a multitude of ways. For further information on recovery, consult the Scottish Recovery Network at http://www.scottishrecovery.net/ or Rethink http://www.rethink.org/.

The traditional view of psychosis as a progressively deteriorating condition with a slow decline over many years is challenged by new evidence suggesting a plateau effect where both positive and negative symptoms tend to stabilise about 2–5 years after onset. Some deficits in services have been addressed by improved early intervention services. The TIPS (Melle *et al.* 2005, Fjell *et al.* 2007, Joa *et al.* 2008, 2009) study examined early intervention programmes and duration of untreated psychosis (DUP) and found early intervention has a positive effect on both symptoms of psychosis and suicidal behaviour, although such programmes need to be tailored to the particular needs of young people (Melle *et al.* 2004).

9.7 Prevention and early intervention

Early detection has been described as one of the cornerstones of early intervention (Reading *et al.* 2005) and has the aim of shortening the duration and intensity of treatment, reducing hospital admissions and preventing relapse (Craig *et al.* 2004). We know that intensive intervention at an early stage can reduce symptoms of psychosis (Petersen *et al.* 2005). Attempts have been made to identify and suggest interventions for people at ultra high risk of psychosis (UHR) including atypical medication (olanzapine, aripiprazole), typical medication (haloperidol), selective serotonin reuptake inhibitors (SSRIs), omega-3 fatty acids, family work, psychoeducation, cognitive–behaviour therapy (CBT), skills training, psychoeducation and family interventions. There is evidence that some interventions may be helpful, although further research is needed (de Koning *et al.* 2009).

Engaging young people in early intervention services presents particular difficulties. Young people may be reluctant to seek help because of stigma, lack of knowledge about where to go and a fear of what may happen should they actually seek help. Other issues include the child's social environment – as communities subject to vandalism, crime and violence may place young people in a context where it is difficult to engage with services. The ethnic background of the young person may affect their ability to engage. Poverty can be a real issue for some asylum seekers and refugees, and may be compounded by issues of discrimination and stigma.

Engagement is central to any children and young people's service. To achieve engagement, workers need to have both excellent interpersonal and professional skills. Helping young people engage involves creative, innovative and stigma-free approaches. Staff involved in services may use text messages to keep contact with young people, and in preference to hospital visits may meet in cafés or local leisure facilities. Peck and Greatley (1999) have described the importance of not only engaging with, but advocating for, young people as central to the success of early intervention services.

 Activity

Make a list of other factors that may prevent a young person seeking help. What might help young people to engage?

At the time of writing, there are both competing health/social care needs and economic pressures on resources. If early intervention is to continue to develop, evidence of the positive difference it can make to people's lives needs to be established. In Lester *et al.*'s (2009) study, a range of strategies were employed at a time of financial constraint; these included restricting age criteria, discharging people earlier than the service ideal, imposing waiting lists and spending less time on community work.

9.8 Assessment

A thorough assessment of a child or young person presenting with a possible psychosis is essential. Information should usually be obtained from different sources. History taking should involve the young person and their parents/carer, and may include other family members, school or other relevant people. Assessment involves the investigation of the relationship between the illness, the person and the person's lived experience (Jenkins and Barrett 2004).

Assessment should include all areas of a child or young person's life. Enquiries should be made about family history of mental health problems, the child's previous and current personality – how they were and are socially, emotionally, cognitively and educationally. Relationships within a family should be explored including any changes within or to the family. Meeting the whole family can be helpful as siblings may have helpful insights into family functioning, and different perspectives of the same problem may be useful. Timing of changes, such as when they occurred and what was happening at the time, might provide a context for such changes.

Questions to ask may include how has the psychosis affected the child or young person's sense of self, their development and personality? What is it like for them at home? How do family members and carers view what has happened? A risk assessment is essential; children and young people who experience a psychosis may be at risk of harming themselves in response to hallucinations, delusions or because of low mood. Young people with a psychosis are at increased risk of suicide. Risk of harm to others must also be assessed as delusional thoughts or hallucinations may be influencing the young person to harm others. Such behaviour and experiences can be very distressing for both the young person and their family. Careful, thoughtful plans need to be in place to support the young person and their family.

Assessment of children can be problematic, e.g. they may have difficulty in identifying feelings or naming symptoms. Speaking about their experiences may be frightening, or unsettling. A young person developing a psychosis may be reluctant to share their experiences with others, they may feel suspicious or paranoid, and if previous experiences of treatment have been poor this may affect engagement. There may be attention or concentration problems, hallucinations, substance misuse, language or cultural barriers. As Jenkins (1998) has argued, culture influences every area of psychosis from identification, definition and meaning, through to the effect that gender and ethnicity have on the experience, its course and its outcome. Young people from the British African-Caribbean population are more likely to be admitted as inpatients, more likely to be detained under the mental health and are more likely to be admitted to medium secure mental health units (Commander et al. 1997, Lelliott et al. 2001, Audini and Lelliott 2002, Tolmac and Hodes 2004). Taking account of a young person's cultural background and reflecting on your own attitudes are essential if young people are to be treated equitably.

Activity

Why might young people from the British African-Caribbean population be treated differently?
   How might you address the cause of this difference?

Assessment of psychosis with young people who have an learning/intellectual disability presents particular challenges, particularly in young people with severe learning/intellectual disability (Clarke 1999). Assessment can be difficult because of interviews and questionnaires which rely on a level of verbal fluency which may not be present in the young person being interviewed. Misdiagnosis and diagnostic instability can be particular problems (Friedlander and Donnelly 2004).

A physical assessment is important in early onset psychosis because some physical illnesses, including auto-immune and metabolic disorders, systemic and central nervous system infections, and cerebrovascular abnormalities, may mimic or produce psychotic symptoms. While only occasionally found, it is still important to exclude their presence. Caution should also be exercised as some physical investigations are invasive and may consequently impede the engagement of the young person. The examples listed above are not exhaustive and an assessment should identify physical problems where present. Recommended physical investigations are:

- urine and blood drug screen
- full blood and urine examination
- liver function tests
- CTI or MRI scan.

Given the association with substance misuse and psychosis, establishing if a young person is misusing substances is essential. Young people may use substances such as cannabis and alcohol to alleviate their symptoms. It is thought up to 60% of young people with a psychosis may use substances (Lambert *et al.* 2005). Abstinence is unlikely to be a realistic goal for young people; however, reduction of substance use is achievable and associated with improved outcomes.

The method of assessment needs careful consideration as different methods may produce different results. In a study looking at psychotic-like experiences (PLEs), Laurens *et al.* (2007) found that 63.4% of boys and 53.5% of girls reported experiencing at least one PLE. Previous studies, such as Poulton *et al.* (2000), reported much lower rates of similar experiences (14.7%). In line with earlier studies, Laurens *et al.* (2007) found that parents were less likely to report that their children were experiencing difficulties than the children themselves. Questionnaires may be more acceptable to some children. Assessment is easier face-to-face; however for young people in remote and rural areas, alternative methods may be required. Stain *et al.* (2008) found that telepsychiatry using video link interviews was reliable, and reviewed favourably by young people.

An assessment may take several sessions to complete and be carried out in different settings such as Child and Adolescent Mental Health Services, home, school or where the young person feels more comfortable. Helping the young person talk about, and make sense of their experiences may help engagement, and over time help the young person think about the future.

9.9 Interventions

As we have seen, there is growing evidence to suggest that intervention should begin as early as possible. However, there may be young people who are thought to be developing a psychosis but who are not. There is an argument that children we suspect to be in the prodromal phase should not be treated as if they were experiencing a psychosis. This should be balanced with the knowledge that some young people are particularly vulnerable to treatment being delayed, including young people who have learning disabilities, are homeless or have alcohol and substance misuse problems.

Early intervention is usually multifaceted, complex and may include individual therapy, family interventions, psychosocial interventions, psychoeducation, social skills training, work with the school or employer, antipsychotic treatment and reintegrating the young person back into their community. Joining with the young person to help them do the ordinary things that may have become extraordinarily difficult, such as going to the cinema, eating out, going to a leisure centre or keeping appointments, can be an important aspect of recovery.

Working alongside children and young people involves thinking about how the young person may be experiencing problems and reflecting on how you present yourself to them, listening to the young person's point of view and attempting to understand how psychosis uniquely affects them. Targeting help towards social problems and psychological distress is likely to be more welcome and assist engagement than focusing primarily on medication. Connecting with the young person is essential if any progress is to be made.

Most young people treated for psychosis will receive antipsychotic medication, so engaging young people will involve explanation of the need for and effects of such medication. Education about side effects and discussing how these might be reduced are strategies which may help engagement. Regular, careful reviewing and monitoring of effects and side effects is essential. Recent research suggests that children may be at a greater risk than adults of weight gain and prolactin elevation when prescribed antipsychotics (Fedorowicz and Fombonne 2005) as well as of cardiovascular side effects (McIntyre and Jerrell 2008). It has also been suggested that ethnicity may play a part in response to medication (Patel *et al.* 2006). In young people experiencing their first-episode, olanzapine may be tolerated for longer than typical antipsychotic medication (Lieberman *et al.* 2005, Johnsen and Jørgensen 2008).

9.10 Drug treatment

Antipsychotic medication is the most common intervention with children and young people who are experiencing a psychosis, and they are generally thought to be an effective treatment. The use of medication is based on the hypothesis that psychosis is caused by increased dopamine activity in the brain and that antipsychotics block dopamine receptors thereby reducing the influence of dopamine. It is also thought that too much glutamate may influence the dopamine system to become overactive. McKenna (2007) argues that 'schizophrenia' is a neurochemical disorder and that it would be surprising to find that dopamine is not implicated in some way. As McKenna (2007) outlines, drugs which are not dopamine antagonists have not been effective in reducing symptoms of 'schizophrenia'.

The prescription of antipsychotic medication is influenced by a number of factors, not least the country in which the young person is receiving treatment. In the USA, between 1.5 and 2.2 times more antipsychotic medication is prescribed than in Germany or the Netherlands (Zito *et al.* 2008). Olfson *et al.* (2006) reported a greater than fivefold increase in antipsychotic prescriptions from 1993 to 2002. Only 14.2% prescriptions in Olfson *et al.*'s (2006) study were for 'psychotic disorders'; the remaining prescriptions were for disruptive behaviour disorders (37.8%), mood disorders (31.8%), learning disabilities and pervasive developmental disabilities (17.3%).

 Activity

What are the benefits of being prescribed second-generation (atypical) medication compared with first-generation (typical) medication?

9.11   Effectiveness of medication

Most studies into the effectiveness of antipsychotic medication are with adults. Evidence from trials with children and young people is slowly emerging. Much has been made of the difference between first- (FGAs) and second-generation antipsychotics (SGAs), with early reports that SGAs were more effective, and had fewer side effects than FGAs. The view of the superiority of all SGAs has recently been challenged, with some studies showing patterns of greater improvement in symptoms and quality of life measures when taking FGAs compared to SGAs (Jones *et al.* 2006). An important consideration in Jones *et al.*'s study was that the second-generation drugs used did not include clozapine which has been proven to be a more effective SGA. Lieberman *et al.* (2005) reported little difference between the SGAs studied and perphenazine (an FGA introduced more than 40 years previously).

It has been argued that some SGAs are more effective than others. Leucht *et al.* (2009) analysed 150 randomised trials, and found that different 'SGAs' produced very different results. When SGAs were compared as a whole group to FGAs, they were more expensive, no more effective, and had a similar profile of side effects. The use of first-generation haloperidol (which in comparison to other FGAs is associated with a greater degree of adverse reactions) in these comparison studies meant that these were often biased in favour of second-generation drugs. Tyrer and Kendall (2009) concluded that the term 'SGAs' should be abandoned because the drugs as a group do not warrant the distinction.

Both FGAs and SGAs are effective at reducing symptoms such as hallucinations, delusions, thought disorder and ideas of reference in the short term in most people. Medication should be commenced on a low dose, with small increases made every few weeks. Polypharmacy should be avoided. A careful collaborative strategy makes it more likely the young person will continue with the medication. Where possible the choice of drug should be negotiated with the young person and their family, including a discussion about the merits and potential side effects of the proposed medication. McGorry (2006) argues that there should be a period of at least 48 hours where the young person is free from antipsychotic medication, and only benzodiazepines prescribed. This period allows time to carry out physical investigations, enhance the engagement process, help build a trusting relationship and explain treatment options. Following this period, antipsychotic medication should be introduced, with the aim of reducing the length and severity of this phase.

If medication is started too early, it may make a diagnosis more difficult. Once started, it usually takes several weeks to achieve a response and months for remission to occur. Increasing doses of antipsychotic beyond certain thresholds does not produce benefits – rather it increases the risk of side effects.

9.12 Side effects

Side effects and adverse events are common when taking antipsychotic medication; some young people can tolerate side effects, while others discontinue the medication. Some studies report adverse reactions of up to 68% (Alacqua *et al.* 2008). As many as 19% of young people may discontinue medication within 1 month of commencing treatment and approximately half experience adverse events. Discontinuation rates range from 19% to 59% (Rugino and Janvier 2005, Valicenti-McDermott and Demb 2006). Lieberman *et al.* (2005) examined the effectiveness of antipsychotic drugs with 1,493 people in 57 sites in the USA and found that 74% of adults discontinued their medication before 18 months; their reasons for discontinuing were inefficacy, intolerable side effects or other reasons. They found that olanzapine had the lowest discontinuation rates but was associated with greater weight gain.

A separate but relevant consideration is the long-term effects on children and young people of taking antipsychotic medication, an area rarely considered in research studies. Psychotropic medication has been found to have an effect beyond the period of taking the drug – a process called neural imprinting (Andersen and Navalta 2004). Neural imprinting is a particular issue for children and young people and is worthy of increased research focus.

Talking about difficult things

Helping young people manage what might be bewildering, new and unsettling experiences is important in their recovery. The importance of listening to someone who is distressed cannot be overstated. Even someone who appears to have difficulty paying attention, is experiencing thought disorder, pressure of speech or delusions, can benefit from another person being willing to take the time to listen and understand their experience – although it can be difficult to know what to say when listening to experiences which run counter to one's own, especially when these experiences are difficult to believe or understand.

Beliefs are opinions which we consider to be true; these beliefs might be forcibly challenged by alternative interpretations – yet we still hold these beliefs to be true. When these beliefs take on a major importance, and are outwith the cultural experience of the young person, they are called delusions. Delusions were once considered to be unshakeable beliefs; however this view is changing, and delusions are now considered to be on a spectrum, with delusions being amenable to change (Garety and Hemsley 1994). Coupland and Cuss (2007) argue that delusions can serve a protective purpose and counsel against challenging delusions unless they are distressing or have the potential to cause harm – putting the young person in contact with other young people coping with similar experiences can bring about change through effective group work.

It usually is not helpful to argue with young people that they are experiencing delusions; however, helping them consider alternative balanced views may help them to consider the impact of their beliefs. It is thought that delusional thinking might arise from trying to rationally explain something which seems unexplainable and may be a result of abnormalities in perception, while other explanations include the idea that people who experience delusions are likely to jump to conclusions. A CBT approach that helps the young person manage their distress by developing coping strategies, such as generating, considering and employing alternative views, may be helpful (Morrison *et al.* 2008).

 Activity

Consider something which you believe to be true which can be challenged by scientific evidence. Why do you think you still hold this opinion despite evidence to the contrary? How do you feel when you are challenged?

Romme (1998) demonstrated that it was not the hallucination per se that made life difficult for the voice hearer, it was how hallucinations were construed and managed. Not all people who hear voices are diagnosed as 'mentally ill', and Romme (1998) and Honig *et al.* (1998) reported 'non-patients' were more likely to report positive experiences with their voices, mainly because the content of what the voices said was positive. Patients' voices were more critical and frightening to the voice hearer.

A major consideration therefore in managing voices is how the voice is experienced and whether they are considered problematic. Other explanations for voices should be considered, and the context in which voices occur may be influential, e.g. it is very common to experience voices after the loss of a close relative. How and when the voices occur is relevant: are the voices worse when the young person is on their own? Or in crowded places? Or do they occur more often when there is an oncoming event?

A number of different strategies have proved successful in managing or minimising the effects of auditory hallucinations. Distraction techniques, such as reading aloud, talking with someone else, listening to the TV/radio, naming objects, listening to music through headphones, using ear plugs, humming a single note, may be helpful. Other techniques are related to taking control such as summarising what the voice is saying, self-monitoring, saying 'stop' or talking back to the voice. Peer relations are clearly important in adolescence: knowing someone else shares similar problems can be a comfort for young people; therefore groups can be helpful, whether they are psychoeducational, activity based or Hearing Voices groups such as those which build on the work of Romme and Escher (1993, 2000). The importance of putting people in touch with each other can help – unless such groups are arranged, a young person is unlikely to meet someone else who experiences similar problems. Putting young people in contact with others of a similar age who are coping with similar experiences can help reduce a sense of isolation. Newton *et al.* (2007) found groups to be a safe place to explore shared experiences which helped young people to manage their auditory hallucinations.

9.13 Talking therapies

Psychological therapies, including social skills training, cognitive approaches, family interventions and psychoeducation, are increasingly used in all stages of psychosis. The following section will outline some of these approaches. However, there is little evidence of such interventions being used with young people with learning disabilities, although there is slowly emerging evidence of CBT approaches being used with adults with mild to moderate learning disabilities. Brown and Marshall (2006) outline the need for a modified CBT approach to be employed with people with learning disabilities and for CBT training to be part of the development of registered nurses working with people who have learning disabilities.

Cognitive–behavioural therapy

There is growing evidence from adult studies that individual CBT helps people manage their psychosis (Rector and Beck 2002, Gumley *et al.* 2006, Farhall *et al.* 2007, Wykes *et al.* 2008) and NICE (2009) recommends CBT is used in the acute phase of intervention. Using CBT in groups is a more recent approach and has produced mixed results. Penn *et al.* (2009) compared group CBT with enhanced supportive therapy (ST), and found ST resulted in a greater reduction in negative beliefs about their voices at

1-year follow-up. Group CBT appeared to improve people's overall symptoms, but not the intensity of their voices, while ST showed improvement in people's ability to manage their auditory hallucinations. Drury *et al.* (2000) found people receiving group CBT recovered more quickly; however, apart from a reduction in delusional beliefs, initial gains were not maintained at 5-year follow-up.

There is evidence that CBT may help some young people with hallucinations when used with individuals, groups and families. Drury *et al.* (1996a, b) found that CBT helped young people to manage their distress, and consider alternative meanings for their beliefs. Wragg and Whitehead (2004) reported a single case study indicating there was some improvement in the young person's symptoms of psychosis, depression and anxiety but not in their self-esteem.

Personal therapy

Personal therapy (PT) is an individually tailored programme involving behavioural techniques such as modelling, rehearsal, practice, feedback and homework assignments (Hogarty 1995, 2002). It has been suggested that PT can slow down relapse and helps young people with psychosis to adjust.

Cognitive psychotherapy in early psychosis

Cognitive psychotherapy in early psychosis (COPE) is a specific approach which aims to help young people in their recovery from psychosis (Jackson *et al.* 2001). COPE lasts around 9–12 months, and consists of four components:

1. *Assessment and engagement*, which involves establishing an alliance, developing a contract and establishing a formulation.
2. *Adaptation*, which involves helping the young person understand the meaning of their experiences and promoting a sense of mastery over them.
3. *Managing secondary problems* which can occur with psychosis, such as post-traumatic stress disorder (PTSD), anxiety, panic attacks or substance misuse, which means identifying and challenging underlying cognitions, role-plays and teaching coping skills.
4. A *termination* phase where a relapse plan is developed.

Early studies of COPE found little advantage over treatment as usual in symptoms of psychosis and quality of life (Jackson *et al.* 2001); however, there was some evidence to suggest that COPE may help people integrate their experiences of psychosis. More recently, Jackson *et al.* (2005) found no significant advantage for COPE over routine care.

Systematic targeting of prolonged psychosis

Systematic treatment of persistent psychosis (STOPP) is a cognitive–behavioural based intervention for young people who have been experiencing psychosis for longer than 3 months. The intervention was developed by the Early Psychosis Prevention and Intervention Centre (EPPIC) and has been the subject of further research (Herrmann-Doig *et al.* 2002).

There are four phases in STOPP:

1. *Developing a collaborative working relationship*: which includes the development of a formulation to help the young person understand what is happening to them.
2. *Exploring and coping with psychosis*: developing ways of coping with the symptoms of psychosis.
3. *Strengthening the capacity to relate to others*: helping young people to stay in social contact with others and helping the young person manage their self-esteem.
4. *Finishing and moving on*: thinking about the future.

Cognitive therapy based to promote adjustment and recovery following a first episode of psychosis

Cognitive therapy based to promote adjustment and recovery following a first episode of psychosis (CARF) uses a modular approach to reduce the effect of emotional problems associated with psychosis such as depression, low self-esteem and trauma. CARF helps the reappraisal of the effects of loss, changed view of self and the sense of embarrassment/humiliation which can accompany psychosis, and has been reported as helpful in managing PTSD (Jackson and Birchwood 2006).

 Activity

Identify three components of talking therapies used for young people with early onset psychosis.

9.14 Promoting resilience, staying well and recovery

Numerous factors seem to promote recovery and prevent relapse. Having strong social supports is important; including a stable, safe and structured environment. A sense of purpose seems to help, as well as an ability to confide worries and experiences to someone else. Being able to understand what has happened and having realistic expectations of life lead to better coping. Physical well-being plays a part in mental well-being, so healthy eating, physical activity and addressing physical ill-health are important. The Gloucestershire Recovery in Sports team (GRIP) reports the successful use of exercise and sport for young people/young adults and carers (Adams *et al.* 2007).

Elevated stress levels, enduring positive and negative symptoms, depression, substance misuse and personal relationships that tend towards conflict may affect recovery. Being absent from school or work for longer than 2 years can make a return to employment/education difficult, and employment is known to have beneficial effects. In a small follow-up study, Reichert *et al.* (2008) found that most young people had been readmitted to hospital at least twice, and most were living at home or in supported accommodation, and were either unemployed or in supported employment.

How people manage their experiences of psychosis may affect recovery, so whether people 'seal over' or 'integrate' their experiences may influence recovery (Mcglashan *et al.* 1975). People who *seal over* manage their experiences by avoidance, or develop strategies to help them forget or see the experience as separate from themselves. People who *integrate* try to make sense of their experience as part of themselves and are thought to be more likely to seek understanding of, and support with their experiences (Jackson and Birchwood 2006).

After initial treatment, symptoms may subside fairly rapidly with medication, the speed may be confusing for family members. Deciding when to reintegrate into school, work or social life is complex; for some young people a prompt return is helpful, while this approach may precipitate a further episode of psychosis in others. However, a stepped approach is helpful to most people. Young people may benefit from ongoing cognitive, psychotherapeutic and skills-based therapies in a supportive environment. Affirmation cards which are positive and affirming reminders of the goodness and strength of people can be helpful to some people, particularity if a picture or photograph is included on the card (Coupland and Cuss 2007). Affirmation cards include statements such as 'I am a valued person' and 'I am unique and creative'.

Around 80–90% of people recover within 1 year; however, up to 80% may relapse within 5 years (Barnes and Drake 2007). The risk of relapse is much higher if medication is discontinued; although young people can remain well after discontinuing medication (Chen *et al.* 2008), it is recommended that young people continue to take medication for at least

6–12 months (Coghill *et al.* 2009) and when discontinuation is considered the withdrawal should be over months.

9.15 Involving the family

Families/carers are an important resource for young people in all stages of psychosis. There is sometimes a difficult balance to maintain between involving the family and respecting confidentiality. Most young people experiencing a first episode of psychosis will be living at home. Even if they are living away from home, it is likely that they will have left recently, so family/carer involvement may still be relevant. The family or unit the child is living in is important because of the perceived influence of high expressed emotion (EE). EEs are negative communications which are angry, critical or over-involved. Hahlweg *et al.* (1989) found whether someone was in a high EE household was a more important predictor of relapse than taking medication. However, Asarnow and Asarnow (1994) argue that there is no indication that high EE occurs with early onset psychosis. Butzlaff and Hooley (1988) reports the strongest relationship for the influence of high EE is with people with an enduring illness and the effects are worse for eating disorders and mood disorders than for psychosis. Whatever the benefits of avoiding high EE environments, involvement of the family or carer is important. Families can provide valuable support and assist the young person in making sense of their experiences. The needs of the family who are experiencing first-episode psychosis need to be carefully considered and addressed.

Families and carers may feel marginalised by services. Developing strategies which encourage family/carer involvement in decision making alongside their relative can reduce the sense of marginalisation. There are a number of interventions aimed at supporting familes where a child is experiencing a psychosis, of which two examples will be discussed. Most family interventions focus on managing emotions, education about psychosis and problem-solving. There are families where explaining the intervention is enough, families where psychoeducation about psychosis is needed and families where something change needs to be addressed if the young person is to be supported to remain at home and for recovery to be promoted. However, despite evidence that family interventions are helpful they are not always routinely used in early intervention (Fadden 1997, 2006, Brent and Giuliano 2007).

Family intervention is an approach which includes psychoeducation and CBT (Midence 2006) and has evidence to support its effectiveness

(Pitschel-Waltz *et al.* 2001, Pharoah *et al.* 2003). It is important from the outset that families are informed that interventions are there to support both the young person and the family. Families are likely to feel open to criticism or blame and this should be addressed by clear explanations of the purpose of family involvement. The emotional climate in which the child is living has an effect on their recovery, but this does not mean that the family are to blame rather they may have to make adjustments to managing what is often a new challenge. Psychoeducation plays an important part in this, as offering explanations for changes in young people's behaviour can help the family adapt and make changes to support the young person.

Behavioural family therapy (BFT) is an established intervention which focuses on providing information to families, establishing early signs/relapse prevention, education about psychosis and developing communication skills (Falloon *et al.* 1996, Campbell 2004). The primary aim of BFT is to reduce the rate of relapse by improving communication and problem-solving. Families are observed in the process of problem solving and feedback given through the use of video-taped sessions. Experiences of psychosis are normalised and explanations are explored which avoid the use of jargon. Two goals of therapy are obtained from each family member aged 8 years and older. Expressing feeling and making requests can be difficult when a family member is experiencing a psychosis; therefore, there is a focus on expressing pleasant and unpleasant feelings, and making positive and negative requests. BFT uses a problem-solving approach, with structured family meetings, using a chairperson and secretary from the family, who through negotiation develop a list of things to do. There are 12–20 sessions with booster sessions at later dates.

Askey *et al.* (2007) reviewed studies of family interventions for first-episode psychosis and made a number of recommendations: That early intervention teams should have a family focus which is engaging, inclusive, optimistic and have a positive outlook. Psychoeducation should be appealing to young people and be jargon free. How families view their role and how they perceive psychosis will affect how they engage with service and understand what is happening; services should keep this in mind and acknowledge the sense of isolation and loss families may feel. Interventions should have a problem-solving focus and be offered when requested by families. These recommendations provide a framework for the development of developmentally appropriate services designed to meet the needs of children, young people and their families.

Activity

Think about the importance of early intervention work with families – identify three goals of early intervention for families.

9.16 Conclusion

Early onset psychosis presents a major challenge to the psychological and emotional development of children and young people. Similar challenges are faced by services in providing age appropriate and timely interventions which continue to be innovative and of high quality. Young people may experience only one episode of psychosis and face no further challenges. However, some young people will experience enduring problems and need to be supported by family, friends and specialist services. Being able to recognise when relapse is a possibility is key to its prevention – this would help us to think about how young people can be supported and the effects of relapse be minimised. A similar focus needs to remain on early intervention and early prevention.

Services for young people have improved considerably over the last few decades. For improvement to be maintained in the present economic climate, evidence will have to be gathered and alliances built to defend these important services, which appear vulnerable, probably because they are at the boundary between young people and adult services. The WHO and the International Early Psychosis Association developed a consensus statement with a 5-year programme of action which sets out to improve access and engagement, raise community awareness, promote recovery, family engagement and the training of practitioners (Bertolote and McGorry 2005). The values which underpin this consensus statement are respect for the abilities and qualities of all involved, recovery, partnership, participation, cost-effective interventions and the involvement of family and friends – values which should be used as a framework for thinking about how to work alongside children/young people and their families.

Recommended reading

Adams, S., Bishop, L. and Bellinger, J. (2007). Recovery through sport in first episode psychosis. In: Velleman, R., Davis, E., Smith, G. and Drage, M. (eds). *Changing Outcome in Psychosis Collaborative Cases from Practitioners, Users and Carers.* Oxford: BPS Blackwell.

Andersen, S. L. and Navalta, C. P. (2004). Altering the course of neurodevelopment: a framework for understanding the enduring effects of psychotropic drugs. *Journal of Developmental Neuroscience* 22, 423–440.

Askey, R., Gamble, C. and Gray, R. (2007). Family work in first-onset psychosis: a literature review. *Journal of Psychiatric and Mental Health Nursing* 14, 356–365.

Bertolote, J. and McGorry, P. (2005). Early intervention and recovery for young people with early psychosis: consensus statement. *British Journal of Psychiatry* 187 (Suppl. 48), 116–119.

Boeing, L., Murray, V., Pelosi, A., McCabe, R., Blackwood, D. and Wrate, R. (2007). Adolescent onset psychosis: prevalence, needs and service provision. *British Journal of Psychiatry* 190, 18–26.

de Koning, M. B., Bloemen, O. J. N., van Amelsvoort, T. A. M. J., Becker, H. E., Nieman, D. H., van der Gaag, M. and Linszen, D. H. (2009). Early intervention in patients at ultra high risk of psychosis: benefits and risks. *Acta Psychiatrica Scandinavica* 119, 426–442.

Emerson, E. and Hatton, C. (2007). Mental health of children and adolescents with intellectual disabilities in Britain. *British Journal of Psychiatry* 191, 493–499.

Jackson, H. and Birchwood, M. (2006). Trauma and first episode psychosis. In: Larkin, W. and Morrison, A. P. (eds). *Trauma and Psychosis: New Directions for Theory and Therapy*. London: Routledge.

Kelleher, I., Harley, M., Lynch, F., Arseneault, L., Fitzpatrick, C. and Cannon, M. (2008). Associations between childhood trauma, bullying and psychotic symptoms among a school-based adolescent sample. *British Journal of Psychiatry* 193 (5), 378–382.

Laurens, K. R., Hodgins, S., Maughan, B., Murray, R. M., Rutter, M. L. and Taylor, E. A. (2007). Community screening for psychotic-like experiences and other putative antecedents of schizophrenia in children aged 9–12 years. *Schizophrenia Research* 90, 130–146.

McGorry, P. D., Killackey, E. and Yung, A. (2008). Early intervention in psychosis: concepts, evidence and future directions. *World Psychiatry* 7, 148–156.

Newton, E., Larkin, M., Melhuish, R. and Wykes, T. (2007). More than just a place to talk: young people's experiences of group psychological therapy as an early intervention for auditory hallucinations. *Psychology and Psychotherapy: Theory, Research and Practice* 80, 127–149.

Read, J., van Os, J., Morrison, A. P. and Ross, C. A. (2005). Childhood trauma, psychosis and schizophrenia: a literature review with theoretical and clinical implications. *Acta Psychiatrica Scandinavica* 112, 330–350.

Romme, R. and Morrison, M. (2007). The harmful concept of schizophrenia. *Mental Health Nursing* 27 (2), 7–11.

Tiffin, P. A. (2007). Managing psychotic illness in young people: a practical overview. *Child and Adolescent Mental Health* 12 (4), 173–186.

Websites

Rethink – A campaigning organisation for better treatment of people with psychosis:

http://www.rethink.org/

The Early Psychosis Prevention and Intervention Centre:
http://www.eppic.org.au/

The Sign Guidelines on Psychosocial Interventions:
http://www.sign.ac.uk/guidelines/fulltext/30/index.html

TIPS an early intervention in psychosis project supported by a number of different countries:
http://www.tips-info.com/eng/

Psychosis Sucks – a Canadian website managed by Fraser Health Authority which has information for young people and families:
http://www.psychosissucks.ca/epi/index.cfm?action=links

Asylum: an international magazine for democratic psychiatry, psychology, education and community development incorporating the newsletter of psychology politics resistance (PPR):
http://www.asylumonline.net/

Chapter 10

ADHD

Lorna Jones[1] and Anne Claveirole[2]

[1] ADHD Team, NHS Lothian Child and Adolescent Mental Health Services, Edinburgh, Scotland
[2] School of Nursing, Midwifery and Social Care, Edinburgh Napier University, Edinburgh, Scotland

10.1 Introduction

Attention deficit hyperactivity disorder (ADHD) has been the subject of considerable controversy and debate since the 1970s. The debates have centred on the causative factors of ADHD and the use of stimulant medication as treatment, particularly on a long-term basis, but the very existence of this diagnostic category has also been questioned.

In this chapter, we will reflect on the experience of young people, their families and schools, review the pros and cons of ADHD as a diagnostic category, and analyse its prevalence, risk and resilience factors before discussing its assessment and common interventions. You are encouraged to read about the current debates because they are often raised by families, teachers and professional colleagues.

> **Learning outcomes**
>
> After studying this chapter, you should be able to:
>
> 1. Empathise with the experience children, families and schools have of ADHD.
> 2. Understand the scientific foundation of the diagnostic category called ADHD and the debates that surround it.
> 3. Identify the symptoms associated with ADHD in children and young people.

Understanding Children and Young People's Mental Health, first edition. Edited by Anne Claveirole and Martin Gaughan. Published 2011 by John Wiley & Sons Ltd. © 2011 John Wiley & Sons Ltd.

4. Discuss the complex interplay of genetic and environmental factors contributing to ADHD and its outcomes.
5. Carry out and formulate the systematic assessment of a child/family with suspected ADHD under supervision.
6. Demonstrate understanding of the arguments for and against the use of stimulant medication in the treatment of ADHD.
7. Plan appropriate interventions for a child diagnosed with ADHD at home, school and elsewhere, in partnership with those involved with the family's care.

10.2 What is ADHD?

The term ADHD covers three types of behaviours observed in children: *impulsivity*, which means acting too quickly and without thinking; *hyperactivity*, meaning constant and restless moving and *inattention*, which is the inability to focus one's attention on anything for long. These behaviours are often – but not always – associated in the same child, each to a different extent. Efforts to link this cluster of behaviours to a biological cause have not yielded sufficient results to indicate a physiological illness; therefore the disorder, like many other diagnostic categories, is only defined at a behavioural level (NCCMH 2009). Importantly, ADHD symptoms are not pathological per se, they refer to behaviour traits that are spread across the population in a continuum from none to severe; they do not constitute a qualitatively different category of human experience (Haslam *et al.* 2006, Sonuga-Barke 2006).

10.3 The experience of ADHD

ADHD is a frustrating condition for everyone involved. This is especially true for the child experiencing it. Studies have shown that children and young people with ADHD have a poor quality of life.

Children and young people with ADHD giving evidence for the national clinical practice guideline (NCCMH 2009) said they felt different from other children. Receiving a diagnosis made it easier to identify help for them but they felt stigmatised to need treatment for their behaviour (Kendall *et al.* 2003). Young people can feel that they are always in trouble and no one understands them. They struggle to understand themselves: to figure out why they repeat the same behaviour again and again, despite knowing it is wrong and being punished for it. They begin to believe they are 'bad' children. Some also think they are stupid for not being able to comprehend why they are so forgetful or why they cannot focus and learn in the same way as other children. Young people encountered in clinical practice have described their experience as having a head full of bees or living in a fog. They can become angry and depressed because they feel they are told off for things over which they have little control. In contrast, others love the energy, the 'get up and go' they have – the adrenaline rush that goes with having no fear. However, energy, impulsiveness and adrenaline bursts often lead to them being socially excluded. They find it hard to make friends and to keep them (Green *et al.* 2005). Routine and a stable environment help them manage, as do close friendships and continuity in therapeutic relationships (NCCMH 2009).

Parents describe living with a child who has ADHD as being like living with a tornado. They have little time for themselves or for their other children and they have to pick up the pieces left by their whirlwind child. They endure a variety of emotions, from frustration, worry and embarrassment to fierce protectiveness. They are frequently judged by others, including their partners and other family members. They often feel at a loss about what to do next because nothing seems to work. Families welcome support from agencies like health centres, schools and social services because medication is not enough (Steer 2005).

Teachers are faced with having to manage a child who performs best in a one-to-one situation, among a class of 25–30 children. The child's behaviour can include not staying in his seat, shouting out or interrupting; to complete any work, this child requires an adult by his side (Harpin 2005) (boys with ADHD outnumber girls by 3:1 or 4:1).

/ **Activity**

The following activities may help you to understand what it is like to have ADHD.

Think about the impact the following may have on thoughts, feelings and ability to carry out the task at hand and discuss it with a partner:

1. Sit in a room with one or more televisions on, each displaying a different channel; put the radio on loudly in the background. Try to focus on what another person in the room is saying to you or try to complete a task such as reading a book.
2. Try to remember an impulsive thing you once did or said and its impact on you, others and what you were supposed to be doing.
3. For many children with ADHD, movement aids concentration. Try to focus on a conversation or television programme whilst trying not to blink. Do this for at least 1 minute.

> 4. We all have times when we find it difficult to concentrate or do something impulsive. Children and young people with ADHD experience this many times a day.
> 5. Discuss how ADHD might impact on self-esteem, functioning and relationships with others over the longer term.

10.4 ADHD as a diagnostic category

This is an area which has caused fierce controversy: some specialists claim that ADHD is a neuro-developmental disorder of genetic origin, the existence of which is as valid and reliable as the link between smoking and cancer (Barkley and 78 Co-endorsers 2002); others insist that no demonstrable physical disability has yet been identified (Timimi and 33 Co-endorsers 2004). Experts continue to disagree but the comprehensive evidence gathered on behalf of NICE and published in 2009 suggests that it is not robust enough to describe ADHD as a neuro-developmental disorder of genetic origin (NCCMH 2009).

Most diagnostic categories for mental disorders are social constructions which lack an evidence base for biological markers. Such social constructs help clinicians to differentiate between normal and abnormal behaviours in groups of people and to seek scientific understanding (Sonuga-Barke 1998, 2006). This is the case for ADHD which fits within a continuous range of behaviours where it represents the extreme of normal variations rather than a distinct category (Haslam *et al.* 2006).

ADHD is a diagnosis taken from the American Psychiatric Association's diagnostic manual (text revised) - DSM-IV-TR - (2000) which has two subcategories: ADHD-I (inattentive) and ADHD-H (hyperactive–impulsive). ADHD (combined type) includes both types. Symptoms must have been present for 6 months before age 7, be inconsistent with expected developmental level, maladaptive and cause problems across two or more settings (NCCMH 2009). ICD-10, the WHO diagnostic manual (1992), lists hyperkinetic disorders of childhood. They are based on more stringent criteria and all three types of behaviours must be present. Therefore it describes a more severe subgroup than the DSM-IV-TR combined type. European guidelines for diagnosing hyperkinetic disorders were updated in 2004 (Taylor *et al.* 2004).

Some children are more seriously affected than others, but a child's impulsivity, inattention and hyperactivity also interact in a unique way with internal variables like the child's personality, academic ability and social skills, and external variables such as the family, school, peers, health services or socio-economic circumstances. Other mental health difficulties are often associated with ADHD.

The behaviours which constitute ADHD being on a continuum, there is no objective way of deciding where they cease to be normal, so that a line has to be drawn arbitrarily (Coghill 2006). However, clinicians are guided by a careful examination of each individual case and an important consideration is the degree of impairment ADHD behaviours cause to the child's daily activities. There are cultural differences in the extent to which inattention, hyperactivity and impulsivity are felt to be a problem. Inattention on its own is often overlooked because it is less disruptive to the environment than hyperactivity, even though it can be as much of an impairment to the child's own well-being as hyperactivity would be. The tolerance of the adults who surround the child plays a part in the referral picture; some children who show all the symptoms of ADHD may never be referred.

ADHD has a negative impact on a child's interpersonal, social and academic performance, on the family and the school and consequently, on the child's self-esteem. In spite of the blurred and somewhat arbitrary boundaries of this diagnostic category, it is useful because it provides a starting point to intervene in the lives of people whose behaviour causes serious psychosocial difficulties (Coghill 2006). It is also a starting point for genetic, neurological and sociological research. The outcomes of undiagnosed and untreated ADHD include a propensity to serious accidents, educational and work under-achievement, damage to family life and relationships (conflict, divorce, low productivity and isolation), increased risk of substance misuse and criminal activities, and a poor quality of life.

10.5 Prevalence

ADHD is a worldwide phenomenon but cultural differences in the way it is defined and symptoms are measured mean that the international prevalence figures vary widely across studies, from 20% to 1%. This is unlikely to reflect the true picture of childhood ADHD and is more likely to be due to variations in the way the statistics have been obtained (NCCMH 2009). Polanczyk et al. (2007) put it to around 5%. Because of the more stringent criteria, a diagnosis of hyperkinetic disorder (ICD-10) is less common. ADHD is seen in all social classes and ethnic groups, but unevenly so (see Section 10.8). There is no clear evidence that it is increasing (Buitelaar and Rothenberger 2004, Collishaw et al. 2004, Green et al. 2005).

Boys outnumber girls by a ratio of 4:1 (SIGN 2001). In their study of the prevalence of DSM-IV disorders, Ford et al. (2003) found that nearly 4% of boys and under 1% of girls between the ages of 5 and 15 had ADHD in the UK. In North America the figures are higher.

10.6   Risk factors

The causes of ADHD are poorly understood and remain an area of controversy. The dominant consensus in European health care is that ADHD is a heterogeneous disorder which results from a complex interplay of genetic and environmental factors (Taylor *et al.* 2004, NCCMH 2009); more research is needed to understand how this interplay works. Environmental influences play an important part; they can be biological, often in interaction with the genetic input, psychosocial and cultural. None of the risk factors associated with ADHD are either necessary or sufficient to cause it but each contributes to the overall risk. Different clusters of risk factors may lead to different sub-types (NCCMH 2009).

Genetic factors

Genes seem to influence the formation of ADHD behaviours not only in clinical subgroups but across the whole population. A systematic review of 20 twin studies suggests that ADHD behaviours have a heritability of 60–90% (Faraone *et al.* 2005). This compares with autistic spectrum disorders which have a heritability of 90%, the highest of the multi-factorial mental disorders of childhood (Rutter 2005). High heritability does not rule out environmental contributions, particularly gene–environment interaction (Durston *et al.* 2006). Several genes are likely to be involved, each adding to the chances of developing ADHD.

Environmental factors of biological origin

Neurobiology

A diagnosis of ADHD does not necessarily imply a neurological abnormality (NCCMH 2009). However, a lot of research has focused on the neurological basis of ADHD and a picture is emerging of the different brain sections involved, each playing a small part. MRI and PET technologies have made it possible to study the brain structure and functioning of children with ADHD and to compare it with control groups (Arnsten 2006). Findings suggest that the neurotransmitters dopamine and noradrenaline under-stimulate certain parts of the brain, namely the pre-frontal and parietal cortex, the basal ganglia and the cerebellum. Under-stimulation caused by ineffective neurotransmission may lead to poor regulation of the behaviour these centres control. Stimulant medication would then increase the concentration of dopamine and noradrenaline and partially redress the situation. There is some evidence to suggest that different types of ADHD may involve different parts of the brain (Casey *et al.* 2007).

Neuropsychology

Children with ADHD show problematic cognitive behaviours: they are distractible, they appear forgetful and they are organisationally deficient. Distractibility can be described as being unable to prioritise the information received from the environment. Children without ADHD can filter out background noise (such as someone mowing the grass outside a classroom) because it is irrelevant to the task in hand, whereas children with ADHD find it difficult to tune out unimportant information. Therefore their attention is solicited in several directions at once and their focus is constantly shifting.

Children with ADHD also appear to be unable to remember information for long. This leads to organisational problems. Linked to this are difficulties with sequencing events: either to remember what came first earlier or to anticipate what will happen next. Difficulties with sequencing ahead can lead to doing things without thinking of the consequences.

Overall, children who have ADHD appear to have deficits in higher-order cognitive skills called the executive function which includes the ability to plan, organise and problem-solve, reflect, self-monitor, time-manage and prioritise (Brown 2005, Goldberg *et al.* 2005).

Cognitive functions which control and regulate behaviour, such as those just described, have been the object of neuropsychological studies in the hope of tracing them back to defective neural mechanisms (Barkley 1997, Sergeant *et al.* 2002). How to interpret the results of these cognitive-experimental studies, however, remains controversial (NCCMH 2009).

Pre- and perinatal factors

ADHD can be associated with low birthweight and complications during pregnancy or birth. There is also evidence of a link between ADHD and maternal smoking, as well as misuse of drugs and alcohol during pregnancy. These activities are thought to alter the brain chemistry of the foetus (Milberger *et al.* 1997, Thapar *et al.* 2003).

Trauma and illness

ADHD can also be associated with physical trauma to the brain and nervous system in infancy, e.g. lack of oxygen, head injury, febrile convulsions and severe viral infections such as meningitis (Milberger *et al.* 1997).

Diet

The role of diet in ADHD, particularly that of additives, preservatives and e numbers which may cause hyperactivity or increase it in children who have ADHD, is the subject of much debate. Some parents take the initiative of applying dietary restrictions to their children. There is some evidence of a link between artificial food colourings and preservatives and hyperactivity in the general population (Bateman *et al.* 2004). A recent study also found a link between food additives and levels of ADHD behaviours in children, significant in some cases (McCann *et al.* 2007). There was no indication, however, that these effects were long term.

The other much discussed aspect of diet centres around fatty acids deficiency, particularly the omega-3 and -6 (Richardson and Puri 2000). The brain needs fatty acids and a sufficient supply is often lacking. Testosterone may impair uptake of fatty acids in boys (Richardson 2004). Further research is necessary.

Diet may play a part in the management of ADHD: this will be discussed again later. However, changing a child's diet does not seem completely to eradicate symptoms of ADHD in the majority of cases.

Toxicity

Lead and other heavy metal toxicity has been thought to cause symptoms of ADHD but this has not been confirmed.

Environmental factors of psychosocial origin

Psychosocial factors can be the sole or main cause of ADHD (NCCMH 2009). Children reared in Romanian orphanages for at least 6 months before being adopted in Britain were shown to develop ADHD-like behaviours and impairments (Stevens *et al.* 2008). A substantial minority of these children seemed to have suffered some form of deprivation-related neural damage (Rutter and O'Connor 2004).

Although ADHD is found in all social classes and ethnic groups, it is not spread equally across them; socio-economic deprivation, abuse and neglect are associated with higher levels of ADHD (Famularo *et al.* 1992, McLeer *et al.* 1994), as are parental conflict and parental mental health problems (Biederman *et al.* 2006). It does not appear to be spread equally among ethnic groups either: analysis of the 2004 census data in Great Britain found that the prevalence of hyperkinetic disorders was low among all non-white groups. This was also found in the 1999 census data and has been observed in clinical practice (Green *et al.* 2005). We do not know how to explain it.

Rutter *et al.* (1975) showed that it is the accumulation of risk factors (e.g. socio-economic adversity *and* parental mental ill health *and* institutional upbringing) rather one risk factor on its own which affects children's development and the advent of mental health problems (see Chapter 1). Biederman *et al.* (2006) used Rutter's adversity indicators to demonstrate that, in this respect, ADHD is no different from other mental health problems.

ADHD behaviours and negative parenting styles also act as mutually reinforcing feedback mechanisms: the impulsive, hyperactive behaviour of children with ADHD make positive and consistent parenting difficult, but conversely, parents' lack of consistency and family conflicts have an impact on children's behavioural control (Bauermeister *et al.* 2005). This is why parent training and support plays an important part in the management of ADHD.

Environmental factors: the role of culture

Some controversies related to the ADHD diagnostic category have already been raised. Sociological science has been the main critic of the concept of ADHD as a psychiatric disorder: a sociological analysis of the concept of ADHD looks at it as a social construct rather than a biological one (Timimi 2005, Lloyd *et al.* 2006, Gray 2008). Some aspects of this critique are mentioned here because it is necessary to keep reflecting critically on health care policy and practice.

In a culture like ours where health is highly valued, the medical paradigm can be understood as a powerful way of making sense of people's behaviour, particularly when diagnostic categories lack biological markers to identify disease (Lloyd *et al.* 2006). However, giving medical labels to children's difficult behaviours has some drawbacks. Being identified as having ADHD labels a child as different and makes him vulnerable to exclusion from his peer group. Children and young people reporting their experience of having ADHD have described this as a problem for them (NCCMH 2009).

The most radical critique suggests that ADHD is a collective rather than an individual problem; it sees in ADHD a cultural symptom: a sign that all is not well in modern Western culture. According to this perspective, vulnerable children display cultural distress in the form of ADHD behaviours. Changes in the culture are necessary if children with ADHD are to be helped. Individual management of ADHD only victimises the child further without attending to the causes of the problem (Armstrong 2006).

The cultural component of ADHD diagnostic and treatment practices must explain why they are so varied across and within countries. This can be judged from (1) the huge variations between countries in the consumption of methylphenidate (for which data is reliably collected by the United Nations International Narcotics Control Board and Inter-continental Marketing Services (IMS) Health and (2) the five- to sevenfold increase in prescription between 1999 and 2003 worldwide (twofold in England between 1998 and 2004, according to NICE, 2006). The reason for these variations is not known, but it suggests that diagnostic and treat-ment trends are heavily influenced by social and cultural factors. Under-standing national differences in approaches to ADHD as well as practitioners and prescribers' thinking would be helpful (Singh and Rose 2006). Unless we develop a more objective construct of ADHD, we run the risk of attributing to children the consequences of social situations and cultural forces (Singh and Rose 2006).

10.7 Resilience: factors affecting outcome

Good outcomes and the success of a treatment programme will be enhanced by personal, family and environmental factors (Carr 2006). Good physical health, moderate levels of ADHD behaviours, supportive parents, low family stress other than ADHD, good relationships with peers and a positive school experience all go to contribute to better outcomes. Those who are most successful at managing ADHD have developed positive coping strategies to help them with day-to-day life. Children and families who understand ADHD and see it as a challenge to overcome rather than a disability or an embarrassment tend to embrace strategies more readily.

Poor outcomes are more likely when ADHD behaviours are severe, oppositional defiant and antisocial behaviours have developed, anxiety and depression, other family difficulties and social disadvantage are present, and the family and health care support is inconsistent (Coghill et al. 2006).

Children with ADHD often make friends easily but find it difficult to keep them they can be tempted to hang out with the wrong crowd because 'bad friends are better than no friends'; thus they risk exclusion from school and involvement with the criminal justice system. Because of their impulsive and overactive behaviours, children and young people with ADHD are more prone to accidents. They are also at risk of being victims of crime due to their poor awareness of danger and their lack of impulse control.

Do children grow out of ADHD? The condition was thought to be a dis-order of childhood which did not exist in the adult population. We now know that it is not the case, although ADHD symptoms seem to decline with time (Harpin 2005). Faraone et al. (2006) found that 65% of the children affected carried some, if not all, of their symptoms into adulthood, although only 15% still met the full criteria by the time they reached the age of 25. There is a risk of later maladjustment, such as isolation, unemployment, a poor quality of life and secondary mental health difficulties (for instance anxiety and depression). Those who have been hyperactive and impulsive are more likely to develop an antisocial adjustment (NCCMH 2009).

10.8 Assessment

ADHD is a medical diagnostic category for use by the medical profession who has been trained to use it. However, no professional usually diagnoses ADHD on his/her own; it requires a multi-modal, multi-professional and multi-agency approach (NCCMH 2009). In a specialist clinic, the assessment may be lead by a psychiatrist, a paediatrician, a specialist nurse or a clinical psychologist. This part of the chapter focuses on the assessment of ADHD in an NHS context as recommended by national guidelines (NICE 2006, NCCMH 2009).

No biological or psychological test can confirm a diagnosis of ADHD. A diagnosis relies on observations and descriptions of the child or young person's behaviour. Standardised tools based on the diagnostic criteria can help but much of the assessment is based on carefully interviewing parents and teachers and observing the child.

Aims of assessment

The assessment aims to find:

- The extent and severity of the core ADHD behaviours
- The consistency of the ADHD behaviours across settings
- The origin and developmental course of the ADHD behaviours
- The presence and extent of associated problems, including other mental health disorders (co-morbidity)

Many children are referred to services for assessment because of their impulsive and overactive behaviour, but only a portion of them will have ADHD because young children in particular do not have words to talk about their experience, so that a change in their behaviour is all that can alert adults that all is not well. Therefore, an important task of the assessment is to differentiate between genuine ADHD and 'look-alike' problems like reaction to a life-event, anxiety, depression or autistic spectrum disorder (see Box 10.1). However, ADHD often overlaps with these other difficulties. It may not be possible to discriminate between one diagnosis and another in

Box 10.1 ADHD Look-Alike Problems

- Autism spectrum disorders
- Learning disability including specific learning difficulties
- Anxiety
- Depression
- Attachment difficulties
- Developmental delay
- Fine motor and/or co-ordination difficulties

a preschool child because a number of learning and developmental difficulties could explain the symptoms. In this case, the family may be offered support and advice on how to manage the child's behaviour and assessment be postponed until the child goes to school.

The inattentive sub-type of ADHD is less troublesome to parents and teachers than hyperactive and impulsive behaviour; therefore, it may not be noticed or referred. It has been suggested that girls may be more vulnerable to it than boys.

An assessment includes:

- An interview with the child or young person with their family
- An interview with the child or young person alone
- A medical assessment
- Collection of information from school and other relevant settings
- Rating scales
- Psychological and psychometric assessment

Interview with the child or young person with their family

This is usually the first stage of the assessment. It is good practice to have an interview plan so that all the important issues can be systematically explored. These are:

- The range of problem behaviours which have triggered the referral and their history (see Table 10.1)
- What has been tried to solve them
- The family and its social background
- The child's health and the family's health
- The child's development (see Table 10.1)
- The child's education and learning ability
- Parenting approaches

Table 10.1 Assessment Interview with the Child and Family: Questions to Address Regarding Child Development and Diagnostic Criteria

Child Development	Diagnostic Criteria
• Prenatal maternal health	• Quality of the child's concentration and concentration span, distractibility and daydreaming
• Physical and social influences during pregnancy such as substance misuse or stress	• Organisational skills and memory
• Maternal post-natal mental and physical health such as post-natal depression	• Ability to wait and take turns, interrupting
• Description of health during infancy and *developmental milestones* including information about sleep, appetite, hearing and vision	• Safety issues such as crossing the road, talking to strangers, wandering off, climbing, awareness of dangers
• Evidence of physical or emotional trauma	• Activity levels, ability to be quiet
	• School-based difficulties

■ Other difficulties, particularly look-alike conditions (see Box 10.1): this may be the object of the medical assessment (see below)

Parents can tell many stories about their child's problematic behaviours. It is important to search for exceptions to these statements too, and to find positive aspects of the child to discuss.

An assessment interview can take 2 or 3 hours: two sessions may be necessary. It is important also to see the child or young person separately; the parents too may welcome such an opportunity for themselves.

Interview with the child or young person alone

The aim of this is to obtain the child's perspective of their difficulties and to assess the child's insight. This interview can help to assess the child's comprehension, social skills and concentration span.

Medical assessment

If the main assessment interview is not carried out by a medical practitioner, a medical assessment needs to take place to:

■ rule out medical problems that may cause ADHD-like symptoms, such as a hearing impairment, epilepsy, thyroid dysfunction or iron deficiency anaemia

- identify physical signs of genetic conditions which increase the risk of ADHD
- diagnose co-existing physical, neurological and developmental disorders
- take a baseline of the child's physical measurements: height, weight, blood pressure and pulse
- eliminate cardiovascular problems before prescribing medication.

Information from school and other relevant settings

It is important to talk to people who know the child in settings other than the clinic because children with ADHD can sit and concentrate in intimidating new environments longer than in familiar settings. They are also more likely to struggle with mundane and repetitive tasks, and with tasks requiring perseverance. This is why observing the child at school in the classroom is useful. It also allows the assessor to note other difficulties such as writing, social skills, tics and anxiety. Reading annual school reports is useful: they provide evidence of the problems and their duration.

Information from other professionals or organisations (e.g. a speech and language therapist or the social services) involved with the child can help.

It is important to remember that the condition may present differently in adolescence. The most common difference is that overactive behaviour may be confined to fidgeting or an inner sense of restlessness.

Rating scales

Rating scales help to assess mental health, social and behavioural problems. Some assess these broadly, others are specific to ADHD. Regarding the latter, the Conners Rating Scales (Conners 1997) are commonly used in clinical practice. They are standardised questionnaires based on the DSM-IV criteria; there are three versions, one for teachers, one for parents and one for adolescents.

The advantage of standardised instruments is their potential for making comparisons with the general population and specific clinical groups. Their disadvantage is their limited inter-rater reliability. They are also less sensitive and specific in their assessment than the diagnostic interview; therefore, they can only be expected to contribute to the overall assessment (NCCMH 2009).

Examples of other commonly used rating scales can be found at www.adhd.net and the Brown Attention Deficit Disorder Scales at www .tpc-international.com.

Psychological and psychometric assessment

It is important to assess global and specific learning disabilities. Some specific learning difficulties (e.g. dyslexia) can contribute to a child's inability to concentrate. Global learning disabilities (below average IQ) need to be taken into account when planning intervention. A psychologist may assess other cognitive impairments affecting memory, attention and mental organisation. Observing the child during these tests gives further insight into concentration span, impulse control, activity levels and perseverance.

The role of occupational therapy

Occupational therapists can contribute to the diagnosis and treatment of ADHD difficulties regarding gross and fine motor skills (e.g. co-ordination and handwriting) which often affect children who have ADHD.

Children with ADHD can have sensory processing difficulties (tuning out of background noise for example) which can lead to fidgeting and poor concentration. The role of the occupational therapist in the assessment and treatment of ADHD is described in detail by Chu and Reynolds (2007a, b).

 Activity

Select a child or young person you have contact with in your professional role who has a diagnosis of ADHD. Consider the following:

What procedure was followed to diagnose this child? What are his/her prominent behaviours/symptoms?

What would this child say his/her problems are? What would the family say the child's problems are?

Are there difficulties present in addition to ADHD?

10.9 Interventions

The management of ADHD behaviours is another area of controversy, particularly the use of stimulant medication. In this section, a multi-modal approach is presented, in keeping with the latest guidelines for NHS interventions (NCCMH 2009). This includes educational, social, psychological and pharmacological dimensions. The aim of intervening is to improve the impairments caused by ADHD and to prevent the development of negative long-term outcomes.

Following a diagnosis of ADHD, it is helpful to appoint someone to manage the case and co-ordinate the care of the child. This health care professional will liaise with the family, other members of the treatment team and outside agencies, for instance the school.

Psychological interventions

Psychological interventions include a range of cognitive and behavioural approaches focused on the child and/or the parents. The most useful are based on social learning theory. They can be used to assemble a comprehensive package to address the problems associated with ADHD.

Psychological interventions take longer to work than medication: NCCMH (2009) estimates a minimum of 8–10 weeks if a therapy (such as cognitive–behaviour therapy (CBT), social skills training or parent training) is delivered every week, whereas optimum medication dosage can be adjusted in 6 weeks. This can discourage parents from trying them, together with the fact that there is often a waiting list for psychological treatment.

Overall, parents' ratings suggest that psychological interventions for children who have ADHD have moderately beneficial effects, both as an alternative to medication and as a complement (NCCMH 2009). As a treatment package, they are more expensive than medication alone.

Therapies based on social learning theory

CBT helps to understand the links between thoughts, feelings and behaviours and to change them for the better. Therapy can also focus on thoughts or feelings or behaviour alone. Behaviour modification techniques are particularly useful to target ADHD behaviours. They use rewards to change a child's behaviour and occasionally sanctions for dangerous or disruptive behaviour; timeout is also used to take a child away from social reinforcers which encourage undesirable behaviour (such as receiving too much attention). These techniques are recommended for school-age children and young people with moderate impairments (in combination with social skills training or on their own depending on the child's needs). An emphasis on cognitions is more useful for older children and adolescents than for young children. Cognitive approaches can be used in self-instruction manuals where they help a young person to develop a planned and systematic way of thinking ahead, reflecting back and planning.

Social skills training involves teaching social interaction skills: non-verbal skills can be practiced, such as posture, eye contact and smiling as well as focused social strategies like anger management and assertiveness skills.

All these therapies can be done in groups or individually. Older adolescents may prefer individual therapy.

Parent interventions

Parent training is also based on social learning theory. The main goal is to teach principles of child management to parents: how to make use of positive attention and good communication to enhance their relationship with their child and how to use behavioural modification techniques. It also addresses problems specific to particular parents, such as lack of confidence, low self-esteem, depression or isolation. Two well-known and evidence-based parent training programmes of this type are Matt Sanders' 'Triple P' (Positive Parenting Programme) from Australia (Hoath and Sanders 2002) and Carolyn Webster-Stratton's USA-based 'The Incredible Years' (Jones *et al*. 2007).

Psychoeducation: parents and families need information about ADHD, both in writing and in discussion with health care staff; they often feel that they cannot manage the child's difficulties and they need support to help them cope. Parent support groups can provide a focus for mutual support and for ongoing information sessions (Johnston and Mash 2001).

Parent training is the first line of treatment for preschool children. For schoolchildren with moderate impairment, parents can be offered parent training and/or psychoeducation.

Problem-solving approaches and family therapy may be used. Person-centred individual and group psychotherapy can help with low self-esteem, anxiety and depression.

Behaviour management at home and at school

Structure, consistency and routine are foundations for the behaviour management of all children. These principles are particularly important with a child who has ADHD to convey predictability and help him anticipate what is coming next. They apply at home and at school.

Children with ADHD often become accustomed to negative communication and punishment, which are ineffective in shaping their behaviour. Like most of us, they respond better to positive reinforcement and praise but behaviour modification techniques must be adapted to their needs. Children who have ADHD have difficulty learning from their mistakes spontaneously and they often repeat the same behaviour again and again, despite the consequences. To have an impact, rewards work best if they are immediate; they must also be short term so that they can be repeated as frequently as the behaviour requires. Grounding a child for a week will not prevent him from repeating the same behaviour within a short period of time. Encouraging the child to visualise a task, with positive reinforcement at each stage, can help him recall what needs to be done. Instructions are best broken up and given one or two at a time; they may need to be repeated many times.

Here are a few interventions which can be used to reduce the impact of ADHD behaviours and their associated difficulties. Interventions must be appropriate to the child and the situation. What works one day may not work the next: those working with children who have ADHD must be flexible and have a toolkit of strategies to use.

Classroom-based strategies

Children with ADHD have been shown to fall behind academically from primary school onwards, with inattention being particularly related to academic under-achievement (Merrell and Tymms 2005, NCCMH 2009).

NCCMH (2009) recommends more education about ADHD being made available to trainee teachers, as well as guidance about how to support children who have ADHD. They also recommend that health care professionals make contact with a child's nursery or school to explain the diagnosis and level of impairment, the care plan and the child's educational needs (provided the parents agree that this contact be made). Behavioural interventions should be provided to children and young people who have ADHD in the classroom by teachers who have been trained to do it.

Children with ADHD respond best to short-term realistic targets for their behaviour. Their day can be broken down into mornings and afternoons and positive incentives given accordingly. Visual aids are helpful such as a timetable. In secondary schools, support sheets kept by the student, where each teacher writes a comment on his behaviour at the end of a teaching session, can help a young person focus his efforts. Communication books between home and school help children manage their behaviour, but they must focus on positive as well as negative behaviour.

Simple strategies, such as placing the child near the teacher's desk and away from doors and windows, can reduce distractions and allow for closer monitoring of concentration. Breaking tasks down into manageable chunks, repeating instructions again and again, providing frequent prompting and refocusing the child on the task are necessary. A child may be more attentive to a visual and practical presentation.

A hyperactive child requires frequent breaks to move: some teachers send children on bogus errands to facilitate this. The use of fidget toys and doodle books for periods of listening can be useful.

Homework is often difficult for children and young people with ADHD and home–school liaison is paramount. Teachers who are flexible, supportive and imaginative make a difference. There are some excellent books for teachers regarding the management of ADHD in the classroom (see recommended resources).

Home-based/parenting strategies

Children with ADHD wear down the skills of the best of parents: it is important not to judge those who appear to struggle. Parents' behaviours, like those of their children, are shaped by positive and negative reinforcement. When a child with ADHD does not respond to parents' efforts to use positive parenting techniques, these parents may resort to increasingly punitive strategies or give up all together.

Parents are advised to prepare a toolkit of strategies to accommodate a variety of behaviours and occasions. For example, a trip to the cinema can be planned, from buying tickets in advance to prevent queuing, to going at the last minute to prevent sitting through adverts, and allowing breaks for movement by taking the child out or bringing fidget toys. Remaining calm and accepting that you may not be able to see the whole film also helps.

An emphasis on organisation from an early age is useful: teaching the child to write things down, to have a set place for keys, shoes and school bags and to use sticky notes as reminders of homework or appointments.

Children who have ADHD often have lots of energy; it is important to ensure that it is channelled in a positive way. Many are talented at sport and other activities but they require close supervision and need to be kept safe.

The stress of caring for a child with ADHD can have pronounced effects on family life and the parental relationship. Parents of children with ADHD often have a reduced quality of life and are highly stressed, leaving them susceptible to mental health difficulties. Encouraging parents to attend support groups to meet other parents and exchange stories and ideas can decrease their sense of isolation.

Pharmacological treatment

This section follows closely the NCCMH (2009) guideline for the NHS in the UK. See also Taylor and colleagues' update regarding the diagnosis and treatment of hyperkinetic disorder in Europe (Taylor *et al.* 2004).

Medication is not recommended as a first line of treatment for children and young people who have moderate ADHD impairments. It is best kept for those with severe ADHD behaviours and impairments, those with moderate ADHD who have refused non-pharmacological interventions and those for whom behaviour and cognitive interventions have not been

effective enough. There is good evidence that carefully monitored medication at the correct dose frees a child of the many frustrations which come
from having ADHD. However, the medications known to have a clinical
effect on ADHD seem to reduce symptoms and improve functioning only
for as long as they are present in the body. They do not cure ADHD
behaviours. And while these short-term positive effects are supported by
evidence, longer-term benefits are less clear and some research even suggests possible dangers (MTA Co-operative Group 2004, Timimi 2006).
Therefore, pharmacological treatment should always be part of a comprehensive package of interventions including psychological, educational and
behavioural dimensions.

Available medications

Methylphenidate and dexamfetamine are central nervous system stimulant class B schedule drugs to be prescribed under the supervision of a
specialist. They take effect within 20–60 minutes of the first dose and have
a therapeutic effect of short duration (approximately 4 hours for methylphenidate and 6 hours for dexamfetamine). To have a continuous effect
through the day, prescriptions need to be repeated two or three times,
although slow release preparations now exist (see Table 10.2).

More recently, a third drug, atomoxetine, has been licensed in the UK for
the treatment of ADHD. It is a selective noradrenaline reuptake inhibitor,
not a stimulant; therefore its prescribing and storage conditions are less
strict. It is taken in one or two doses through the day and must be taken
every day to be effective. A therapeutic benefit can take 6–12 weeks to
develop.

Methylphenidate and atomoxetine are the only medications for which
there is randomised controlled trial (RCT) evidence of clinical effectiveness in schoolchildren with ADHD, with methylphenidate being the
more effective of the two. No RCT demonstrates the effectiveness of dexamfetamine in children with ADHD, although a few lower-quality trials do.
It is a more potent stimulant that methylphenidate and is only recommended for hyperkinetic disorder (the most severe type of ADHD) when
other medications have been tried and failed.

Anti-psychotics are not recommended. There is no evidence of the
effectiveness of pharmacological treatment in preschool children.

Prescription and management of treatment

Medication should only be prescribed by a medical specialist with expertise and experience of ADHD, after a comprehensive assessment and

Table 10.2 Medications Commonly Used to Treat ADHD and Their Properties

Active Ingredient	Brand Names	Category	Duration of Therapeutic Effect	Frequency of Administration
Methylphenidate hydrochloride (licenced for children aged 6+)	Ritalin, Equasym, Medikinet	Immediate release neuro-stimulant	3–4 hours	2–3 times daily
Methylphenidate hydrochloride	Concerta XL	Long-acting neuro-stimulant	8–12 hours	Once daily (a.m.)
Methylphenidate hydrochloride	Equasym XL Medikinet XL	Long-acting neuro-stimulant	6–8 hours	Once daily (a.m.)
Dexamfetamine (licenced for children aged 3+)	Dexedrine	Immediate release neuro-stimulant	4–6 hours	2–3 times daily
Atomoxetine (licenced for children aged 6+)	Strattera	Selective nor-adrenaline reuptake inhibitor	24 hours	1–2 times daily

diagnosis. The choice of one medication rather than another is guided by several factors which the assessor has to weigh up. It is important to explain the medication to the child or young person, the parents and the school and to enlist their help to give ongoing feedback about which dose is the most effective at home and at school while the dose is being stabilised.

The advantage of short-term formulation stimulants is that they can be targeted precisely at times in the day when the child needs them most, e.g. at school, but not in the evenings or at weekends when psychological approaches may be enough. However, having to take a schedule drug at school during the day is potentially stigmatising for children and a big responsibility for schools, hence the advantage of slow release preparations.

When pharmacological treatment has been prescribed, it must be monitored carefully for side effects. Stimulants can cause sleeplessness (initial insomnia often settles but not always), irritability, rebound hyperactivity and loss of appetite; they can slow physical growth (MTA Co-operative Group 2004) and affect the cardiovascular system (Biederman et al. 2006, Nissen 2006, Winterstein et al. 2007). Routine monitoring includes recording blood pressure and pulse, height and weight and keeping a growth chart. A comprehensive list of side effects can be obtained from the current issue of the British National Formulary (BNF). If side effects reach a significant degree, the medication should be discontinued.

There are concerns regarding the effects on the developing brain, nervous and cardiovascular systems of long-term exposure to stimulant medication. Further high-quality research is urgently required in this field to obtain reliable evidence. In the meantime, treatment should be suspended periodically to assess the child's condition without medication (NICE 2006).

Limitations of pharmacological treatment

The use of psychostimulants remains controversial and there are concerns about prescribing such medication to children. (SIGN 2001: 1).

Given in the correct dose and taken orally as prescribed, stimulant medications have been shown to be relatively safe. It is nevertheless worrying to give neuro-stimulant medication to children, particularly young ones, because such psychotropic drugs have an impact on brain structure and function. Methylphenidate is not licensed for use in children younger than 6, but dexamfetamine, the stronger of the two, is licensed for children as young as 3 who have severe ADHD behaviours and impairments.

It is also important to remember that some children do not respond to medication, or have too mild a response for it to be therapeutic, and that some do not tolerate its side effects. Many children also have residual problems due to ADHD that medication does not improve, such as low self-esteem or poor interpersonal relationships. Finally, some professionals, parents and young people simply object to using psychotropic medications; in these cases, it may help to spend time explaining the advantages of a prescription but there is no point in persisting if it is not going to be adhered to. Therefore it is important to integrate medication into a multi-modal treatment approach.

Diet

Research regarding the effect of omega-3 and -6 supplements on ADHD behaviours is ongoing, but the evidence in favour of dietary supplements or against specific foodstuffs like artificial additives is not conclusive at present and a specific diet cannot be recommended (NCCMH 2009).

It is important that children and young people who have ADHD eat a balanced diet and drink enough fluids. As with all children, highly coloured and sweet food with refined sugars and artificial additives should be a small part of the diet. The effect of some foodstuffs is idiosyncratic, so that parents can be advised to exclude food which they think makes their child more overactive. The government recently produced guidance regarding food additives linked to hyperactivity and behavioural problems in children (Food Standard Agency, updated July 2010; see http://www .food.gov.uk/safereating/chemsafe/additivesbranch/colours/hyper/). In the vast majority of cases, excluding certain foods does not dramatically improve ADHD behaviours in the longer term.

 Activity

How do routines help you in your day-to-day life? What happens if there is an unexpected break to the routine? How do you feel? Does it impact on the task at hand?

Think about what happens to your routine when on holiday, how do you react to this? An example might be not being aware of what day it is.

10.10 Conclusion

ADHD is a mental health disorder characterised by three problematic behaviours: impulsivity, inattention and hyperactivity. In some children, inattention predominates; in others, hyperactivity while many suffer from a combination of both. The causes of ADHD are not fully understood; it is thought to be a disorder of heterogeneous origin, resulting from a complex interplay of genetic and environmental factors with biological, psychological and cultural components. It is a frustrating condition for the child, the family, the school and any other setting involved with the child because it impairs many of the child's normal and developmentally important experiences such as relationships, education, family life and ultimately self-esteem. ADHD needs to be carefully assessed by medical specialists in children and young people's mental health settings. The best treatment programmes are multi-modal and include a combination of psychological, behavioural and pharmacological management measures. Although it may improve with time, most children take their ADHD difficulties into adult life.

Case study

Jordan is an 8-year-old boy who has been referred to Child and Adolescent Mental Health Services by his general practitioner. The referral letter states that Jordan lives at home with his mother, Sue, aged 35. Jordan's father has minimal contact with him. Sue took Jordan to the doctor after the school reported that he was not finishing his work, was disruptive and did not seem to respond to consequences. He was up out of his seat a lot without permission and was getting into fights in the playground. The school thought Jordan was not achieving his academic potential. At home, Sue found it difficult to manage Jordan's behaviour and described being at the end of her tether with him.

Jordan has been allocated to you for an initial assessment appointment.

■ What information would you seek to obtain from Sue and Jordan at the appointment?
■ What might you expect to observe?

At the appointment, Sue tells you that Jordan has always been a difficult child. He 'ran before he could walk' and once he started talking he wouldn't stop. He won't do as he is told and punishments do not seem to work. Jordan was always in trouble at nursery for not listening to instructions and running away from teachers.

Jordan is described as having lots of energy. He fidgets even when he watches television. He has no road sense. Sue finds homework time particularly stressful and states that Jordan knows the answers but won't write anything down; when he does his writing is very messy. She feels he can't concentrate on activities for more than 5 or 10 minutes at a time. He is forgetful and frequently loses things. The developmental history details frequent ear infections as a toddler and Jordan broke his arm at age 3 when he fell off a wall. Sue feels that Jordan often engages in dangerous behaviours and doesn't think of the harm he could do to himself.

Jordan has a good appetite and sleeps well. He doesn't like certain textures against his skin and is described as very clumsy.

Jordan was described as being similar to his father who had a difficult time at school and has found it difficult to maintain employment as an adult due to his behaviour and poor time keeping. Sue and Jordan's father separated when Jordan was 2 years old.

Jordan states he likes school but the teacher picks on him and he gets into trouble for things he hasn't done. When asked about friends, he lists many but his mother states that he falls out with them regularly. He finds writing boring and likes to play football. He thinks he needs help being able not to talk in class. During the appointment, Jordan interrupts his mother frequently whilst she is talking and plays noisily in the corner.

- What symptoms are being displayed that would lead you to further assess Jordan for ADHD?
- What plans would you make with the family at this assessment appointment?
- Are there any other assessments you would like to be completed?
- Who else would you like to speak to about Jordan?

Once you have completed your assessment of Jordan, you discuss the case with a child and adolescent psychiatrist who confirms that Jordan fulfils the criteria for a diagnosis of ADHD.

- What support and interventions would you recommend for Jordan?
- How might you support Sue?

Recommended reading

Attwood, J. (2001). *Supporting Children with ADHD*. Questions Publishing Company.

Barkley, R. A. (2000). *Taking Charge of ADHD: The Complete Authoritative Guide for Parents*. New York: The Guilford Press.

Cooper, P. and Ideus, K. (1996). *Attention Deficit Disorder: A Practical Guide for Teachers*, 2nd edition. London: David Fulton Publishers.

Hartmann, T. (2000). *Thom Hartmann's Complete Guide to ADHD: Help for Your Family at Home, School and Work*. Nevada: Underwood Books.

Rogers, B. (2002). *Classroom Behaviour: A Practical Guide to Effective Teaching Behaviour Management and Colleague Support*, 2nd edition. UK: Paul Chapman Educational Publishing.

Shader, R. I. (2006). Facts and public policy: Should I keep my child on ADHD drugs? *Journal of Clinical Psychopharmacology* 26 (3), 223–226.

Smith, A., Shenton, O., and Rice, J. (1996). *Accelerated Learning in the Classroom*. Network Educational Press.

Chapter 11

AUTISTIC SPECTRUM DISORDERS

Gillian Marshall-McConnell[1] and Anne Claveirole[2]

[1] Scottish Society for Autism, Glasgow, Scotland
[2] School of Nursing, Midwifery and Social Care, Edinburgh Napier University, Edinburgh, Scotland

11.1 Introduction

This chapter aims to provide an insight into the complex world of autistic spectrum disorders (ASDs). As the number of people diagnosed with ASDs increases, you are likely to come across young people on the autistic spectrum. The chapter focuses on high functioning autism – autism without delay in language and cognitive development.

We will start by clarifying what the names used for this disorder mean and what the differences are between autism, ASD and Asperger's syndrome, and we will describe the core difficulties of children with ASDs. We will examine the changing profile of ASD incidence and its possible meaning. We will consider risk factors and possible causes, discuss the assessment process and the strategies involved in supporting children with ASDs and their families.

> **Learning outcomes**
>
> After studying this chapter, you should be able to:
>
> 1. Identify the differences between autism, ASDs and Asperger's syndrome.
> 2. Understand the main difficulties experienced by children affected by ASD.

Understanding Children and Young People's Mental Health, first edition. Edited by Anne Claveirole and Martin Gaughan. Published 2011 by John Wiley & Sons Ltd. © 2011 John Wiley & Sons Ltd.

3. Appreciate the current level of evidence available regarding possible contributions from genetic and environmental factors to the causation of ASDs.
4. Discuss the difficulties parents/carers may experience during the early development of a child with ASD.
5. Know the criteria for diagnosing children with ASD and understand the diagnosing process.
6. Design a care plan for a child with ASD with the support of the family and other relevant professionals.
7. Work more effectively with children affected by ASD and their families.

11.2 Definition and classification

Classical autism is now seen as a condition at the severe end of a continuum of disorders which all have symptoms in common. This continuum is called the autistic spectrum and ASDs are disorders with autistic-type symptoms (see Fig. 11.1). The autistic spectrum is wide and encompasses varying degrees of disability. In the 10th edition of the *International Classification of Diseases* (ICD-10), ASDs are classified as part of the umbrella group of 'pervasive development disorders' (World Health Organization (WHO) 1992). At one end of the autistic spectrum is classical or Kanner's autism (also called childhood autism), at the other end, is Asperger's syndrome.

Autism was first recognised as an independent category of disorders in the 1940s. In 1943, Austrian psychiatrist Leo Kanner, who had emigrated to the USA in 1924, described *Early Infantile Autism* (Kanner 1943). Until then, such children were thought to be 'emotionally disturbed' and/or 'mentally retarded' and the word autism had only been used to describe the isolation of patients with schizophrenia (Frith 1991). At about the same time, but in German, Hans Asperger, an Austrian paediatrician, wrote a

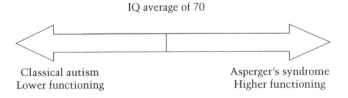

IQ average of 70

Classical autism   Asperger's syndrome
Lower functioning   Higher functioning

Figure 11.1 The autistic spectrum.

paper describing what he called *Autistic Psychopathy* (Asperger 1944 in Frith 1991). Both Kanner and Asperger were independently describing a new syndrome, although Asperger was probably focusing on more able children displaying milder autistic traits (Frith 1991). Kanner's work had an immediate impact and even though autism had not been previously identified, case descriptions were soon found that fitted the autistic category. Asperger's work, by contrast, was not taken into account in the English-speaking world until Lorna Wing discussed it in *Psychological Medicine* in 1981 (Wing 1981). Yet in 1801, French scientist Dr Itard's description of the wild boy of Aveyron is now thought to have been a case of childhood autism.

The more severe ASDs often include global and long-lasting learning disabilities, in which case they are described as 'low functioning'; Asperger's syndrome is a high functioning ASD. The degree of a person's disability may change during their lifetime, depending on the support they receive as a young child or from the time of their being diagnosed.

Core difficulties of ASDs

ASDs are diagnosed on the basis of core behavioural features, not biological aetiology, because the latter is still unclear (Jordan 1999). No single behaviour indicates autism on its own but a cluster of behaviours, related to three areas of psychological functioning commonly referred to as 'the triad of impairments' (Wing and Gould 1979), leads to a diagnosis of ASD.

ICD-10 (WHO 1992) and the 4th edition of the *Diagnostic and Statistical Manual* (DSM-IV) (American Psychiatric Association (APA) 1994) state that for a diagnosis of ASD to be given, the following features must be present:

1. Restriction of reciprocal social interactions
2. Restriction of reciprocal communication (verbal and non-verbal)
3. Restriction of imagination as reflected in a repertoire of behaviours

All three elements must be present for a diagnosis of ASD to be confirmed and abnormalities in development must have been present before the age of 3 years. The full diagnostic criteria can be found in Peeters and Gillberg (1999: 28–29) or in the ICD-10 and DSM-IV diagnostic manuals.

Although there are strict diagnostic criteria for ASDs, misdiagnosis is common, due to similarities with other disabilities, such as dyspraxia, aphasia, attention deficit disorder (ADD) and psychotic illnesses such as schizophrenia.

Differences between autism and asperger's syndrome

Here are descriptions of the two opposite ends of the autistic spectrum, childhood autism and Asperger's syndrome. Children affected by either one of these disorders display the three core features listed earlier but to varying degrees. Many children fall somewhere between the two with regard to the presence and severity of their symptoms.

Childhood autism (also called Kanner's syndrome)

Children with autism do not appear to be aware of the existence of others or they seem aloof and indifferent to other people. Kanner selected five diagnostic criteria from the common characteristics he described in his paper (Frith 1991: 93):

1. *A profound lack of affective contact with other people,*
2. *An anxiously obsessive desire for the preservation of sameness,*
3. *A fascination for objects which are handled with skill in fine motor movements,*
4. *Mutism, or a kind of language that does not seem intended to serve interpersonal communication,*
5. *The retention of an intelligent and pensive physiognomy and good cognitive potential manifested, in those who can speak, by feats of memory or, in mute children, by their skill on performance tests especially the Seguin form board* (a tool used to assess visual discrimination and to match eye–hand co-ordination).

Kanner described language difficulties, e.g. echolalia (the repetition of speech without real understanding of what has been said). This is more a difficulty in understanding speech than a problem with speech production. It may be a mechanism by which the child learns language through memorising and repeating words, and trying to find out how they fit into our language system.

Look for example at the following dialogue:

Mother: Do you want milk?
Child: Do you want milk, yes.

The answer will eventually be yes without the repetition of the question.

Between 70% and 80% of children with a diagnosis of classical autism have an intelligence quotient (IQ) of 70 or under (Fombonne 2005b). Of those with a higher IQ, most fall in the 70–100 range (Peeters and Gillberg 1999).

Kanner described other abnormalities, which he did not place among his diagnostic criteria (Frith 1991). Children with autism do not show a willingness to be picked up as babies, and often have poor eye contact. Many are clumsy and have difficulty in physical motor tasks, such as walking down stairs. They may show stereotypical movements of their limbs, e.g. hand flapping, finger flicking and rocking. Some respond to sensory stimuli in unexpected ways, such as fear or fascination (see section on theory of mind). While some children are unable to imitate or be involved in pretend play, others can mimic exact accents, words or movements. Children with autism can have problems with feeding, which can lead to real problems for parents attempting to make them eat a wide and healthy range of foods. At times they eat non-edible objects as well.

The most prominent feature of children with autism is probably their behaviour. They display high levels of anxiety, most commonly expressed as temper tantrums and challenging behaviour, without, at times, any apparent reason. They seem to react negatively to any effort to make them feel better, leaving parents and carers feeling useless.

Asperger's syndrome

Unlike children with classical autism, those with Asperger's syndrome do not have visibly obvious problems. These children tend to have higher IQs than non-autistic children and are generally of high intelligence. They can usually talk, and can speak fluently by the age of 5, even if language development was slow to begin with. They often speak very formally, and at times sound overly adult. Metaphorical figures of speech, like 'pull your socks up' or 'don't bite my head off' do not make sense to them because they take the literal meaning from what is said. So you have to be careful: you may find the child pulling their socks up or looking at you strangely!

Children with Asperger's syndrome may find it difficult to initiate a conversation or, if you manage to engage them, it may be one-sided, with them continually talking about their hobby or interest. Their speech may be delivered in a flat monotoned way, lacking expression or facial gestures. Their gaze is often classed as 'abnormal' with a 'fixated quality'. Both children and adults with Asperger's syndrome can offend people with their blunt and open way of talking. They do not mean to do this but are unable to interpret social cues. Inappropriate behaviour and misunderstanding of emotions can isolate them further. They may become involved in criminal activities as a way of getting themselves accepted by others.

Like children with autism, children with Asperger's syndrome are often unable to attribute mental states to others; this is due to the absence of what is called a theory of mind – we will come back to this in a later section. It leads them to believe that you know what they know without them having to tell you. As this is a misunderstanding, it can cause them anxiety and frustration and make you feel helpless.

Because of all these difficulties, children with Asperger's syndrome do not fit well in social situations where people have no knowledge of the disorder and they find it difficult to build relationships and make friends. This causes them and their family a great deal of anxiety and they often experience mental health problems, such as depression, later in life. Public awareness of the condition is uncommon and support systems are lacking.

People with Asperger's syndrome can look superficially as if they are well adapted to social interaction (which is not the case in classical autism), but in many ways they are egocentric and isolated.

ASDs vary considerably from person to person. Rita Jordan states that 'there is no one behaviour that is autistic, and it is the total pattern of our behaviour, plus the reasons that underlie it that indicate autism' (Jordan 1999: 3). In this chapter, we will focus on high functioning ASDs because low functioning ASDs are best dealt with in the wider context of learning disabilities, which is not the object of this book.

 Activity

From your reading of this chapter and other recommended reading, note the main differences between a young person who has autism and one who has Asperger's syndrome.

11.3 Prevalence

ASD was once thought to affect only the middle classes but it was then recognised that they simply had better access to diagnostic centres. It is now acknowledged that ASDs cut across all social, geographical and ethnic groups, yet Baird *et al.* (2006) found that identification of ASD in children of less educated parents was lower, which is a cause for concern.

The number of people with ASD has been hard to establish. The National Autistic Society (2009) mentions 1 in 100 (=100/10,000) for the UK but estimates are usually much more conservative, with Fombonne's review of existing surveys published in English to date (2005) suggesting 60/10,000 or 0.6% for all pervasive developmental disorders (PDDs) and 16/10,000 for ASD (0.16%). Differences in diagnostic criteria and in study methods can bring threefold variations in prevalence rates (Fombonne 2005a). Nevertheless, Fombonne asserts that 0.6% puts PDDs, including

ASDs, 'among the most prevalent conditions of childhood' (p. 7), with greater numbers being detected than in the past.

A study of 56,946 nine- to ten-year-old children in South Thames (Baird *et al.* 2006) reports 116/10,000 for all ASDs, with 39/10,000 for childhood autism and 77/10,000 for other ASDs. This suggests the considerably higher figure of 1.16% children with ASD than that quoted in Fombonne's 2005 review (0.16%); yet the authors caution against assuming that the incidence of ASD is rising, even if a true rise cannot be ruled out. The increase is likely to be at least partially due to a broadening of diagnostic criteria over time.

Autism is significantly more common in males than females by a ratio of approximately 4:1 for all ASDs (Fombonne 2005b). Various reasons are suggested as to why this may be. It is possible that the symptoms of autism manifest themselves differently in girls and therefore go unnoticed or are classed as learning disability rather than autism. There is also a hormonal hypothesis (Baron-Cohen 2002) which we will mention in the next section.

11.4 Risk factors/causation theories

The consensus is that ASDs are multi-factorial neuro-developmental disorders. There is overwhelming evidence that they have a biological basis with a strong genetic component, although the process is not understood yet. Factors other than genetic are environmental, but in ASDs the environmental evidence has been insufficient so far to allow firm conclusions (Rutter 2005). The aim of current research is to uncover the causal pathway, likely to involve several interacting causes. We need to understand better the genetic and environmental determinants of brain structure and function in development, and relations between the brain, cognition, behaviour and symptomatology (Deeley and Murphy 2009).

Genetic liability is established through twin studies whereas research into brain abnormalities progresses through the use of MRI and PET scans. Brain functions are compared between people with ASD and neuro-normal controls to study how certain brain networks support a range of cognitive functions (Deeley and Murphy 2009).

Potential environmental factors in ASDs are of great interest to people with ASD themselves, their families and the media, as you can see on the websites of interest groups, and there are many hypotheses. Some are strongly held, but the strength of scientific evidence varies as do the views of the researchers and experts. We advise you to read some of this evidence for yourself and to reflect on the relationship between different scientific fields (such as medicine, nutrition or pharmacology) and interest groups (such as people with ASDs, families, teachers or health care staff).

Genetics factors

Twin studies have shown that heredity is the best established risk factor for ASD because there is a 60% concordance rate between identical twins as against 5% between non-identical ones. This gives ASD a hereditability of 90%: the highest of all the multi-factorial mental disorders of childhood (Rutter 2005).

The genetic liability goes beyond the diagnostic categories to include autistic-like difficulties which are too mild to score on the ICD-10 criteria. These clusters of autistic-type characteristics are called phenotypes and they also concord very highly in identical twins. There is likely to be between three and twelve susceptible genes for autism, acting synergistically. Most siblings of people with ASD do not have ASD in spite of its high heritability (only 6% do, which appears low, but is much higher than in the general population), it is because they do not have all the required genes (Rutter 2005). Intensive research is going on to identify the susceptible genes.

Following on from this, a study of 3,000 twin pairs of 7–9 year olds (Happe *et al.* 2006) reported modest to low correlations between the three core areas of impairment (see above), which implies that separate genes contribute to each and that the triad of impairments is likely to be underpinned by abnormalities in several rather than one brain region.

Pre- and perinatal factors

This area is a typical example of expert divergence regarding the evidence. Complications leading to brain damage in pregnancy, delivery and the post-natal period are said to be more common in children with autism than in the general population. In her original paper on ASD, Lorna Wing noted that almost half of her cases had a history of pre-, peri- and post-natal conditions which may have caused brain damage (Wing 1981). Other experts have supported this hypothesis (Happe *et al.* 1996, Ghaziuddin *et al.* 2002) and research into this link continues. However, Rutter (2005) finds that the studies are small and the associations they show between perinatal complications and ASDs varied, so that there is no actual evidence that these associations are causal. Both variables (perinatal complications and ASD) may share a genetic predisposition or the complications may be a response to a genetically abnormal foetus (Rutter 2005). The conclusion of medical scientists is that perinatal complications are consequences rather than causes of ASDs.

Endocrine factors

Simon Baron-Cohen is professor of developmental psychopathology at the University of Cambridge and director of the Autism Research Centre (http://www.autismresearchcentre.com/). He has suggested that foetal testosterone levels are related to gender-linked aspects of cognition and behaviour, including the development of autistic traits (Baron-Cohen 2002). This would make autism an extreme manifestation of male-typical characteristics. The Autism Research Centre is currently investigating this possibility (Auyeung *et al.* 2009).

Heavy metal toxicity

Research has been undertaken focusing on heavy metals, such as mercury and lead, which are known to be neurotoxins. Exposure to mercury during early development can cause developmental problems. It has been suggested that mercury poisoning may be implicated in the aetiology of ASDs because symptoms of intoxication with mercury are similar to ASD symptoms (Medical Research Council, MRC, 2001). However, a randomised controlled trial of mercury levels in ASD and control groups of children showed no elevation in mercury levels in children with ASD (MRC 2001). Lead poisoning has also been suggested but no evidence has yet been found (Rutter 2005).

A link between autism and some vaccines was argued on the basis that some contained a mercury base, thimerosal (which has since been discontinued). However, the impact of thimerosal as a cause of mercury intoxication would be notable in epidemiological evidence and this is not the case (Rutter 2005).

Measles, mumps and rubella vaccine

The possibility was raised a few years ago that the measles, mumps and rubella (MMR) immunisation might be a risk factor for ASD. Some parents claimed that their child was developing normally until they received the vaccine which was followed by a diagnosis of autism. They put forward the view that a regressive form of autism, through which previously acquired social and communicative skills were lost, had occurred, which would explain the rise in recently diagnosed ASDs. A study reported supporting evidence in a Lancet article (Wakefield *et al.* 1998). However, the study (which only included 12 children, the selection of which was biased) has since been discredited. Andrew Wakefield was accused of professional misconduct with regard to his research and investigated by the British Medical Association (BMA) in 2007. In May 2010, he was struck off the medical register.

Studies investigating a link between the MMR vaccine and ASDs have unanimously found that this was not proven (MRC 2001, Rutter 2005). The epidemiological evidence also disproves the link: if the MMR vaccine were linked to ASDs, there would be an increase in ASDs in countries that introduced the vaccine, which is not the case, and in a country like Japan where it was stopped, the rate of ASDs would fall but this has not happened (Rutter 2005). Rutter stresses that epidemiological evidence does not allow small numbers of cases to be detected, therefore it is possible that a link exists for a few children. The existence of regressive autism has not been disproved (Rutter 2005).

Some parents are requesting that their child be given the vaccine at three different times, rather than in combination. This is not available in the NHS but some clinics offer it privately.

Metabolic factors

The Autism Research Unit (ARU) at the University of Sunderland undertakes and publishes research on autism as a metabolic disorder under the direction of pharmacist Dr Paul Shattock. Intestinal abnormalities have been found in some children with ASD. It is not clear yet whether these affect all children with ASD, or whether they are more common than among children with no ASD. Research focuses particularly on intestinal permeability (also called leaky gut syndrome) and the benefits of gluten and casein free diets to avoid excess opioids in the blood (Shattock *et al.* 2001). This would reduce the behaviours associated with ASD, at least in some children (see http://centres.sunderland.ac.uk/autism/).

  Activity

Consider the different reasons which are given for the causes of ASDs – which one/s make the most sense to you and why?

11.5 Associated problems

This section describes the additional difficulties people with autism may experience, including other medical diagnoses, which is referred to as co-morbidity.

Sensory system dysfunction

Children with ASD have unusual responses to sensory stimuli (Bogdashina 2003). Their sensory experiences may be different from those of neurotypical people (sensory stimuli may look, sound, taste, smell or feel different to a child with ASD) or they may interpret sensory stimuli differently. Perception may involve hyper- or hyposensitivity, variations in volumes, etc. Consequently, a person with ASD will develop a different kind of knowledge about the world, which neuro-normal people may struggle to recognise. These differences can explain strange behaviour, such as head banging, poking of eyes, hitting ears and spinning objects. Children with ASD probably do not realise that their perception is different from that of other children and that their behaviour (motor clumsiness, withdrawal from touch, refusal to eat/wear/touch certain textures, tastes or colours) does not make sense to those around them (Bogdashina 2003).

Brain abnormalities

PET and MRI scanning have revealed areas of low activity in the brain of people with ASDs but this is not specific to them so further work is required. Neurotransmitters may be involved but there is limited evidence so far.

Psychological abnormalities

Cognitive theories start from the child's behaviour and look to mental/ cognitive processes for an explanatory mechanism. Cognitive psychologists hope to find links between these and brain abnormalities. These cognitive abnormalities have the status of theory rather than research evidence but they help to guide brain research and generate hypotheses. They are also helpful to organise interventions. How far they apply to all people with ASD, and how significant a component of each syndrome is, remains to be worked out.

A defective theory of mind

Being human gives us the ability to have a 'theory of mind', i.e. 'to reflect on one's own and others' mind' (Baron-Cohen 2001). It is the ability to appreciate that others have mental states, i.e. intentions, desires, beliefs and emotions of their own that we can infer from their behaviour. It is about reading and understanding other minds. And it is an ability that appears to be defective in most people with ASDs. Children of about 4 years normally can tell the difference between mental actions like thinking, dreaming and knowing, and physical actions like eating and running. Children with autism have difficulty with this. They also find pretend play and make-believe games problematic (Baron-Cohen 2001). Children with Asperger's syndrome who have high IQ may develop the ability but typically later than the normal developmental age (Happe 1995).

Baron-Cohen *et al.* (1985) provide an example of the theory of mind deficit using the 'Sally Anne test'. This experiment consists of two dolls, one named Sally who has a basket and the other Anne who has a box.

Sally puts a marble in her basket and then leaves the room. Whilst Sally is out of the room, Anne takes the marble out of Sally's basket and places it in her box. Sally then returns to the room and the children are asked where they think Sally will look for her marble. In Baron-Cohen et al.'s research (1985), a group of children with ASDs and a mental age of 4+ years were studied, with a control group of children of the same age and ability with Down's syndrome and a group of typically developing children. The results showed that almost 80% of the children with ASDs failed the test in comparison with 14% of the children with Down's syndrome. This is due to the lack of theory of mind in the children with ASDs: they believed that, because they knew that the situation within the test had changed, i.e. Anne had moved the marble from Sally's basket to her own box, Sally should have known this too without having to be told. As a consequence, children with ASDs have difficulties in predicting people's behaviour, which leads to fear and avoidance of others; and difficulties in reading other people's intentions and understanding their emotions, which in turn leads to a lack of empathy and to not explaining their own behaviour.

Impaired executive function

The executive function refers to a set of high-level skills which include the ability to plan, organise and problem-solve, to reflect and self-monitor, to manage time and prioritise, to behave flexibly and use new strategies and to understand complex or abstract concepts (Attwood 2007). These abilities are based in the frontal lobes of the brain (MRC 2001) and there is growing evidence that deficits in the executive function are typical of ASDs and other disorders like attention deficit hyperactivity disorder (ADHD) (Goldberg et al. 2005), although children with high functioning autism may not be so impaired in this area as those with classical autism.

Weak central coherence

This is a psychological theory developed by Utah Frith and Francesca Happe (1994) regarding the way children with ASDs process information. They describe central coherence as the ability to draw meaning from the mass of information in everyday life by extracting what is useful and discarding unnecessary detail, so as to perceive the 'big picture'. A child with autism is likely to attend to the separate parts, get lost in the detail and lose the meaning of the situation. For example, when we look at a photograph of children playing on a beach, we perceive the general impression and not the colour of their clothes or the number of towels. Weak central coherence leads to a fragmented view of the world and makes for difficulties in the classroom. The most complex and chaotic information to organise is probably emotional and social. Attwood (2007) suggests that many of the strange behaviours of children with ASD are explained by their efforts to draw order out of constant chaos: the love of routine and rituals, the dislike of change, the absorption in special interests, rules and laws (laws of science or religion and the legal system).

Medical conditions/co-morbidity

Researchers are interested in definite diagnosable medical conditions associated with ASD because it is hoped that some causal implication may be demonstrated. Co-morbidity affects 10% of the ASD population and Rutter (2005) states that this is high enough to indicate that every case be thoroughly investigated.

Medical conditions often diagnosed in children with ASDs include:

- *Epilepsy*: The high rate of epilepsy found in approximately one-third of children with autism was an early indication that ASDs were biological disorders (MRC 2001). One in five or six preschool children with autism develops epilepsy in the first few years of life, and another 20% will develop it as they get older. This is not the case for the children with Asperger's syndrome, whose number is similar to that of the general population.
- *Sensory impairments of vision and hearing*: One in five people with ASD has reduced vision and will need to wear glasses. Many young children will display some abnormal eye movements. One in four people has a degree of hearing impairment and a few are completely deaf. This area can be difficult to diagnose because people with ASDs and non-autistic people hear differently.
- *Fragile X syndrome*, which affects 2–3% of the ASD population (Chakrabarti and Fombonne 2001).
- *Tuberous sclerosis*, which is found in 1–3% (Harrison and Bolton 1997).
- *Cerebral palsy, Down's syndrome, neurofibromatosis, congenital rubella and phenylketonuria.*

Mental health problems (Ghaziuddin 2005)

Anxiety disorders and depression are common in children with Asperger's syndrome as they grow up. These problems are secondary to those associated with Asperger's. Children who have Asperger's syndrome have the desire to communicate, and often feel real sorrow at not finding friends or a spouse. It can be more difficult to diagnose symptoms of depression in less able children because of difficulties of language and comprehension.

Other problems

The following problems can be seen in children with ASD:

■ *Clumsiness* of movement, which can lead to misdiagnosis of dyspraxia.
■ *Hyperactivity* especially in early childhood.
■ *Strange behaviours*: At least one-third of children with ASD show bizarre and ritualistic eating habits, aggressive behaviour, mood swings and aggressive outbursts. They also display a high pain threshold, and it may be difficult to realise when they are injured since they do not cry out in pain.
■ *Language impairment*: Many children with autism have some form of language impairment. Most people with Asperger's syndrome or higher functioning autism have the ability to speak, but they cannot always understand the purpose of talking or what we say to them.
■ *Hyperlexia*: Many young children with ASD learn to read at an early age without any formal teaching, in spite of the language development delay. This is known as hyperlexia. They may also be very gifted artists, musicians or mathematicians without being taught any of the skills required.

 Activity

Look at a child with ASD you know or work with: compare the child's behaviour with the above list and determine whether they show any signs of these associated problems. If relevant, relate them to the child's care plan.

Making use of what you read in the previous section, suggest reasons why you think people with ASD display challenging behaviours.

Perhaps try the 'Sally Anne test' (explained in the section on theory of mind) with the child you know and note the results. Compare this with the Baron-Cohen results.

11.6 Development

From the difficulties we have identified, it is clear that the development of children with ASDs and their families is not going to be straightforward. We recommend that you read autistic adults' accounts of their childhood, such as Donna Williams's (1992) and Temple Grandin's (1995), to see how they describe their experience.

ASDs are usually present from the beginning of the child's life. Some children affected by ASD appear to have followed the expected development path until around 18 months to 2 years, when regression occurs. The existence of this late onset or regressive ASD is difficult to demonstrate because it is difficult to be sure that early development was normal (Rutter 2005). The most likely explanations are the following:

- Some parents may find it difficult to acknowledge that there is anything wrong with their child.
- Diagnosis of the condition may be delayed due to lack of knowledge or awareness on the part of the professionals.
- Especially in the case of children with Asperger's syndrome, islets of ability can shadow the early signs of the disorder.

No single pattern of childhood behaviour or development identifies a child with ASD.

The first year

The most common characteristics parents describe about their child when very young are either babies that are good, quiet and undemanding or, in complete contrast, demanding babies who resist contact and feeding and any form of touch or eye contact.

Babies with ASDs rarely use eye contact, facial expression or gestures as normally developing children do. They do not always relate to their parents, something which parents find difficult to cope with. It makes them wonder what they are doing wrong. These problems can lead to delay in the child's ability to recognise their parents until they are about 3 or 4.

Children with ASDs react differently to neuro-typically developing children. They are not interested in games such as peek-a-boo and do not develop finger pointing till later years. Many babies do not react to their name being called but they may react to certain noises or language. Some babies are hyperactive from their first few months, while others show the complete opposite and look lethargic. As the child grows older, you may find that they lead you to what they want without looking at you or interacting in any way.

Preschool years

It is usually during this stage of development that parents realise something may be wrong. The child with ASD may have developed no speech or use only a few words, repeating them over and over again. The child may not persevere in learning to talk because they have no understanding of the context in which to use the words, and therefore do not see the point of talking. Thus, about half of children diagnosed with ASD never speak. If children do develop speech, it often becomes echolalic, but unlike neuro-typical children who learn from echoing adults, children with ASD can do this for years. They may also reverse personal pronouns, e.g. using you for I and we for you.

The basic communication problem is these children's inability to understand the meaning of language. This may be the underlying reason why they repeat things said to them, as they can often understand words on their own, but not in a sentence or in a different context.

The child may show little to no interest in other people and use them only when they need something. Then, stereotypical behaviour is likely to be displayed. When surrounded by too many people, the child may scream and start hitting themselves, or may be seen standing with their back to a group of people.

School years

Major differences in communication become more obvious as the child gets older and starts school. This applies to children with classical autism or Asperger's syndrome. Most children find it easier to understand written words and visual images than the spoken word because many think in pictures (see Grandin 1995). This can be the best way to communicate with children or adults with ASD. Their school years tend to be the most difficult period of these children's lives, particularly for children with Asperger's syndrome who are aware of what is happening around them and that they are different. They will continue to face challenges throughout their lives, albeit in different ways, as they get older. Mark Haddon's book, *The Curious Incident of the Dog in the Night-time* (2003), paints a useful picture of what life is like for 15-year-old Christopher who has a high functioning form of autism.

Self-abusive behaviour is not uncommon in both children and adults affected with ASD. When you are working with a child on the autistic spectrum, it is important to remember that behaviour is a form of com-munication and to look for the underlying trigger rather than judge the child for the behaviour he or she has shown.

 Activity

What do you think are the developmental challenges young people on the autistic spectrum face – what are the areas they might need extra support with?

11.7 Assessment and diagnosis

Reaching a diagnosis involves using a combination of screening instruments and interviews. Different tests are used for autism and for Asperger's syndrome because tests for the latter need to be sensitive to more subtle characteristics than generic autism tools (Attwood 2007). Every characteristic of the disorder included in the diagnostic criteria must be checked. In Asperger's syndrome, areas of unusual abilities should be assessed as well. A useful guide to a systematic assessment is Wing *et al.* (2002)'s Diagnostic Interview for Social and Communication Disorders (DISCO), which clinicians need to be trained to use.

A diagnosis should be made as early as possible in the child's life because it is a passport to help and support for the family, at the time and in the future. If a child is not diagnosed until later, this may affect his opportunities. The diagnostic procedure can take some time and those involved with the child need to be aware of the stigma which accompanies the diagnosis of ASD.

Several professionals are likely to be involved in the pre-diagnostic and diagnostic stages. Who they are depends on the age of the child. They would include a general practitioner (GP), a paediatrician, a psychiatrist or clinical psychologist, a speech and language therapist, an educational psychologist and a specialist service like the Scottish Society for Autism or the National Autistic Society.

The number of people involved in the assessment and the lack of a standardised diagnostic procedure can lead to differences of opinion among professionals and the possibility of misdiagnosis. There is more than one route to diagnosis, and many parents will go directly to a private specialist in their search for answers.

Taking a family history and looking for genetic traces is important since this is the most common contributing factor; so is examining the child's early development for symptomatic behaviour. A good developmental history is crucial to the process. Some professionals are unhappy about labelling a child autistic, although it can be very difficult for parents to access services for their child without a medical diagnosis.

Diagnostic manuals and criteria such as ICD-10 (WHO 1992) and DSM-IV (APA 1994) are work in progress. Asperger's syndrome was included in their most recent editions for the first time and there is a consensus that DSM-IV contains a number of errors which make it difficult to distinguish between autism and Asperger's syndrome; DSM-IV also gives precedence to autism in a way which some experienced diagnosticians think is not true to the clinical picture (Attwood 2007). Attwood recommends

Gillberg's diagnostic criteria for Asperger's syndrome (Gillberg 1991, 2002) as 'those that most closely resemble the original descriptions of Asperger' (Attwood 2007).

Attwood (2007) also stresses that the distinction between high functioning autism and Asperger's syndrome is not clear and that there are no criteria for a differential diagnosis. In this chapter, we have used both to cover the same meaning.

PDD is the broadest category for autistic-type syndromes. These disorders are described as 'a group of disorders characterised by qualitative abnormalities in reciprocal social interactions and in patterns of communication, and by a restricted, stereotyped, repetitive repertoire of interests and activities' (WHO 1992). Childhood autism and Asperger's syndrome are more precise sub-categories. Children who do not meet the full criteria for one of them can be diagnosed as having a PDD, or a 'pervasive developmental disorder not otherwise specified' (PDDNOS).

Misdiagnosis

Obsessive compulsive disorder (OCD) has features similar to those of autism. The ritualistic and compulsive behaviours of OCD cannot always be distinguished from the fixed routines and repetitive behaviours of a child with ASD. However, children with OCD do not usually encounter the problems with communication or interaction that children on the autistic spectrum do.

Fragile X syndrome is associated with slow development and social and communication problems. Confusion in diagnosis arises because a higher rate of people on the autistic spectrum have fragile X syndrome than in the general population.

Asperger's syndrome (especially in adults) is sometimes misdiagnosed as semantic pragmatic disorder, schizoid personality disorder, atypical depression and occasionally schizophrenia.

Activity

Consider factors which might lead to a child being misdiagnosed – what do you think are the types of behaviour or problems that might be confused with ASD?

11.8 Management of care

Once a child has been diagnosed, the appropriate care and education plan must be put in place. Children with Asperger's syndrome and other ASDs have great potential if they are diagnosed early enough and if they receive the right support. They are all different and each child's idiosyncrasies must be taken into account when developing care plans: there is no one-size-fits-all solution. These plans must be flexible.

Stability and consistency are extremely important in the lives of children with ASD and the care plan must reflect this. The child should be included in this planning as much as possible. This can be achieved by incorporating their particular means of communication into the process, whether this be visual prompts, signs or a picture, e.g. PECS (picture exchange communication system, see www.pecs.org.uk). Fear and anxiety are high in children on the autistic spectrum and it is adults' job to reassure them as much as possible. Getting to know the child before the care planning meetings begin can help.

It can be difficult to ensure that the child, the parents and the care staff share an understanding of what is being discussed and it is important to use every means available to help. The child may not understand the questions we ask, so it is better not to ask closed questions because a yes or a no answer does not make the child's understanding clear or enable the enquirer to gain a true picture. Asking the child to repeat what he has understood may help, as well as the adult repeating what she has understood.

Including as many professionals to help in the care of the child is essential. Speech therapists, occupational therapists, educational psychologists and specialist paediatricians are excellent people to contribute in the plan. They may not all need to be at the meeting at the same time, but their input at some point, be-it home visits or via written reports at care planning meetings, is vital.

There are many ways of helping children with ASD. Below are examples of principles (support of inter-subjectivity) and resources (Treatment and Education of Autistic and Communications-Handicapped CHildren, TEACCH) which have been used. Interventions must be matched to individual children's needs, which vary greatly. You will need to do your own research if you want to know more about what is available.

Information about ASDs for GPs and other primary care staff is available on the NHS Education for Scotland website (http://www.nes.scot.nhs.uk/asd/).

Support of inter-subjectivity

Trevarthen's research focuses on the communicative abilities of typical infants and their need to engage actively with attentive others for their brains to develop essential functions. This has led him to postulate that interventions with children whose ability and motivation to communicate is impaired should start with supporting the basics of inter-subjective communication. Trevarthen suggests verbal and non-verbal exercises (including music making), which include timing, turn-taking, prosody (the rhythm and stress of speech as in poetry), reciprocal imitation and jointly focused attention (Trevarthen and Aitken 2001).

TEACCH

An important evidence-based programme devised for children and adults with ASDs is TEACCH (Mesibov *et al.* 2004). It includes interventions for people with ASD, training for staff and a research programme (http://www. teacch.com/).

The TEACCH programme was started at the University of North Carolina in 1966 by Dr Eric Schopler at a time when autism was thought to be an emotional disorder caused by poor parenting, something which his early research led him to disagree with.

The TEACCH programme is based on a set of core values which transcend the specific components of the programme. The main value is an effort to describe and understand ASD ways of viewing life as different but no less valid than neuro-typical ones. They call this the culture of autism. TEACCH is based on collaboration between parents and professionals. It aims to decrease the distance between children and adults on the autistic spectrum and the rest of society. The programme itself includes assessments, educational strategies and therapeutic interventions, many of which are now used in Britain. If you would like to learn more about TEACCH, follow the references given above. You will also find information on the website of the National Autistic Society.

When working with a child who is on the autistic spectrum, we must be willing to give without necessarily getting anything back in return. It is important not to be disappointed or self-critical when this happens. The progress the child makes from our hard work will compensate for this, and the end result is worth waiting for!

  Activity

What are the most important elements of support which need to be in place for:

1. A child with autism
2. A teenager with Asperger's syndrome.

Family support

Never underestimate the difficulties parents can face when they have a child diagnosed with ASD. Parents and carers need to be offered the support they need as part of the ongoing care of the child. They usually require a lot of support from professionals because of the complex nature of ASD. Many had no prior knowledge of ASD and when their child is diagnosed, they do not know which way to turn.

One of the first questions parents ask concerns what they have done to make their child autistic; another is about the future the child will have. Fear is uppermost in their minds. It is our job to support them in this and give them the facts. We need to be aware of the stresses and tensions experienced by the families of children with ASD, and of the fact that rigidity and routine can make their lives very difficult. The breakdown of the family unit is not uncommon in these circumstances.

In many cases, extra pressure is placed on siblings who can become secondary carers, or do not receive the attention they need because the child with ASD requires so much. Parents' lives start revolving around ASD, to the detriment of friends and the activities they pursued before their child was born. Understandably, there is a desire for information, support mechanisms or treatment, and some parents are willing to try anything they think may help them or their child. Parents should be encouraged to be cautious when looking at educational and treatment programmes as some are better validated than others. Parents need the best information available as well as training and support in all issues relating to ASD.

Two helpful information booklets by the Scottish Intercollegiate Guidelines Network (SIGN, 2008), one for parents and one for young people, are available from the NHS Evidence website.

Parents: http://www.library.nhs.uk/CHILDHEALTH/ViewResource.aspx?resID=282030

Young People:

http://www.library.nhs.uk/childHealth/viewResource.aspx?resID=282029

 Activity

What methods could you use to support a family who have a 5-year-old child with autism who is in mainstream school?
   What kind of support would an older sibling need in such a family?

11.9 Conclusion

People on the autistic spectrum must be included in every possible way in today's society but only in ways that work for them. Otherwise the distress and failure they face can do more long-term damage than exclusion itself. Early intervention strategies that provide for different areas of the child and family's life are crucial for the success of the child's future development and to preserve the family's integrity.

Recommended reading

Attwood, T. (2007). *The Complete Guide to Asperger's Syndrome*. London: Jessica Kingsley Publishers.

Frith, U. (1991). *Autism and Asperger's Syndrome*. Cambridge: Cambridge University Press.

Haddon, M. (2003). *The Curious Incident of the Dog in the Night-time*. London: Jonathan Cape.

Peeters, T. and Gillberg, C. (1999). *Autism – Medical and Educational Aspects*, 2nd edition. London: Whurr Publishers.

Williams, D. (1998). *Autism – An Inside-Out Approach*. London: Jessica Kingsley Publishers.

Wing, L. (1996). *The Autistic Spectrum: A Guide for Parents and Professionals*. London: Constable.

Useful websites

The National Autistic Society:
www.nas.org.uk
The Scottish Society for Autism:
www.autism-in-scotland.org.uk
The Autism Research Unit at the University of Sunderland:
http://centres.sunderland.ac.uk/autism/
The National Centre for Autism Studies at the University of Strathclyde:
http://www.strath.ac.uk/autism-ncas/
The Autism Centre for Education and Research at the University of Birmingham:
http://www.education.bham.ac.uk/research/acer/index.shtml
A private website but interesting:
www.autism-resources.com/

Chapter 12

MISUSE OF SUBSTANCES

Liz Brodie[1] and Jayne Reed[2]

[1] School of Nursing, Midwifery and Social Care, Edinburgh Napier University, Edinburgh, Scotland
[2] Community Drug Problem Service, NHS Lothian, Edinburgh, Scotland

12.1 Introduction

Young people today experience a wide range and diversity of substance misuse problems. Since the early 1990s, the extent of substance misuse has been of increasing concern to those involved with the welfare of children. We know that substance use affects young people in a multitude of ways, with wider implications for society. Substance misuse may impact on young people's future development; when as adults and parents they are faced with their own occupational, social, health and economic challenges. This chapter will outline a definition of substance misuse and the impact and prevalence of misuse. Vulnerability factors will be discussed and the importance of early interventions summarised. The chapter will conclude with a review of assessment and treatment.

Adult treatment services tend to focus on dependence issues, while young people's services have to focus on wider issues due to the interruption of developmental processes. Even a single episode of substance use can result in accidental harm, intoxication, victimisation, mental health problems or death (Crome 2004). For some young people, engagement in a regular pattern of substance use will result in disruption of education, relationship problems and risks to their longer-term physical and emotional health. A small percentage will develop dependent misuse with an accompanying constellation of longer-term physical, social and emotional difficulties. The range of substances misused by young people is similar to

Understanding Children and Young People's Mental Health, first edition. Edited by Anne Claveirole and Martin Gaughan. Published 2011 by John Wiley & Sons Ltd. © 2011 John Wiley & Sons Ltd.

that of adults; however, the use of volatile substances is more common among children and young people.

Most adult substance misuse and dependence begins in early adolescence. Criminal behaviour in adulthood can be predicted at ages 13–15 years and has a strong if poorly-understood relationship with substance misuse (Farrington 1996 cited in MacDonald and Marsh 2005). Adult mental health problems and a wide spectrum of social disruption are related to early onset substance misuse. One of our aims must be to develop interventions to delay first use and to interrupt the pathways to more extensive patterns of harmful use. It can take several years before individuals recognise their substance misuse is problematic and seek help. Young people are less likely than adults to present to services with substance misuse as their primary problem (McArdle 2004). As young people most vulnerable to substance misuse become even more vulnerable by engaging in this activity, we need to be aware of the risk factors, early signs and range of relevant interventions appropriate to the complexity of their needs.

Learning outcomes
1. Discuss the impact of individual and social/environmental factors and their influence on the development of substance-using behaviours.
2. Define the range of substance-using behaviours of young people today.
3. List the range of harms experienced by young people who misuse substances.
4. Analyse relationships between vulnerability, risk and resilience.
5. Analyse elements of good practice in assessment, intervention and liaison in the facilitation of recovery.

12.2 Substance use and substance misuse

The Health Advisory Service (2001: 17) defines substance use as 'controlled, occasional, unproblematic and recreational' and substance misuse as 'harmful, problematic or dependent'. The current ICD-10 (World Health Organization, WHO, 1992) coding does not distinguish between substance misuse in adults and children/young people, which is an issue in need of attention, given the unique developmental challenges young people face. ICD-10 does however address the difference between substance use and substance dependence. These distinctions are presented in Boxes 12.1 and 12.2.

Box 12.1 WHO's Definition of Harmful Substance Use

A pattern of psychoactive substance use that is causing damage to health. The damage may be physical (as in cases of hepatitis from the self-administration of injected psychoactive substances) or mental (e.g. episodes of depressive disorder secondary to heavy consumption of alcohol).Data from WHO (1992: 74–75).

Box 12.2 WHO's Definition of Dependence Syndrome

A cluster of behavioural, cognitive, and physiological phenomena that develop after repeated substance use and that typically include a strong desire to take the drug, difficulties in controlling its use, persisting in its use despite harmful consequences, a higher priority given to drug use than to other activities and obligations, increased tolerance, and sometimes a physical withdrawal state.

The dependence syndrome may be present for a specific psychoactive substance (e.g. tobacco, alcohol, or diazepam), for a class of substances (e.g. opioid drugs), or for a wider range of pharmacologically different psychoactive substances. Data from WHO (1992: 75–76).

Substance use in young people can be considered as a normal part of risk-taking and rebellion (Ghodse in Crome *et al.* 2004) and only a very small minority of those who engage in experimentation go on to experience problems. Substance misuse does not exist as an independent problem but as part of a cluster of other difficulties which need to be addressed if outcomes are to be favourable (Bushell *et al.* 2002; NICE 2007a).

12.3 Prevalence

Establishing how many children and young people are using substances is difficult as underreporting is common in this area. Although statistics broadly indicate that serious substance misuse among young people has remained fairly static over the last decade, there is widespread concern about the increase and pattern of alcohol consumption among under 16 year olds in the UK and Western Europe (Frischer *et al.* 2004). In 2005 in England, 22% of pupils reported drinking in the previous week and the average reported weekly consumption among this group was 10.4 units. Binge drinking increased in the UK and other European countries throughout the 1990s (Viner and Taylor 2007) with 27% of young women and 36% of young men aged 16–24 binge drinking at least once a week; 90% of students will have tried alcohol by the time they leave school and 30% of adolescent males report problem drinking (Lask *et al.* 2003).

While the statistics for substance misuse have remained stable, they still constitute a problem with an estimated 70,000 problem drug users between ages 15 and 24 in England and Wales, and 24% of vulnerable young people reporting frequent use of illicit drugs over the past year compared to 5% of less vulnerable groups (Roe and Becker 2005). Growing up in a family where one or both parents have dependent substance misuse increases young people's own risk of developing substance misuse problems. It is estimated that between 2% and 3% of children younger than 16 years old in England and Wales are living with parental drug or alcohol misuse (ACMD 2003).

 Activity

In the next section we will be considering different patterns of substance misuse. Before reading this section, reflect on your views of substance misuse by rating the different types of substance misuse and making notes of your view on their potential harm and acceptability to society.

12.4 Patterns of use and misuse in children and young people

Alcohol and tobacco

There is considerable debate about the role tobacco, alcohol and cannabis play as 'gateway' substances. There appears to be a clear correlation between early smoking and other subsequent substance use; in addition, cannabis can be viewed as a gateway to early smoking. Early use of alcohol is generally experimental and most of the problems experienced by young people are as a result of binge drinking patterns and intoxication.

Volatile substances

Volatile substance use, including glues, thinners, lighter fluid and aerosols, is highest in the under-15 age group. The main risks are accidental death through intoxication and physical health problems due to heavy use. Exacerbation of underlying health problems and developing harmful patterns of other substance misuse is a risk in this group.

Cannabis

Concerns about cannabis as a gateway to more complex poly drug use and later 'hard' drug use have been replaced in recent years by the focus on the relationship of cannabis use to serious mental health problems. While there is a high prevalence of cannabis use in young people, we need to distinguish between the light or occasional use experienced by the majority of young people and the heavy daily use of a small minority. Much of the recent focus has centred on cannabis use and its association with an increased vulnerability to psychosis in predisposed individuals. Baker and Velleman (2007) remind us that no less important is the relationship between anxiety, depression, youth suicide and cannabis use. The increased potency of cannabis is seen to be partially responsible for its role in the development of mental health problems. There is evidence that experimental or light users do not develop further substance misuse problems or mental health problems. Increased vulnerability and social dysfunction will influence the transition to heavy use (Melrose *et al.* 2007). Withdrawal from cannabis may lead to a decrease in appetite, weight loss, sleep problems, craving, irritability and vivid dreams (DOH 2007). Heavy users will attribute both positive and negative meanings to their cannabis use, which will in turn influence whether they continue to use or stop.

Opiates

Although the percentage of young people who use opiates is small, the exponential increase in resultant risk behaviour and vulnerability to a range of harms makes it a priority for recognition and intervention. Dependent use of opiates, particularly if injected, carries increased risk of physical harm. Young people who use heroin, methadone or other opiates can be vulnerable to exploitation, unplanned pregnancy, involvement in crime, increased exposure to blood-borne viruses, and are at greater risk of becoming homeless. Tolerance to opiates can reduce very rapidly and young people who resume use at previous level after a period of abstinence can be at greater risk of overdose.

Stimulant use

The use of stimulants in young people (amphetamine, cocaine, crack cocaine) is low and often part of a wider poly-drug-using pattern. However, the disinhibition associated with stimulants can increase exposure to a range of psychosocial problems, and withdrawal from heavier use can precipitate significant psychological symptoms resulting in self-harm, suicide, violence, agitation or depression (DOH 2007).

Poly drug use

This represents the most common pattern of substance misuse behaviour among more vulnerable young people. Apart from the substances mentioned earlier, others include benzodiazepines, ecstasy or hallucinogens. The use of benzodiazepines in young people, either in a binge or dependent fashion, is of particular concern. They are often perceived to be innocuous, but through their disinhibiting effects (particularly when used with alcohol and opiates) they can increase the risks of overdose, crime, violence and sexual exploitation.

 Activity

Consider factors which may make children and young people vulnerable to substance misuse – identify three factors you think may have the most influence.

12.5 Vulnerability and resilience

The role of substance misuse in children and young people and its wider relationship with mental health is complex, but it is clear that a pre-existing mental health problem and being socially excluded are the more prominent risk factors for problematic substance misuse. Individual and environmental factors contribute to both vulnerability and higher risk. Individual vulnerability factors are presented in Box 12.3.

Box 12.3 Factors Which Make Children and Young People Vulnerable to Substance Misuse

- High levels of impulsivity
- Lack of self-concern
- Anxiety
- Low self-esteem
- Eating disorders
- Risk-taking
- Concentration difficulties
- Post-traumatic stress disorder
- Depression
- Loss
- Behaviour problems
- Self-harm
- Problems of attention
- Trauma
- ADHD
- Poor sense of self-worth
- Abusive parenting
- Negligent parenting

12.6 Environmental and family factors

Early family experiences which can influence the development of substance misuse in young people include attachment problems, domestic disharmony and social and economic deprivation (Lask *et al.* 2003, Ghodse in Crome *et al.* 2004). Parental substance misuse and parental mental health problems may also increase vulnerability. Women using drugs during pregnancy are at increased risk of developing postnatal mental health problems, which may affect attachment with the child. The demands of substance dependence and having an infant with neonatal abstinence syndrome can also negatively affect the formation of a secure attachment. McKeganey et al. (2003) state that young people brought up in substance misusing households have the belief that substance misuse and the associated behaviours such as lack of self-concern and exposure to high-risk situations are normal behaviours.

It is suggested that the response of services to children of alcohol-using parents may be slower due to the more tolerant perception of alcohol use that society holds (Russell 2006) and such children may be at greater risk of remaining hidden and developing their own problems with substance misuse. Children who have experienced insecure attachments, severe discipline, feeling unloved or inadequate, constant criticism or denigration and parents who are unavailable through substance misuse are likely to grow up with little sense of self-worth. In such settings, children are likely to develop impaired cognitive skills, poor social behaviour, criminal involvement and substance misuse.

Serious substance misuse in the UK and other areas of the Western world is concentrated in areas of high social deprivation, inadequate housing, poverty and low employment. Poor educational involvement and achievement can contribute to an atmosphere of low expectation, which may increase the drift into substance misuse (Pearce and Hillman 1998). Where such conditions exist, easy availability of illicit drugs may be a compounding factor. Young people who are homeless or excluded from school, looked after children, those involved in sex work and those from some black and minority ethnic groups may also be at risk of substance misuse (NICE 2007a).

Peer pressure to become involved in substance misuse is often seen as a problem; however, this is more complex than simply being pressured by friends. Young people make choices about their peers, which reflect their needs for affiliation and identity. Crome (2004) states that peers using substances will be an influencing factor and factors such as social exclusion or alienation may be linked with this.

Resilience

Substance-using patterns can change spontaneously as young people mature; even young people at high risk can move away from a problematic pattern if they are able and motivated to make lifestyle changes and find appropriate supports. The recognition and promotion of protective factors is particularly consistent with the recovery focus with its emphasis on developing strengths rather than maintaining a problem-based focus (Scottish Executive 2006). Protective features are thought to be both individual and environmental. Being above-average intelligence, engaged academically, engaged in a leisure activity and having a positive temperament are indicative of resilience. Living with both parents and positive relationships within the family can promote resilience. Relationships outwith the family can also play a part such as having a positive significant relationship with a teacher or a youth worker. Having positive peer networks, skills training and improved parental expectation are additional protective factors. Peer relationships may also have a part to play in the reduction and cessation of substance use and we should take this into account in assessment.

12.7 Early intervention and recognition

Early recognition of the range of risks to the young person is not only essential for prevention, but can provide a framework for a pathway out of substance misuse (Bushell *et al.* 2002). Recent clinical guidelines stress that service failure to address other risk factors can work against the benefits of other interventions (DOH 2007). It is widely acknowledged that recognition of risk factors for early use provides a key opportunity for effective engagement in the prevention of more complex and entrenched patterns. Early interventions may also be a way of enabling young people to accomplish developmental tasks. Abstinence should be encouraged, and when not possible offer age-appropriate harm reduction strategies. An atmosphere of hope and optimism should be promoted.

 Activity

Substance misuse can often be a secret activity, engagement may therefore be difficult. Reflect on the steps you would take to engage a young person who you think may have a substance misuse problem.

12.8 Assessment

Young people in contact with health agencies should be screened to identify whether further assessment for substance abuse is required.

Screening consists of a short structured interview or a standardised tool, which should be applicable to all young people and be capable of use by a wide range of professionals (HAS 2001). The broad categories of screening and assessment may be distinguished by their intensity, the assessor's expertise and the intent and ability of the service to address the problem (Leccese and Waldron 1994). The screening process determines the need for a comprehensive assessment, which is an in-depth examination of the severity and nature of the problem and additional difficulties. Assessment methods must be multifaceted, collaborative and comprehensive if they are to facilitate understanding of the physical, psychological and social aspects of the young person's difficulties (Winters and Stinchfield 1995).

Specialist substance misuse assessments must complement existing assessments. The Common Assessment Framework for young people (DfES 2006) and the Asset (Youth Justice Board 2006) are standardised shared assessment tools, which include identification of the need for specialist assessment or intervention. The key principles of the specialist assessment process are:

- Assessment is part of the care
- Assessment is an ongoing process
- Young people and their parents or carers should participate
- The goals and process of assessment must be clear (National Treatment Agency for Substance Misuse) (NTA 2007: 4)

Assessment is an ongoing process and young people may take time to engage in a therapeutic relationship (NTA 2007). Substance use may often be hidden and young people may find it difficult to talk about their problems. However, many young people find it helpful to discuss their difficulties with a non-judgemental practitioner. Assessment is an intervention in itself and should be used to support young people to reflect on their own situation and identify their strengths and needs (NTA 2007).

 Activity

What are the advantages and disadvantages of involving the family of a young person in a plan to help the young person with their substance misuse problem?

The inclusion of parents and carers can make a significant difference to assessment. Parents can offer different perspectives on young people's difficulties and be active partners in facilitating change. However, parental involvement may be unhelpful if they are putting the young person at risk

(NTA 2007). Many young people are parents themselves and as the welfare of the child is paramount it is vital to assess the needs of their children. Serious and chaotic substance use is not compatible with effective parenting, as substance use can take priority over parenting responsibilities. Identifying the needs of the family, developing effective care plans, providing regular reviews and interagency support can ensure potential harm is reduced and families stay together (Scottish Executive 2006).

 Activity

Callum and Siobhann have developed a dependence on heroin. They are attending your service for help with their dependence – Siobhann is 20 weeks pregnant and both she and Callum are keen to do the best they can for the baby, while recognising that they find it difficult to be abstinent from heroin. What would you advise Siobhann and Callum about the pregnancy and substance use – what plan of action would you consider?

A comprehensive assessment should include the following:

- *Risk assessment* of the young person's substance use should be completed and interventions prioritised which minimise identified harms. The presence of more than one of the risk factors identified earlier increases the overall risk.
- *Demographic and contact details* should be collected at the point of contact and reviewed regularly: name, date of birth, address and type of accommodation, phone numbers, details of parental responsibility, cultural, ethnic and spiritual details, involvement with other agencies and referrer and GP details.
- *Identification of non-substance misuse needs* is crucial. A holistic assessment if not already conducted should be completed by the specialist substance misuse service. If an assessment exists elsewhere, it is important to access this and avoid duplication. Permission from the young person will be required to obtain this.
- *Substance misuse history* such as how it developed and the impact on lifestyle. Type of substance, age of first use, current and past patterns, frequency, duration and levels of use, routes of administration, combinations of substances used, injuries related to misuse and a history of previous attempts to change substance use should be considered.
- *Social impact of substance misuse.* Assessing the context and patterns of the young person's substance misuse will provide a greater understanding

of its impact, risks and triggers. These factors may help to decide appropriate interventions.

- *Health impact of substance misuse.* Substance use can both contribute to physical and psychological health and exacerbate any underlying or existing problems. Physical problems include breathing, heart conditions, pregnancy, sexually transmitted infections and blood-borne infections. Mental health difficulties include anxiety, depression, self-harm, suicidality, paranoia, psychosis and attention deficit hyperactivity disorder (ADHD).
- *Physical assessment* may be required – parental consent should be sought depending on the age of the young person. Tests (when indicated) may include drug toxicology, inspection of injection sites, blood tests and immunisations. If pharmacological treatment is indicated, physical dependence, tolerance, compliance with, and allergies to other medication, height and weight should all be assessed. A mental state assessment may also be indicated.
- *Assessing injecting behaviour* includes wound care, discussion of alternatives to injecting and reduction of frequency, safer techniques, overdose prevention/management and the legal implications of injecting. Under 18 year olds should be encouraged to stop completely, if this is not possible advice about harm reduction should be given. When injecting equipment is distributed, small amounts should be given to encourage regular contact (NTA 2007).

Assessment should be the first step towards a care plan where goals are set and interventions planned. Care plans should address physical, psychological and social functioning, criminal involvement, and child protection issues; to meet these needs interagency working is required (NTA 2007).

12.9 Intervention

Most young people who use substances (even problematically) reduce or stop using without any external help (HAS 2001). Intervention, when required, has the potential for quick progress and improvement due to the shorter duration of substance use and developmental changes in adolescence (DOH 2007).

To promote best practice, key principles have been designed for planning and delivering services for young people which are outlined in Box 12.4.

Box 12.4 Principles for Promoting Best Practice in Services for Children and Young People

> - A child or young person is not an adult.
> - The overall welfare of the individual child or young person is of paramount importance.
> - Services need to respect parental responsibility when working with a young person.
> - Services should recognise and co-operate with the local authority in carrying out its responsibilities towards children and young people.
> - A comprehensive range of services needs to be provided.
> - Services must be child centred.
> - Services should aim to operate, in all cases, according to the principles of good practice.
> - The views of the young person are of central importance, and should always be sought and considered.
> - A holistic approach is vital at all levels, as young people's problems tend to cross professional boundaries.
> - Services must be competent to respond to the needs of the young person.
>
> Source: Inspired from the Standing Conference on Drug Abuse (SCODA) and the Children's Legal Centre (CLC) (1999).

Due to lack of direct relevant research, interventions are often adapted from adult addiction or child and adolescent mental health sources (HAS 2001, Crome *et al.* 2004). Interventions must take into account the unique developmental needs of each young person and their cognitive, emotional and social development. Age, gender, sexual orientation, disability, ethnicity, cultural background and motivation must all be considered. Interventions should incorporate the young person's familial, cultural and environmental background. Parental and family support is often significant when working with young people. Young people receiving care in multiple settings require their treatment to be co-ordinated with statutory and non-statutory agencies working closely together (Aarons *et al.* 2001), facilitated by good communication between services (NICE 2007).

Using interim goals may be a way of reducing immediate harm and improving stability. Harm minimisation is now an accepted approach as many young people relapse. A further aim may be to help the young person move towards abstinence; however, unless detoxification is clearly indicated, young people benefit greatly from a period of stabilisation (DOH 2007). Key outcomes of an intervention are outlined in Box 12.5.

Box 12.5 Key Outcomes of an Intervention

Reducing drug use	Improving family relationships	Improving social relationships
Improving psychological well-being	Reducing the physical harm associated with drug use	Encouraging the uptake of other health and social services

Source: Inspired from Scottish Executive (2002c).

 Activity

Emily is 15 years old and is drinking a half litre bottle of gin every day. Her parents have been in contact with your service and want to know what is happening with her. They have been involved in family meetings but are not aware of the details of Emily's work on her alcohol problem. How would you proceed? Does your organisation have policies and procedures about information sharing and confidentiality – if so how do they help you to proceed?

Legal framework

Working with young people under the age of 16 presents ethical and moral challenges, particularly in relation to confidentiality and information sharing. Young people have a right to have their views taken into account and a right to consent to their own care but must demonstrate that they are competent and fully understand the consequences of the proposed treatment (The Age of Legal Capacity Act 1991 and The Children [Scotland] Act 1995 in Scotland and Gillick v West Norfolk Health Authority, 1985, and The Children Act 2004 in England).

Pharmacological interventions

The evidence base for pharmacological treatment of young people under 18 years is almost non-existent in the UK and currently medications for substance misuse are not recommended for children (Crome *et al.* 2004, DOH, 2007), therefore practitioners prescribe off-license utilising clinical guidelines.

> **Activity**
>
> Consider the advantages and disadvantages of using medication to treat someone with a substance misuse problem. Do you think there are any contradictions in such an approach – if so what do you think they are?

Young people with multiple dependencies may require a combination of pharmacological treatments. Pharmacological interventions for volatile substance use would be limited to treating physical emergencies. Although young people may experience considerable psychological withdrawal from cocaine, amphetamines or cannabis, substitute treatment is not recommended. Careful monitoring of a young person's mental health may be appropriate as cannabis in particular can contribute to or exacerbate mental health problems. Bingeing on benzodiazepines is more common than dependence in adolescents. Those who require detoxification should be stabilised then medication should be gradually reduced depending on the length and severity of dependence.

Alcohol use in adolescents is also mainly characterised by bingeing rather than dependence. If tolerance and dependence have been demonstrated, the use of chlordiazepoxide (a benzodiazepine which reduces anxiety and prevents withdrawal epileptic fits) is recommended to reduce withdrawal symptoms. Acamprosate (which reduces the craving for alcohol) can be prescribed to manage cravings in conjunction with counselling. Disulfiram or Antabuse (which produces an unpleasant physical reaction when taken with alcohol) can also be used as an adjunct to treatment (DOH 2007). Naltrexone (a narcotic antagonist which blocks the effects of heroin in the brain and can reduce the craving for alcohol), although not licensed in the treatment of alcohol dependence, may be used to reduce the desire to drink to excess.

For opioid dependence, the prescribing of methadone, buprenorphine (a partial opioid agonist analgesic) or lofexidine (which blocks the adrenaline/noradrenaline-related withdrawal symptoms of opiate withdrawal) is recommended for those under 18 years of age but only when there are clearly stated treatment aims. Prescribing should be initiated by a specialist or under specialist supervision. Medication should be consumed under supervision by a family member or a community pharmacist to monitor compliance and treatment effectiveness. Prior to prescribing, opiate use must be confirmed by toxicology, and dependence demonstrated by the presence of opiate withdrawal. Where there are doubts about dependence, lofexidine (a non-opioid medication) can be prescribed for symptomatic relief (DOH 2007).

Although abstinence may be the ultimate goal, maintenance can be considered a goal in its own right as it can facilitate the reduction or cessation of illicit opiate use and may have a positive impact on social difficulties and criminal activity (Lingford-Hughes *et al.* 2004). Careful monitoring of prescribing is required and attention should be paid to a young person's age and size when prescribing (DOH 2007). Methadone is effective as it is long acting, assists with withdrawals and is safe when titrated carefully (Kleber 1999); however, buprenorphine is less toxic in overdose, can be more rapidly increased and is less negatively perceived.

Additional psychological and social support is essential with relapse prevention to sustain long-term change. Naltrexone (an opiate blocker) may be used to support young people who have become opiate free; however, as there is insufficient evidence to evaluate Naltrexone's clinical effectiveness, it is recommended that it should only be commenced only by specialist services (Crome *et al.* 2004). The young person should also be motivated and be fully aware of the implications of medical treatment (DOH 2007).

Psychosocial interventions

The Minnesota 12-step programmes, culturally sensitive counselling, family therapy and behaviour therapy are effective in reducing drug use in young people (Scottish Executive 2002c). Family therapy is recommended as a first-line intervention and multi-systemic therapy should be used if a wider pattern of problems is evident. Structured family therapy is effective in its own right and can also enhance the effectiveness of other interventions. Motivational interviewing is effective and can be used to set goals, facilitate reflection on substance use, and motivation to change (Wolpert *et al.* 2006, NICE 2007). Alternative therapies such as acupuncture, reflexology and aromatherapy are under-evaluated; however, they are increasingly offered as a treatment adjunct (Crome 1999).

Young people with mental health problems and substance misuse share many of the same environmental and psychological risk factors as other young people. Previously interventions focused on medicalisation and stabilisation; however, intervention with problems in isolation may lead to the recurrence of co-morbid problems, therefore combined integrated interventions have become the approach of choice. A long-term approach which includes substance use counselling, social network interventions and addressing housing, employment, recreation, physical health and mental health issues may be helpful (Laudet *et al.* 2004). There is no single treatment programme or modality that can claim to respond fully to young people's needs. Matching an appropriate treatment plan with both the young person's current difficulties and needs should be a goal to maximise the treatment potential and optimise outcomes.

12.10　Conclusion

The social, psychological and physical development of children can be adversely affected by substance misuse, and young people are often stigmatised because of their substance misuse. For young people who are parents, further challenges need to be addressed, and the bonding, attachment and development of the child are likely to be affected by having parents who have an enduring substance misuse problem. Young people therefore need to have support plans and strategies in place at an early stage if they are to be helped to overcome these challenges. Identifying and intervening early before substance misuse becomes problematic is a goal of promotion, prevention and intervention services. However, this is a goal which can be difficult to achieve, as barriers such as the values and attitudes of service providers and the accessibility of services may get in the way. We have discussed the complexity and problematic nature of substance misuse and highlighted the importance of developing an approach which is multidisciplinary, involving joint working across all agencies.

The effects of early deprivation, domestic violence, abuse, poverty and trauma are implicated in the development of longstanding substance misuse problems. Intervention with young people with substance misuse problems relies heavily on the motivation of young people and the availability of emotional and community-based supports to bolster the young person. Substance misuse is a problem with a clear relationship to poverty and sometimes an absence of hope; it is an issue which needs to be addressed by political and societal means. Finally, working with children and young people with substance misuse problems involves examining and reflecting on our own values and attitudes – being open to challenge and change reflects a parallel process for both the young person and adults.

Recommended reading

Crome, I. B., McArdle, P., Gilvarry, E. and Bailey, S. (2004). Treatment. In: Crome, I. B., Ghodse, H., Gilvarry, E. and McArdle, P. (eds). *Young People and Substance Misuse*. London: Gaskell.

Lingford-Hughes, A. R., Welch, S. and Nutt, D. J. (2004). Evidence-based guidelines for the pharmacological management of substance misuse, addiction and co morbidity:

recommendations from the British Association for Psychopharmacology. *Journal of Psychopharmacology* 18 (3), 293–335.

National Treatment Agency for Substance Misuse (2007). *Assessing Young People for Substance Misuse*. London: NTA.

Scottish Executive (2006). *Hidden Harm. Next Steps. Supporting Children – Working with Parents*. Edinburgh: Scottish Executive.

Wolpert, M., Fuggle, P., Cottrell, D., *et al.* (2006). *Drawing on the Evidence: Advice for Mental Health Professionals Working with Children and Adolescents*, 2nd edition. London: CAMHS Publications.

REFERENCES

Aarons, G. A., Brown, S. A., Hough, R. L., Garland, A. F. and Wood, P. A. (2001). Prevalence of adolescent substance use disorders across five sectors of care. *Journal of the American Academy of Child and Adolescent Psychiatry* 40 (4), 419–426.

A Child in Trust (1985). *The Report of the Panel of Inquiry into the Circumstances Surrounding the Death of Jasmine Beckford*. London: London Borough of Brent.

ACMD (2003). *Hidden Harm: Responding to the Needs of Children of Problem Drug Users, Report of an Inquiry by the Advisory Council on the Misuse of Drugs*. London: Home Office.

Adams, S., Bishop, L. and Bellinger, J. (2007). Recovery through sport in first episode psychosis. In: Velleman, R., Davis, E., Smith, G. and Drage, M. (eds). *Changing Outcome in Psychosis Collaborative Cases from Practitioners, Users and Carers*. Oxford: BPS Blackwell.

Adcock, M. and White, R. (1985). *Good Enough Parenting: A Framework for Assessment*. London: British Agencies for Adoption and Fostering.

Amundson, J., Stewart, K. and Valentine, L. (1993). Temptations of power and certainty. *Journal of Marital and Family Therapy* 19 (2), 111–123.

Affinity Healthcare (2008). *New Survey Reveals Almost One in Three Young Females Have Tried to Self-harm*. Press release 25 April 2008. Available at http://www.affinityhealth.co.uk/pdf/SHS.pdf.

Ainsworth, M. D. S. (1979). Infant–mother attachment. *American Psychologist* 34, 932–937.

Ainsworth, M. D. S., Blehar, M., Waters, E. and Wall, S. (1978). *Patterns of Attachment*. Hillsdale, NJ: Erlbaum.

Alacqua, M., Trifirò, G., Arcoraci, V., *et al.* (2008). Use and tolerability of newer antipsychotics and antidepressants: a chart review in a paediatric setting. *Pharmacy World and Science Journal* 30, 44–50.

Allen, J. P., Hauser, S. T., Bell, K. L. and O'Connor, T. G. (1994). Longitudinal assessment of autonomy and relatedness in adolescent–family interactions as predictors of adolescent ego development and self-esteem. *Child Development* 65, 179–194.

Allen, L. (1995). Helping with deliberate self-harm: some practical guidelines. *Journal of Mental Health* 4, 243–250.

Understanding Children and Young People's Mental Health, first edition. Edited by Anne Claveirole and Martin Gaughan. Published 2011 by John Wiley & Sons Ltd. © 2011 John Wiley & Sons Ltd.

Alsaker, F. D. (1996). Timing of puberty and reactions to pubertal change. In: Rutter, M. (ed). *Psychological Disturbances in Young People: Challenges for Prevention*. Cambridge: Cambridge University Press.

Amato, P. R. and Keith, B. (1991). Parental divorce and the well-being of children: a meta-analysis. *Psychological Bulletin* 110, 26–46.

Ambrosini, P., Metz, C., Prabucki, K. and Lee, J. (1989). Videotape reliability of the third revised edition of the K-SADS. *Journal of the American Academy of Child and Adolescent Psychiatry* 28, 723–728.

Andersen, S. L. and Navalta, C. P. (2004). Altering the course of neuro-development: a framework for understanding the enduring effects of psychotropic drugs. *International Journal of Developmental Neuroscience* 22 (5–6), 423–440.

Anderson, J. C., Williams, S., McGee, R and Silva, P. A (1987). DSM-III disorders in preadolescent children: prevalence in a large sample from the general population *Archives of General Psychiatry* 44, 69–76.

Andersson, T. and Magnusson, D. (1990). Biological maturation in adolescence and the development of drinking habits and alcohol abuse among young males: a prospective longitudinal study. *Journal of Youth and Adolescence* 19, 33–42.

Angold, A. and Costello, E. (2000). The Child and Adolescent Psychiatric Assessment (APA). *Journal of the American Academy of Child and Adolescent Psychiatry* 39, 39–48.

Angold, A., Costello, E. J., Pickles, A., Messer, S. C., Winder, F. and Silva, D. (1995). The development of a short questionnaire for use in epidemiological studies of depression in children and adolescents. *Methods in Psychiatric Research* 5, 237–249.

Angold, A., Costello, E. J. and Worthman, C. M. (1998). Puberty and depression: the roles of age, pubertal status and pubertal timing. *Psychological Medicine* 28, 51–61.

APA (1994). *Diagnostic and Statistical Manual of Mental Disorders*, 4th edition (DSM-IV). Washington, DC: APA.

APA (2000). *Diagnostic and Statistical Manual of Mental Disorders*, 4th edition – Text Revised (DSM-IV-TR). Washington, DC: APA.

Arabi, M., Cox, A. and Martins, V. (2007). Foreword. In: Spandler, H. and Warner, S. (eds). *Beyond Fear and Control: Working with Young People Who Self-harm*. Ross on Wye: PPCS Books.

Armstrong, T. (2006). Canaries in the coal mine: the symptoms of children labelled 'ADHD' as biocultural feedback. In: Lloyd, G., Stead, J. and Cohen, D. (eds). *Critical New Perspectives on ADHD*. London: Routledge.

Arnett, J. J. (2002). The psychology of globalisation. *American Psychologist* 57 (10), 774–783.

Arnold, L. and Magill, L. (1998). *The Self-harm Help Book*. Bristol: Basement Project.

Arnsten, A. F. (2006). Fundamentals of attention-deficit/hyperactivity disorder: circuits and pathways. *Clinical Psychiatry* 67 (Suppl. 8), 7–12.

Arseneault, L., Cannon, M., Witton, J. and Murray, R. M. (2004). Causal association between cannabis and psychosis: Examination of the evidence. *The British Journal of Psychiatry* 184, 110–117.

Asarnow, J. R., Tompson, M. C. and Goldstein, M. J. (1994). Childhood onset schizophrenia: A follow-up study. *Schizophrenia Bulletin* 20 (4), 599–617.

Asarnow, R. F. and Asarnow, J. R. (1994). Childhood onset schizophrenia. *Schizophrenia Bulletin* 20, 591–597.

Aseltine, R. H., Jr., Amy, J., Schilling, E. A. and Glanovsky, J. (2007). Evaluating the SOS suicide prevention program: a replication and extension. *BMC Public Health* 7, 161.

Askey, R., Gamble, C. and Gray, R. (2007). Family work in first-onset psychosis: a literature review. *Journal of Psychiatric and Mental Health Nursing* 14, 356–365.

Asperger, H. (1944). Autistic psychopathy in childhood. In: Frith, U. (ed). *Autism and Asperger's Syndrome*. Cambridge: Cambridge University Press.

Attwood, J. (2001). *Supporting Children with ADHD*. Questions Publishing Company.

Attwood, T. (2007). *The Complete Guide to Asperger's Syndrome*. London: Jessica Kingsley Publishers.

Audini, B. and Lelliott, P. (2002). Age, gender and ethnicity of those detained under Part II of the Mental Health Act 1983. *The British Journal of Psychiatry* 180, 222–226.

Auyeung, B., Baron-Cohen, S., Ashwin, E., Knickmeyer, R., Taylor, K. and Hackett, G. (2009). Fetal testosterone and autistic traits. *British Journal of Psychology* 100, 1–22.

Babiker, G. and Arnold, L. (1997). *The Language of Injury: Comprehending Self-Mutilation*. Leicester: BPS Books.

Baird, G., Simonoff, E., Pickles, A., *et al.* (2006). Prevalence of disorders of the autism spectrum in a population cohort of children in South Thames: the Special Needs and Autism Project (SNAP). *The Lancet* 368 (9531), 179–181.

Baker, A. and Velleman, R. (2007). *Mental Health and Drug and Alcohol Problems*. Hove: Routledge.

Balding, J. W. (2005). *Young People in 2004*. Exeter: School Health Education Unit.

Bamberg, M. (2001). Why young American English-speaking children confuse anger and sadness: a study of grammar in practice. In: Nelson, K., Aksu-Koc, A. and Johnson, C. (eds). *Children's Language, Vol. 10: Language in Use, Narratives and Interaction*. Mahwah, NJ: Lawrence Erlbaum Associates.

Baral, I., Kora, K., Yueksel, S. and Sezgin, U. (1998). Self-mutilating behaviour of sexually abused female adults in Turkey. *Journal of Interpersonal Violence* 13 (4), 427–437.

Barber, B. K. (1996). Parental psychological control: revisiting a neglected construct. *Child Development* 67, 3296–3319.

Barber, B. K. (ed) (2002). *Parental Psychological Control of Children and Adolescents*. Washington, DC: American Psychological Association.

Barber, J. G. and Delfabbro, P. H. (2004). *Children in Foster Care*. London: Taylor and Francis.

Barker, P. and Buchanan-Barker, P. (2005). *The Tidal Model: A Guide for Mental Health Professionals*. London: Routledge.

Barkley, R. A. (1997). Behavioural inhibition, sustained attention, and executive functions: constructing a unifying theory of ADHD. *Psychological Bulletin* 121, 65–94.

Barkley, R. A. and 78 Co-endorsers (2002). International consensus statement on attention deficit hyperactivity disorder. *Clinical Child and Family Psychology Review* 5, 89–111.

Barnes, T. R. E. and Drake, R. (2007). Pharmacological strategies for relapse prevention in schizophrenia. *Psychiatry* 6 (9), 351–356.

Baron-Cohen, S. (2001). Theory of mind in normal development and autism. *Prisme* 34, 174–183.

Baron-Cohen, S. (2002). *The Extreme Male Brain Theory of Autism*. Cambridge, UK: Autism Research Centre.

Baron-Cohen, S., Leslie, A. M. and Frith, U. (1985). Does the autistic child have a 'theory of mind'? *Cognition* 21, 37–46.

Bass, C. and Adshead, G. (2007). Fabrication and induction of illness in children: the psychopathology of abuse. *Advances in Psychiatric Treatment* 13, 169–177.

Batchelor, J. and Kerslake, A. (1990). *Failure to Find Failure to Thrive: The Case for Improved Screening, Prevention and Treatment in Primary Care*. Croydon: Whiting and Birch.

Bateman, B., Warner, J. O., Hutchinson, E., *et al.* (2004). The effects of a double blind, placebo controlled, artificial food colourings and benzoate preservative challenge on hyperactivity in a general population sample of preschool children. *Archives of Disease in Childhood* 89 (6), 506–511.

Bauer, N. S. and Webster-Stratton, C. (2006). Prevention of behavioral disorders in primary care. *Current Opinions in Pediatry* 18, 654–660.

Bauermeister, J., Matos, M., Reina, G., *et al.* (2005). Comparison of the DSM-IV combined and inattentive types of ADHD in a school-based sample of Latino/Hispanic children. *The Journal of Child Psychology and Psychiatry* 46, 166–179.

Beautrais, A. L. (2004). *Suicide Postvention. Support for Families, Friends and Significant Others After a Suicide: A Literature Review and Synthesis of Evidence*. New Zealand: Ministry of Youth Affairs.

Bebbington, P. E., Bhugra, D., Brugha, T., *et al.* (2004). Psychosis, victimisation and childhood disadvantage: evidence from the second British National Survey of Psychiatric Morbidity. *The British Journal of Psychiatry* 185, 220–226.

Beck, A. T., Mendelson, M. and Mock, J. (1961). Inventory for measuring depression. *Archives of General Psychiatry* 4, 561–571.

Beck, A. T., Kovacs, M. and Weissman, A. (1979). Assessment of suicidal intention: the scale for suicidal intention. *Journal of Consulting and Clinical Psychology* 47, 343–352.

Beckett, C. (2002). *Human Growth and Development*. New York: Sage.

Bellamy, C. (2005). *The State of the World's Children 2005: Childhood Under Threat*. New York: United Nations' Children's Fund (UNICEF). Available at http://www.unicef.org/publications/files/SOWC_2005_(English).pdf.

Belsky, J. and Nezworski, T. (1988). *Clinical Implications of Attachment*. Hillsdale, NJ: Erlbaum.

Benoit, D. and Parker, K. C. H. (1994). Stability and transmission of attachment across three generations. *Child Development* 65, 1444–1456.

Bentall, R. P. (2003). *Madness Explained*. Allen Lane: Penguin Books.

von Bertalanffy, L. (1968). *General Systems Theory*. New York: Braziller.

Bertelsen, M., Jeppesen, P., Petersen, L., *et al.* (2007). Suicidal behaviour and mortality in first-episode psychosis: The OPUS trial. *The British Journal of Psychiatry* 191, s140–s146.

Bertolote, J. and McGorry, P. (2005). Early intervention and recovery for young people with early psychosis: consensus statement. *The British Journal of Psychiatry* 187 (Suppl. 48), 116–119.

Berzonsky, M. D. and Lombardo, J. P. (1983). Pubertal timing and identity crisis: a preliminary investigation. *The Journal of Early Adolescence* 3 (3), 239–246.

Bhardwaj, A. (2001). Growing up young, Asian and female in Britain: a report on self-harm and suicide. *Feminist Review* 68, 52–68.

Bhugra, D., Desai, M. and Baldwin, D. S. (1999). Attempted suicide in West London. I: Rates across ethnic communities. *Psychological Medicine* 29, 1125–1130.

Biddle, L., Gunnell, D., Sharp, D. and Donovan, J. L. (2004). Factors influencing help seeking in mentally distressed young adults: a cross-sectional survey. *The British Journal of General Practice* 54 (501), 248–253.

Biddle, L., Brock, A., Brookes, S. and Gunnell, D. (2008). Suicide rates in young men in England and Wales in the 21st century: time trend study. *British Medical Journal* 336 (7643), 539–542.

Biederman, J., Spencer, T. J., Wilens, T. E., Prince, J. B. and Faraone, S. V. (2006). Treatment of ADHD with stimulant medications: response to Nissen's perspective in *The New England Journal of Medicine. Journal of the American Academy of Child and Adolescent Psychiatry* 45 (10), 1147–1150.

Birchwood, M., MacMillan, F., Hogg, B., Prasad, R., Harvey, C. and Bering, S. (1989). Predicting relapses in schizophrenia: the development and implementation of an early signs monitoring system using patients and families as observers: a preliminary investigation. *Psychological Medicine* 19, 649–656.

Birleson, P. (1981). The validity of depressive disorder in childhood and the development of a self-rating scale: a research report. *Journal of Child Psychology and Psychiatry* 22, 73–88.

Birmaher, B., Waterman, S. G., Ryan, N. D., *et al.* (1998). Randomized, controlled trial of amitriptyline versus placebo for adolescents with treatment-resistant major depression. *Journal of the American Academy of Child and Adolescent Psychiatry* 37 (5), 527–535.

Birman, D. and Trickett, E. J. (2001). Cultural transitions in first-generation immigrants: acculturation of Soviet Jewish refugee adolescents and parents. *Journal of Cross-Cultural Psychology* 32, 456–477.

Black, D. (1993). A brief history of child and adolescent psychiatry. In: Black, D. and Cottrell, D. (eds). *Seminars in Child and Adolescent Psychiatry*. London: Gaskell.

Block, J. and Robins, R. W. (1993). A longitudinal study of consistency and change in self-esteem from early adolescence to early adulthood. *Child Development* 64, 909–923.

Blum, L. M. (2007). Mother-blame in the Prozac nation: raising kids with invisible disabilities. *Gender and Society* 21 (2), 202–226.

Boeing, L., Murray, V., Pelosi, A., McCabe, R., Blackwood, D. and Wrate, R. (2007). Adolescent onset psychosis: prevalence, needs and service provision. *The British Journal of Psychiatry* 190, 18–26.

Bogdashina, O. (2003). *Sensory Perception Issues in Autism and Asperger's Syndrome: Different Sensory Experience – Different Perceptual Worlds*. London: Jessica Kingsley Publications.

Bonner, R. L. (1990). A 'M.A.P.' to the clinical assessment of suicide risk. *Journal of Mental Health Counselling* 12, 232–236.

Bosman, M. and van Meijel, B. (2008). Perspectives of mental health professionals and patients on self-injury in psychiatry: a literature review. *Archives of Psychiatric Nursing* 22 (4), 180–189.

Bouras, N. and Holt, G. (eds) (2002). *Psychiatric and Behavioural Disorders in Intellectual and Developmental Disabilities*, 2nd edition. Cambridge: Cambridge University Press.

Bowen, M. (1978). *Family Therapy in Clinical Practice*. New York: Aronson.

Bowlby, J. (1944). Forty-four juvenile thieves: their characters and home-life. *International Journal of Psychoanalysis* 25, 19–53, 107–128.

Bowlby, J. (1951). *Maternal Care and Mental Health*. Geneva: WHO monograph series No. 2.

Bowlby, J. (1969). *Attachment and Loss, Vol. 1: Attachment*. New York: Basic Books.

Bowlby, J. (1973). *Attachment and Loss, Vol. 2: Separation: Anxiety and Anger*. New York: Basic Books.

Bowlby, J. (1979). *The Making and Breaking of Affectional Bonds*. London: Tavistock.

Bowlby, J. (1988). *A Secure Base*. New York: Basic Books.

Bradshaw, J. (2005). Child poverty and deprivation. In: Bradshaw, J. and Mayhew, E. (eds). *The Well-being of Children in the UK*. London: Save the Children Fund and the University of York.

Bradshaw, J. and Mayhew, E. (eds) (2005). *The Well-being of Children in the UK*. London: Save the Children Fund and the University of York.

Brain, K. L., Haines, J. and Williams, C. L. (1998). The psychophysiology of self-mutilation: evidence of tension reduction. *Archives of Suicide Research* 4, 227–242.

Bramlett, M. D. and Mosher, W. D. (2001). First marriage dissolution, divorce and remarriage in the United States. *Advance Data from Vital and Health Statistics*. Washington, DC: National Centre for Health Statistics.

Brennan, K. A., Clark, C. L. and Shaver, P. R. (1998). Self-report measurement of adult attachment: an integrative overview. In: Simpson, J. A. and Rholes, W. S. (eds). *Attachment Theory and Close Relationships*. New York: Guildford Press.

Brent, B. K. and Giuliano, A. J. (2007). Psychotic-spectrum illness and family-based treatments: a case-based illustration of the underuse of family interventions. *Harvard Review of Psychiatry* 15 (4), 161–168.

Brent, D., Greenhill, L., Compton, S., *et al.* (2009). The treatment of Adolescent Suicide Attempters Study (TASA): predictors of suicidal events in an open treatment trial. *Journal of the American Academy of Child and Adolescent Psychiatry* 48 (10), 987–996.

Brezo, J., Paris, J., Vitaro, F., Hébert, M., Tremblay, R. E. and Turecki, G. (2008). Predicting suicide attempts in young adults with histories of childhood abuse. *The British Journal of Psychiatry* 193, 134–139.

Brooks-Gunn, J. and Reiter, E. O. (1990). The role of pubertal processes. In: Feldman, S. S. and Elliott, G. R. (eds). *At the Threshold: The Developing Adolescent*. Cambridge, MA: Harvard University Press.

Brooks-Gunn, J. and Warren, M. P. (1985). Effects of delayed menarche in different contexts: dance and nondance students. *Journal of Youth and Adolescence* 14, 285–300.

Brown, M. and Marshall, K. (2006). Cognitive behaviour therapy and people with learning disabilities: implications for developing nursing practice. *Journal of Psychiatric and Mental Health Nursing* 13, 234–241.

Brown, T. E. (2005). *Attention Deficit Disorder: The Unfocused Mind in Children and Adults*. MA: Yale University Press.

Browne, K. and Hamilton-Giachritsis, C. (2007). Child abuse: defining understanding and intervening. In: Wilson, K. and James, A. (eds). *The Child Protection Handbook*, 3rd edition. London: Ballière Tindall Elsevier.

Brunstein Klomek, A., Marrocco, F., Kleinman, M., Schonfeld, I. S And Gould, M. S (2007). Bullying, Depression, and Suicidality in Adolescents *Journal of the American Academy of Child and Adolescent Psychiatry* 46 (1), 40–49.

Bryant-Waugh, R. and Lask, B. (2007). Overview of the eating disorders. In: Lask, B. and Bryant-Waugh, R. (eds). *Eating Disorders in Childhood and Adolescence*, 3rd edition. Hove: Routledge.

Bschor, T. (2002). Masked depression: the rise and fall of a diagnosis. *Psychiatrische Praxis* 29, 207–210.

Buchanan, C. M., Eccles, J. S., Flanagan, C., Midgley, C., Feldlaufer, H. and Harold, R. (1990). Parents' and teachers' beliefs about adolescents: effects of sex and experience. *Journal of Youth and Adolescence* 19, 363–394.

Buchanan, C. M., Maccoby, E. E. and Dornbusch, S. M. (1996). *Adolescents After Divorce*. Cambridge, MA: Harvard University Press.

Buitelaar, J. K. and Rothenberger, A. (2004). ADHD in the scientific and political context. *European Child and Adolescent Psychiatry* 13 (Suppl. 1), 1–6.

Burns, J., Dudley, M., Hazell, P. and Patton, G. (2005). Clinical management of deliberate self-harm in young people: the need for evidence-based approaches to reduce repetition. *The Australian and New Zealand Journal of Psychiatry* 39 (3), 121–128.

Bushell, H., Crome, I. and Williams, R. (2002). How can risk be related to interventions for young people who misuse substances? *Current Opinion in Psychiatry* 15 (4), 355–360.

Butler-Sloss, E. (1988). *The Report of the Enquiry into Child Abuse in Cleveland 1987*. London: HMSO.

Butzlaff, R. L. and Hooley, J. M. (1988). Expressed emotions and psychiatric relapse: a meta-analysis. *Archives of General Psychiatry* 55, 547–552.

Bye, K. (2008). Alcohol and homicide in Eastern Europe. *Homicide Studies* 12, 7–27.

Byng-Hall, J. (1995). *Rewriting Family Scripts: Improvisation and Systems Change*. London: Guildford.

Cameron, R. (2007). Calming down: self-injury and stress control. In: Spandler, H. and Warner, S. (eds). *Beyond Fear and Control: Working with Young People Who Self-harm*. Ross on Wye: PPCS Books.

Campbell, A. S. (2004). How was it for you? Families' experiences of receiving behavioural family therapy. *Journal of Psychiatric and Mental Health Nursing* 11, 261–267.

Canetto, S. S. (1997). Meanings of gender and suicidal behaviour during adolescence. *Suicide and Life-Threatening Behaviour* 27 (4), 339–351.

Canetto, S. S. and Lester, D. (1998). Gender, culture and suicidal behaviour. *Transcultural Psychiatry* 35, 163–191.

Canetto, S. S. and Sakinofsky, I. (1998). The gender paradox in suicide. *Suicide and Life-Threatening Behavior* 28 (1), 1–23.

Cannon, M., Caspi, A., Moffitt, T. E., *et al.* (2002). Evidence for early-childhood, pandevelopmental impairment specific to schizophreniform disorder: results from a longitudinal birth cohort. *Archives of General Psychiatry* 59 (5), 449–456.

Carr, A. (2000). *Family Therapy: Concepts, Process and Practice*. London: Wiley.

Carr, A. (2006). *The Handbook of Child and Adolescent Clinical Psychology: A Contextual Approach*, 2nd edition. London: Routledge.

Carr, A. and O'Reilly, G. (2004). *Clinical Psychology in Ireland, Vol. 5: Empirical Studies of Child Sexual Abuse*. Wales: Edwin Mellen Press cited in Carr, A. (ed) (2006). *The Handbook of Child and Adolescent Clinical Psychology*, 2nd edition. London: Routledge.

Carson, G. C., Claire, I. C. H and Murphy, G. H (1998). Assessment and Treatment of self-injury with a man with a profound learning disability *British Journal of Learning Disabilities* 26 (2) 51–57.

Carter, B. and McGoldrick, M. (1999). Overview. In: Carter, B. and McGoldrick, M. (eds). *The Expanded Family Life Cycle*, 3rd edition. London: Allyn and Bacon.

Carter, G. L., Clover, K., Whyte, I. M., Dawson, A. H. and D'Este, C. (2007). Postcards from the EDge: 24-month outcomes of a randomised controlled trial for hospital-treated self-poisoning. *The British Journal of Psychiatry* 191, 548–553.

Casey, B. J., Nigg, J. T. and Durston, S. (2007). New potential leads in the biology and treatment of attention deficit-hyperactivity disorder. *Current Opinion in Neurology* 20 (2), 119–124.

Caspi, A. and Bem, D. (1990). Personality continuity and change across the life course. In: Pervin, L. A. (ed). *Handbook of Personality Theory and Research*. New York: Guilford.

Caspi, A., Lynam, D., Moffit, T. and Silva, P. A. (1993). Unravelling girls' delinquency: biological, dispositional, and contextual contributions to adolescent misbehaviour. *Developmental Psychology* 29, 19–30.

Cassidy, J. (2000). Adult romantic attachments: a developmental perspective on individual differences. *Review of General Psychology* 4 (2), 107–110.

Cattan, M. and Tilford, S. (2006). *Mental Health Promotion: A Lifespan Approach*. Maidenhead: Open University Press, McGraw-Hill Education.

Cawson, P., Wattam, C., Brooker, S. and Kelly, G. (2000). *Child Maltreatment in the United Kingdom: A Study of the Prevalence of Child Abuse and Neglect*. London: NSPCC.

Centre for Suicide Research (2010). *Rates of Suicide and Open Verdicts in England and Wales 1968–2007: Males*. Source Office of National Statistics. Available at http://cebmh.warne.ox.ac.uk/csr/msui6808.html.

Cepeda, C. (2000). *The Psychiatric Interview of Children and Adolescents*. WA: American Psychiatric Press.

Chakrabarti, S. and Fombonne, E. (2001). Pervasive developmental disorders in pre-school children. *Journal of the American Medical Association* 285, 3093–3099.

Chaplin, T. M., Gillham, J. E., Reivich, K., *et al.* (2006). Depression prevention for early adolescent girls: a pilot study of all girls versus co-ed groups. *The Journal of Early Adolescence* 26, 110.

Chapman, D. P., Whitfield, C. L., Felitti, V. J., Dube, S. R., Edwards, V. J. and Anda, R. F. (2004). Adverse childhood experiences and the risk of depressive disorders in adulthood. *Journal of Affective Disorders* 82, 217–225.

Chavira, D. A., Stein, M. B., Bailey, K. and Stein, M. T. (2004). Comorbidity of generalized social anxiety disorder and depression in a pediatric primary care sample. *Journal of Affective Disorders* 80 (2–3), 163–171.

Chen, E., Hui, C., Lam, M., *et al.* (2008). A double-blind randomized placebo-controlled study of relapse prevention in remitted first-episode psychosis patients following one year of maintenance therapy. *Schizophrenia Research* 98, 11–12.

Child Poverty Action Group – CPAG (2009). *Child Well-being and Child Poverty – Where the UK Stands in the European Table*. London: Child Poverty Action Group. Available at http://www.cpag.org.uk/info/ChildWellbeingandChildPoverty.pdf.

Children Act (1989). London: HMSO.

Children Act (2004). London: HMSO.

Children (Northern Ireland) Order (1995). Belfast: HMSO.

Children (Scotland) Act (1995). Edinburgh: HMSO.

Choose Life (2010). *Choose Life: The National Action Plan to Prevent Suicide in Scotland: Statistics*. Available at http://www.chooselife.net/Statistics/Overview.asp.

Chu, S. and Reynolds, F. (2007a). Occupational therapy for children with attention deficit hyperactivity disorder (ADHD). Part 1: A delineation model of practice. *British Journal of Occupational Therapy* 70 (9), 372–383.

Chu, S. and Reynolds, F. (2007b). Occupational therapy for children with attention deficit hyperactivity disorder (ADHD). Part 2: A multi-centre evaluation of an assessment and treatment package. *British Journal of Occupational Therapy* 70 (10), 439–448.

Clarke, D. (1999). Functional psychoses in people with mental retardation. In: Bouras, N. (ed). *Psychiatric and Behavioural Disorders in Developmental Disabilities and Mental Retardation.* Cambridge: Cambridge University Press.

Clarke, G. N., Hawkins, W., Murphy, M., Sheeber, L., Lewinsohn, P. M. and Seeley, J. R. (1995). Targeted prevention of unipolar depressive disorder in an at-risk sample of high school adolescents: a randomized trial of a group cognitive intervention. *Journal of the American Academy of Child and Adolescent Psychiatry* 34, 312–321.

Claveirole, A. (2005). *Listening to the Voice in Four Scottish Adolescent Mental Health Units: Young People, their Carers and the Unit Cultures.* Unpublished PhD Thesis, Edinburgh Napier University, Edinburgh.

Claveirole, A., Gaughan, M., Hindle, D. and Wrate, R. (2006). *New-to-CAMHS Teaching Package.* HeadsUpScotland: National Project for Children and Young People's Mental Health, Scotland. Available at http://www.nes.scot.nhs.uk/mentalhealth/publications/documents/NewToCAMHS-FINAL.pdf.

Clyde, J. (1992). *The Report of the Enquiry into the Removal of Children from Orkney in February 1991.* Edinburgh: HMSO.

Coghill, D. (2006). The value and limitations of the concepts of ADHD and hyperkinetic disorder in guiding treatment – a clinical perspective. ADHD Consensus Conference to the NICE Guidelines Development Group, October 2006, in NICE (2009) *Attention Deficit Hyperactivity Disorder.*

Coghill, D., Spiel, G., Baldursson, G., *et al.* (2006). Which factors impact on clinician rated impairment in children with ADHD? *European Child and Adolescent Psychiatry* 13 (Suppl. 1), 117–129.

Coghill, D., Bonnar, S., Duke, S., Seth, S. and Graham, J. (2009). *The Oxford Handbook of Child and Adolescent Psychiatry.* Oxford: Oxford Medical Publications.

Cohen, D., Deniau, E., Maturana, A., *et al.* (2008). Are child and adolescent responses to placebo higher in major depression than in anxiety disorders? A systematic review of placebo-controlled trials. *PLoS One* 3 (7), e2632.

Carson, G. C., Claire, I. C. H. and Murphy, G. H. (1998). Assessment and treatment of self-injury with a man with a profound learning disability. *British Journal of Learning Disabilities* 26 (2), 51–57.

Cohen, D., Nicolas, J. D., Flament, M. F., *et al.* (2005). Clinical relevance of chronic catatonic schizophrenia in children and adolescents: evidence from a prospective naturalistic study. *Schizophrenia Research* 76, 301–308.

Colby, A. and Kohlberg, L. (1987). *The Measurement of Moral Judgement.* New York: Cambridge University Press.

Coleman, D. (2006). Interpersonal psychotherapy for depressed adolescents. *Child and Adolescent Social Work Journal* 23 (1), 127–130.

Coleman, J. (1978). Current contradictions in adolescent theory. *Journal of Youth and Adolescence* 7, 1–11.

Collins, K. A. and Dozois, D. J. A. (2008). What are the active ingredients in preventative interventions for depression? *Clinical Psychology: Science and Practice* 15 (4), 313–330.

Collishaw, S., Maughan, B., Goodman, R. and Pickles, A. (2004). Time trends in adolescent mental health. *Journal of Child Psychology and Psychiatry* 45 (8), 1350–1362.

Commander, M. J., Dharan, S. P., Odell, S. M., *et al.* (1997). Access to mental health care in an inner-city health district. I: Pathways into and within specialist psychiatric services. *The British Journal of Psychiatry* 170, 312–316.

Conners, C. K. (1997). *Conners' Ratings Scales Revised.* New York: Multi-Health Systems Inc.

Conrad, P. (2007). *The Medicalization of Society: On the Transformation of Human Conditions into Treatable Disorders.* Baltimore: The John Hopkins University.

Costello, E. J., Erkanli, A. and Angold, A. (2006). Is there an epidemic of child or adolescent depression? *Journal of Child Psychology and Psychiatry* 47 (12), 1263–1271.

Cotgrove, A., Zirinsky, L., Black, D. and Weston, D. (1995). Secondary prevention of attempted suicide in adolescence. *Journal of Adolescence* 18 (5), 569–577.

Coupland, C. and Cuss, T. (2007). Recovery from voice hearing through group work. In: Velleman, R., Davis, E., Smith, G. and Drage, M. (eds). *Changing Outcome in Psychosis Collaborative Cases from Practitioners, Users and Carers.* Oxford: BPS Blackwell.

Craig, T. K., Garety, P., Power, P., *et al.* (2004). The Lambeth Early Onset (LEO) Team: randomised controlled trial of the effectiveness of specialised care for early psychosis. *British Medical Journal* 329, 1067–1071.

Creighton, S. J. (2004). *Prevalence and Incidence of Child Abuse: International Comparisons.* London: NSPCC Research Department.

Crome, I. B. (1999). Treatment interventions – looking towards the millennium. *Drug and Alcohol Dependence* 55 (3), 247–263.

Crome, I. B. (2004). Comorbidity in young people: perspectives and challenges. *Acta Neuropsychiatrica* 16 (1), 47–53.

Crome, I. B., McArdle, P., Gilvarry, E. and Bailey, S. (2004). Treatment. In: Crome, I. B., Ghodse, H., Gilvarry, E. and McArdle, P. (eds). *Young People and Substance Misuse.* London: Gaskell.

Crowell, S. E., Beauchaine, T. P., McCauley, E., Smith, C. J., Vasilev, C. A. and Stevens, A. L. (2008). Parent–child interactions, peripheral serotonin, and self-inflicted injury in adolescents. *Journal of Consulting and Clinical Psychology* 76 (1), 15–21.

Croyle, K. L. (2007). Self-harm experiences among Hispanic and non-Hispanic White young adults. *Hispanic Journal of Behavioral Sciences* 29 (2), 242–253.

Cullberg, J., Wasserman, D. and Stefansson, C. (1988). Who commits suicide after a suicide attempt? An 8 to 10 year follow-up in a suburban catchment area. *Acta Psychiatrica Scandinavica* 77, 598–603.

Curry, J. F. and Reinecke, M. A. (2003). Modular cognitive behavior therapy for adolescents with major depression. In: Reinecke, M. A., Dattilio, F. M. and Freeman, A. (eds). *Cognitive Therapy with Children and Adolescents*, 2nd edition, pp. 95–127. New York: Guilford.

Dagnan, D. and Chadwick, P. (1997). Cognitive therapy with people with learning disabilities: assessment and intervention. In: Kroese, B., Dagnan, D. and Loumidis, K. (eds). *Cognitive Therapy for People with Learning Disabilities.* London: Routledge.

Dahlen, E. R. and Canetto, S. S. (2002). The role of gender and suicide precipitant in attitudes toward nonfatal suicidal behaviour. *Death Studies* 26, 99–116.

Damon, W. and Hart, D. (1988). *Self-understanding in Childhood and Adolescence.* New York: Cambridge University Press.

Daniel, B. and Wassell, S. (2002a). *Adolescence: Assessing and Promoting Resilience in Vulnerable Children 3*. London: Jessica Kingsley Publishers.

Daniel, B. and Wassell, S. (2002b). *The School Years: Assessing and Promoting Resilience in Vulnerable Children 2*. London: Jessica Kingsley Publishers.

David-Ferdon, C. and Kaslow, N. (2008). Evidence-based psychosocial treatments for child and adolescent depression. *Journal of Clinical Child and Adolescent Psychology* 37 (1), 62–104.

Davidson, L. and Strauss, J. (1995). Beyond the psychosocial model: integrating disorder, health and recovery. *Psychiatry* 58, 44–55.

De Bellis, M. D. (2005). The psychobiology of neglect. *Child Maltreatment* 10 (2), 150–172.

de Koning, M. B., Bloemen, O. J. N., van Amelsvoort, T. A. M. J., *et al.* (2009). Early intervention in patients at ultra high risk of psychosis: benefits and risks. *Acta Psychiatrica Scandinavica* 119, 426–442.

De Silva, M. J., McKenzie, K., Harpman, T. and Huttly, S. R. A. (2005). Social capital and mental illness: a systematic review. *Journal of Epidemiology and Community Health* 59, 619–627.

Deeley, Q. and Murphy, D. (2009). Pathophysiology of autism: evidence from brain imaging. *British Journal of Hospital Medicine* 70 (3), 138–142.

Department for Children, Schools and Families (2003). *Every Child Matters*. Available at http://www.dcsf.gov.uk/everychildmatters/.

Department for Education and Skills (2006). *Common Assessment Framework for Children and Young People Manager's Guide*. London: Department for Education and Skills.

Department of Health (2002). *National Suicide Prevention Strategy for England*. London: Department of Health.

Department of Health (2004). *The Ten Essential Shared Capabilities: A Framework for the Whole of the Mental Health Workforce*. London: Department of Health.

Department of Health (2007). *National Service Framework for Older People*. London: Department of Health.

Department of Health (2009). *New Horizons: Towards a Shared Vision for Mental Health*. London: DH Publications.

Department of Health, Social Services and Public Safety (2006). *Protect Life – A Shared Vision – The Northern Ireland Suicide Prevention Strategy*. Belfast: Northern Ireland Department of Health, Social Services and Public Safety.

Derby, K. M., Fisher, W. W., Piazza, C. C., Wilke, A. E. and Johnson, W. (1998). The effects of non-contingent attention for self injury, manding, and collateral responses. *Behaviour Modification* 22(4), 474–484.

DHSS (1974). *Report of the Committee of Inquiry into the Care and Supervision Provided in Relation to Maria Colwell*. London: HMSO.

Dollfus, S., Petit, M., Lesieur, P. and Menard, J. F. (1991). Principal component analysis of PANSS and SANS–SAPS global ratings in schizophrenia patients. *European Psychiatry* 6, 251–259.

Doménech-Llaberia, E., Viñas, F., Pla, E., *et al.* (2009). Prevalence of major depression in preschool children. *European Child and Adolescent Psychiatry* 18 (10), 597–604.

Dowrick, C., Katona, C., Peveler, R. and Lloyd, H. (2005). Somatic symptoms and depression: diagnostic confusion and clinical neglect. *The British Journal of*

General Practice: The Journal of the Royal College of General Practitioners 55 (520), 829–830.

Drury, V., Birchwood, M., Cochrane, R. and Macmillan, F. (1996a). Cognitive therapy and recovery from acute psychosis: a controlled trial. I. Impact on psychotic symptoms. *The British Journal of Psychiatry* 169, 593–601.

Drury, V., Birchwood, M., Cochrane, R. and Macmillan, F. (1996b). Cognitive therapy and recovery from acute psychosis: a controlled trial. II. Impact on recovery time. *The British Journal of Psychiatry* 169, 602–607.

Drury, V., Birchwood, M. and Cochrane, R. (2000). Cognitive therapy and recovery from acute psychosis: A controlled trial five-year follow-up. *The British Journal of Psychiatry* 177, 8–14.

Dudley, A. L., King, N. J., Melvin, G. A., Tonge, B. J. and Williams, N. J. (2005). Investigation of consumer satisfaction with cognitive–behaviour therapy and sertraline in the treatment of adolescent depression. *Australian and New Zealand Journal of Psychiatry* 39 (6), 500–506.

Dudley, R., Siitarinen, J., James, I. and Dodgson, G. (2009). What do people with psychosis think caused their psychosis? A Q methodology study. *Behavioural and Cognitive Psychotherapy* 37 (1), 11–24.

Dummett, N. and Williams, C. (2008). *Overcoming Teenage Low Mood and Depression: A Five Areas Approach.* London: Hodder Arnold.

Dunn, M. S., Goodrow, B., Givens, C. and Austin, S. (2008). Substance use behavior and suicide indicators among rural middle school students. *Journal of School Health* 78 (1), 26–31.

Durlak, J. A. and Wells, A. M. (1997). Primary prevention mental health programs for children and adolescents: A meta-analytic review. *American Journal of Community Psychology* 25 (2), 115–152 cited in SNAP (2000). *Mental Health Promotion Among Young People.* Glasgow: Office for Public Health in Scotland.

Durston, S., Mulder, M., Casey, B. J., *et al.* (2006). Activation in ventral prefrontal cortex is sensitive to genetic vulnerability to attention deficit hyperactivity disorder. *Biological Psychiatry* 60 (10), 1062–1070.

Eckersely, R. (1993). Failing a generation: the impact of culture on the health and well-being of youth. *Journal of Paediatrics and Child Health* 29 (Suppl. 1), S16–S19.

Edwards, J., Harris, M. G. and Bapat, S. (2005). Developing services for first-episode psychosis and the critical period. *The British Journal of Psychiatry* 187, s91–s97.

Eisenberg, M. E. and Resnick, M. D. (2006). Suicidality among gay, lesbian and bisexual youth: the role of protective factors. *The Journal of Adolescent Health* 39 (5), 662–668.

Elkind, D. (1967). Egocentrism in adolescence. *Child Development* 38, 1025–1034.

Emerson, E. and Hatton, C. (2007). Mental health of children and adolescents with intellectual disabilities in Britain. *The British Journal of Psychiatry* 191, 493–499.

Emslie, G. J., Kowatch, R., Costello, L. and Pierce, L. (1995). Double-blind study of fluoxetine in depressed children and adolescents. *42nd Meeting of the American Academy of Child and Adolescent Psychiatrists.* Washington, DC: New Orleans American Academy of Child and Adolescent Psychiatry.

Epstein, J. and Spirito, A. (2009). Risk factors for suicidality among a nationally representative sample of high school students. *Suicide and Life-Threatening Behavior* 39 (3), 241–251.

Erikson, E. H. (1968). *Identity: Youth and Crisis*. New York: Norton.

Erikson, E. H. (1980). *Identity and the Life Cycle*. New York: Norton.

European Commission (2008). *Mental Health in Youth and Education* consensus paper, Directorate-General for Health and Consumers.

Evans, E., Hawton, K., Rodham, K. and Deeks, J. (2005). The prevalence of suicidal phenomena in adolescents: a systematic review of population-based studies. *Suicide and Life-Threatening Behavior* 35 (3), 239–250.

Evren, C., Sar, V., Evren, B. and Dalbudak, E. (2008). Self-mutilation among male patients with alcohol dependency: the role of dissociation. *Comprehensive Psychiatry* 49 (5), 489–495.

Fadden, G. (1997). Implementation of family interventions in routine clinical practice following staff training programmes: a major cause for concern. *Journal of Mental Health* 6 (6), 599–612.

Fadden, G. (2006). Training and disseminating family interventions for schizophrenia: developing family intervention skills with multi-disciplinary groups. *Journal of Family Therapy* 28, 23–38.

Fairbairn, C. (2008). *Cognitive Behaviour Therapy and Eating Disorders*. London: The Guilford Press.

Falloon, I., Mueser, K., Gingerich, S., *et al.* (1996). *Behavioural Family Therapy: A Workbook*, 2nd edition. Buckingham, UK: Buckingham Mental Health Services.

Family and Parenting Institute (2009). *Family Trends: British Families Since the 1950s*. London: Family and Parenting Institute.

Famularo, R., Kinscherff, R. and Fenton, T. (1992). Psychiatric diagnoses of maltreated children: preliminary findings. *Journal of the American Academy of Child and Adolescent Psychiatry* 31, 863–867.

Faraone, S. V., Perlis, R. H., Doyle, A. E., *et al.* (2005). Molecular genetics of attention-deficit hyperactivity disorder. *Biological Psychiatry* 57, 1313–1323.

Faraone, S. V., Biederman, J. and Mick, E. (2006). The age-dependent decline of attention deficit hyperactivity disorder: a meta-analysis of follow-up studies. *Psychological Medicine* 36, 159–165.

Farhall, J., Greenwood, K. M. and Jackson, H. J. (2007). Coping with hallucinated voices in schizophrenia: a review of self-initiated strategies and therapeutic interventions. *Clinical Psychology Review* 27, 476–493.

Farrington, D. (1996). *Understanding and Preventing Youth Crime*. Joseph Rowntree Foundation, Social Policy Findings 93, York: JRF cited in MacDonald, R. and Marsh, J. (eds) (2005). *Disconnected Youth? Growing up in Britain's Poor Neighbourhoods*. Basingstoke: Palgrave.

Faulkner, S. (2007). Eating disorders, dieting and body image. In: Coleman, J. Hendry, L. and Kloep, M. (eds). *Adolescence and Health*. Chichester: John Wiley and Sons Ltd.

Favazza, A. R. (1989). Why patients mutilate themselves. *Hospital and Community Psychiatry* 40 (2), 137–145.

Favazza, A. R. (1992). Repetitive self-mutilation. *Psychiatric Annals* 22 (2), 60–63.

Favazza, A. R. (1998). The coming of age of self-mutilation. *Journal of Nervous and Mental Disease* 186, 259–268.

FDA Center for Drug Evaluation and Research (2004). *Background on Suicidality Associated with Antidepressant Drug Treatment (memorandum)*. Available at www.fda.gov/ohrms/dockets/ac/04/briefing/4006B1_03_Background%20Memo%2001–05–04.htm (accessed 10 July 2009).

Fedorowicz, V. J. and Fombonne, E. (2005). Metabolic side effects of atypical anti-psychotics in children: a literature review. *Journal of Psychopharmacology* 19 (5), 533–550.

Fedyszyn, I., Robinson, J., Matyas, T., Harris, M. and Paxton, S. (2010). Temporal pattern of suicide risk in young individuals with early psychosis. *Psychiatry Research* 175 (1–2), 98–103.

Fergusson, D., Horwood, L., Ridder, E. and Beautrais, A. (2005). Suicidal behaviour in adolescence and subsequent mental health outcomes in young adulthood. *Psychological Medicine* 35 (7), 983–993.

Fergusson, D. M. and Woodward, L. J. (2002). Mental health, educational, and social role outcomes of adolescents with depression. *Archives of General Psychiatry* 59, 225–231.

Fickl, T. (2007). Whose fear is it anyway? Working with young people who dissociate. In: Spandler, H. and Warner, S. (eds). *Beyond Fear and Control: Working with Young People Who Self-harm*. Ross on Wye: PCCS Books.

Fink, M. and Taylor, A. (2008). The medical evidence-based model for psychiatric syndromes: return to a classical paradigm. *Acta Psychiatrica Scandinavica* 117, 81–84.

Finkelhor, D. (1994). The international epidemiology of child sexual abuse. *Child Abuse and Neglect* 18 (5), 409–417.

Fjell, A., Bloch Thorsen, G., Friis, S., *et al.* (2007). Multifamily group treatment in a program for patients with first-episode psychosis: experiences from the TIPS project. *Psychiatric Services* 58 (2), 171–173.

Fleischmann, A., Bertolote, J. M., Belfer, M. and Beautrais, A. (2005). Completed suicide and psychiatric diagnoses in young people: a critical examination of the evidence. *American Journal of Orthopsychiatry* 75, 676–683.

Fleming, T. M., Merry, S. N., Robinson, E. N., Denny, S. J. and Watson, P. D. (2007). Self-reported suicide attempts and associated risk and protective factors among secondary school students in New Zealand. *Australian and New Zealand Journal of Psychiatry* 41 (3), 213–221.

Fliege, H., Lee, J., Grimm, A. and Klapp, B. (2009). Risk factors and correlates of deliberate self-harm behavior: a systematic review. *Journal of Psychosomatic Research* 66 (6), 477–493.

Fombonne, E. (2005a). Epidemiological surveys of autism and other pervasive developmental disorders: an update. *Journal of Autism and Developmental Disorders* 33 (4), 365–382.

Fombonne, E. (2005b). The changing epidemiology of autism. *Journal of Applied Research in Intellectual Disabilities* 18, 281–294.

Fonagy, P., Target, M., Cottrell, D., Phillips, J. and Kurtz, Z. (2002). *What Works for Whom? A Critical Review of Treatments for Children and Adolescents*. New York: The Guilford Press.

Ford, T., Goodman, R. and Meltzer, H. (2003). The British Child and Adolescent Mental Health Survey 1999: the prevalence of DSM-IV disorders. *Journal of the American Academy of Child and Adolescent Psychiatry* 42, 1203–1211.

Ford, T., Goodman, R. and Meltzer, H. (2004). The relative importance of child, family, school and neighbourhood correlates of childhood psychiatric disorder. *Social Psychiatry and Psychiatric Epidemiology* 39, 487–496.

Ford, T., Vostanis, P., Meltzer, H. and Goodman, R. (2007). Psychiatric disorder among British children looked after by local authorities: comparison with children living in private households. *The British Journal of Psychiatry* 190, 319–325.

Fortune, S. A. and Hawton, K. (2005). Deliberate self-harm in children and adolescents: a research update. *Current Opinion in Psychiatry* 18, 401–406.

Fotti, S. A., Katz, L. Y., Afifi, T. O. and Cox, B. J. (2006). The associations between peer and parental relationships and suicidal behaviours in early adolescents. *Canadian Journal of Psychiatry* 5, 698–703.

Foundation for People with Learning Disabilities (2002). *Count Us In. The Report of the Committee of Inquiry into Meeting the Mental Health Needs of Young People with Learning Disabilities*. London: Mental Health Foundation.

Fouskakis, D., Gunnell, D., Rasmussen, F., Tynelius, P., Sipos, A. and Harrison, G. (2004). Is the season of birth association with psychosis due to seasonal variations in foetal growth or other related exposures? A cohort study. *Acta Psychiatrica Scandinavica* 109, 259–263.

Fox, C. and Hawton, K. (2004). *Deliberate Self-harm in Adolescence*. London: Jessica Kingsley Publisher.

Frak, D. (2005). *A Report on the Work of the Recovery Learning Sites and Other Recovery-Orientated Activities and Its Incorporation into the Rethink Plan 2004–08*. London: Rethink.

Fraley, R. C. and Shaver, P. R. (1998). Airport separations: a naturalistic study of adult attachment dynamics in separating couples. *Journal of Personality and Social Psychology* 75, 1198–1212.

Freedman, J. and Combs, G. (1996). *Narrative Therapy: The Social Construction of Preferred Realities*. New York: WW Norton.

Freeman, C. (2002). *Overcoming Anorexia Nervosa: A Self-help Guide Using Cognitive Behavioural Techniques*. London: Robinson.

Freres, D. R., Gillham, J. E., Reivich, K., Shatté, A. J. and Seligman, M. E. P. (2002). Preventing depressive symptoms in middle school students: the Penn Resiliency Program. *International Journal of Emergency Mental Health* 4 (1), 31–40.

Freud, S. (1938). *An Outline of Psychoanalysis*. London: Hogarth Press.

Friedlander, R. I. and Donnelly, T. (2004). Early-onset psychosis in youth with intellectual disability. *Journal of Intellectual Disability Research* 48 (6), 540–547.

Friedman, M., Glasser, M., Laufer, E. and Laufer, M. (1996). Attempted suicide and self-mutilation in adolescence: some observations from a psychoanalytic research project. In: Maltsberger, J. T. and Goldblatt, M. (eds). *Essential Papers in Psychoanalysis*. New York: New York University Press.

Frischer, M., McArdle, P. and Crome, I. (2004). The epidemiology of substance misuse in young people. In: Crome, I. B., Ghodse, H., Gilvarry, E. and McArdle, P. (eds). *Young People and Substance Misuse*. London: Gaskell.

Frith, U. (1991). *Autism and Asperger's Syndrome*. Cambridge: Cambridge University Press.

Frith, U. and Happe, F. (1994). Autism beyond 'theory of mind'. *Cognition* 50, 115–132.

Frombone, E. (1998). Interpersonal psychotherapy for adolescent depression. *Child Psychology and Psychiatry Review* 3 (4), 169–175.

Frosh, S. (1991). *Identity Crisis: Modernity, Psychoanalysis and the Self*. London: Macmillan Education.

Gallup Organisation (2007). *The State of Global Well-being*. New York: Gallup Press.

Gardner, F. (2001). *Self-harm: A Psychotherapeutic Approach*. Hove: Brunner-Routledge.

Garety, P. A. and Hemsley, D. A. (1994). *Delusions: Investigations into the Psychology of Delusional Reasoning (Maudsley Monograph)*. Hove: Oxford University Press.

Gask, L., Dixon, C., Morriss, R., Appleby, L. and Green, G. (2006). Evaluating STORM skills training for managing people at risk of suicide. *Journal of Advanced Nursing* 54 (6), 739–750.

Geller, B., Reising, D., Leonard, H. L., Riddle, M. A. and Walsh, T. (1999). Critical review of tricyclic antidepressant use in children and adolescents. *Journal of the American Academy of Child and Adolescent Psychiatry* 38, 513–516.

Gelles, K. (1991). Physical violence, child abuse and homicide: a continuum of violence or distinct behaviours. *Human Nature* 2, 59–72.

General Register Office for Scotland (2010). Probable Suicides: Deaths which are the Result of Intentional Self-harm or Events of Undetermined Intent accessed 27/07/2010 http://www.gro-scotland.gov.uk/statistics/deaths/suicides/index.html

George, C., Kaplan, N. and Main, M. (1985). *The Attachment Interview*. Berkeley: University of California (Unpublished manuscript).

Ghate, D. and Hazell, N. (2002). *Parenting in Poor Environments*. London: Jessica Kingsley.

Ghaziuddin, M. (2005). *Mental Health Aspects of Autism and Asperger's Syndrome*. London: Jessica Kingsley.

Ghaziuddin, M., Al-Khouri, I. and Ghaziuddin, N. (2002). Autistic symptoms following herpes encephalitis. *European Child and Adolescent Psychiatry* 11 (3), 142–146.

Giedd, J. N., Blumenthal, J., Castellanos, X., *et al.* (1999). Brain development during childhood and adolescence: a longitudinal MRI study. *Nature Neuroscience* 2, 861–863.

Gillberg, C. (1991). Clinical and neurobiological aspects of Asperger syndrome in six family studies. In: Frith, U. (ed). *Autism and Asperger Syndrome*. Cambridge: Cambridge University Press.

Gillberg, C. (2002). *A Guide to Asperger Syndrome*. Cambridge: Cambridge University Press.

Gilligan, R. (2005). Enhancing the resilience of children and young people in public care by mentoring their talents and interests. In: Frost, N. (ed). *Child Welfare – Major Themes in Health and Social Welfare, Vol. III: Child Placement and Children Away from Home*. London: Routledge.

Gilligan, R. (2008). Promoting resilience in young people in long term care – the relevance of roles and relationships in the domains of recreation and work. *Journal of Social Work Practice* 22 (1), 37–50.

Glaser, D. and Prior, V. (1997). Is the term child protection applicable to emotional abuse? *Child Abuse Review* 6, 315–329.

Glaser, D. and Prior, V. (2002). Predicting emotional child abuse and neglect. In: Browne, K., Hanks, H., Stratton, P. and Hamilton, C. (eds). *Early Prediction and Prevention of Child Abuse: A Handbook*. Chichester: John Wiley and Sons Ltd.

Glaser, K. (1967). A masked depression in children and adolescents. *American Journal of Psychotherapy* 21, 565–574.

Goldberg, M., Mostofsky, S., Cutting, L., *et al.* (2005). Subtle executive impairment in children with autism and children with ADHD. *Journal of Autism and Developmental Disorders* 31, 433–440.

Goldstein, T., Axelson, D. A., Mirmaher, B. and Brent, D. A. (2007). Dialectical behaviour therapy for adolescents with bipolar disorder: a 1-year open trial. *Journal of the American Academy of Child and Adolescent Psychiatry* 46 (7), 820–830.

Goodman, R. and Scott, S. (2005). *Child Psychiatry*, 2nd edition. Oxford: Blackwell Publishing.

Goodyer, I., Dubicka, B., Wilkinson, P., *et al.* (2007). Selective serotonin reuptake inhibitors (SSRIs) and routine specialist care with and without cognitive behaviour therapy in adolescents with major depression: randomized controlled trial. *British Medical Journal* 335, 142.

Goodyer, I. M. (1990). *Life Experiences, Development and Childhood Psychopathology.* Chichester: John Wiley.

Goodyer, I. M. and Altham, P. M. E. (1991). Lifetime exit events and recent social and family adversities in anxious and depressed school-age children and adolescents – I. *Journal of Affective Disorders* 21, 219–228.

Gordon, H., Pryor, J. and Reynolds, J. (2001). *Not in Front of the Children? How Conflict Between Parents Affects Children.* London: One plus One Marriage and Partnership Research.

Gordon, R. (2001). Eating disorders East and West: a culture-bound syndrome unbound. In: Nasser, M., Katzman, M. and Gordon, R. (eds). *Eating Disorders and Cultures in Transition.* Hove: Brunner-Routledge.

Gosney, H. and Hawton, K. (2007). Inquest verdicts: youth suicides lost. *Psychiatric Bulletin* 31, 203–205.

Goss, K. and Gilbert, P. (2002). Eating disorders, shame and pride: a cognitive–behavioural functional analysis. In: Gilbert, P. and Miles, J. (eds). *Body Shame: Conceptualisation, Research and Treatment.* Hove: Brunner-Routledge.

Gottesman, I. I. (1991). *Schizophrenia Genesis: The Origins of Madness.* New York: W.H. Freeman and Co.

Gottesman, I. I., McGuffin, P. and Farmer, A. E. (1987). Clinical genetics as clues to the 'real' genetics of schizophrenia. *Schizophrenia Bulletin* 13, 23–47.

Gould, M., Greenberg, T., Velting, D. and Shaffer, D. (2003). Youth suicide risk and preventive interventions: a review of the past 10 years. *Journal of the American Academy Child and Adolescent Psychiatry* 42, 386–405.

Gowers, S. and Bryant-Waugh, R. (2004). Management of child and adolescent eating disorders: the current evidence base and future directions. *Journal of Child Psychology and Psychiatry* 45 (1), 63–83.

Gowers, S., Clark, A., Roberts, C., *et al.* (2007). Clinical effectiveness of treatments for anorexia nervosa in adolescents. *The British Journal of Psychiatry* 191, 427–435.

Graham-Bermann, S. A., DeVoe, E. R., Mattis, J. S., Lynch, S. and Thomas, S. A. (2006). Ecological predictors of traumatic stress symptoms in caucasian and ethnic minority children exposed to intimate partner violence. *Violence Against Women* 12 (7), 663–692.

Grandin, T. (1995). *Thinking in Pictures.* London: Vintage Books.

Gray, C. A. (2008). *Lay and Professional Constructions of Childhood ADHD (Attention Deficit Hyperactivity Disorder): A Discourse Analysis.* PhD Thesis, Queen Margaret University, Edinburgh.

Green, H., McGinnity, A., Meltzer, H., Ford, T. and Goodman, R. (2005). *Mental Health of Children and Young People in Great Britain, 2004. A Survey Carried Out by the Office for National Statistics on Behalf of the Department of Health and the Scottish Executive.* Basingstoke: Palgrave Macmillan.

Green, K. (2007). Finding your own voice social action group with young people. In: Spandler, H. and Warner, S. (eds). *Beyond Fear and Control: Working with Young People Who Self-harm.* Ross on Wye: PPCS Books.

Greene, K., Krcmar, M., Walters, L. H., Rubin, D. L. and Hale, J. (2000). Targeting adolescent risk-taking behaviours: the contributions of egocentrism and sensation-seeking. *Journal of Adolescence* 23, 439–461.

Griesbach, D., Russell, P., Dolev, R. and Lardner, C. (2008). *The Use and Impact of Applied Suicide Intervention Skills Training (ASIST) in Scotland: An Evaluation.* Edinburgh: The Scottish Government.

Grocutt, E. (2009). *Self-harm and Attachment. Managing Self-harm: Psychological Perspectives.* New York: Routledge/Taylor and Francis Group.

Grøholt, B., Ekeberg, O. and Haldorsen, T. (2000). Adolescents hospitalised with deliberate self-harm: the significance of an intention to die. *European Child & Adolescent Psychiatry* 9, 244–254.

Groossens, L. (1995). Identity status development and students' perception of the university environment: a cohort-sequential study. In: Oosterwegal, A. and Wicklund, R. A. (eds). *The Self in European and North American Culture: Development and Processes.* New York: Kluwer.

Grotevant, H. D. and Cooper, C. R. (1985). Patterns of interaction in family relationships and the development of identity exploration in adolescence. *Child Development* 56, 415–428.

Gumley, A., Karatzias, A., Power, K., Reilly, J., McNay, L. and O'Grady, M. (2006). Early intervention for relapse in schizophrenia: impact of cognitive behavioural therapy on negative beliefs about psychosis and self-esteem. *British Journal of Clinical Psychology* 45 (Part 2), 247–260.

Gunnell, D., Shepherd, M. and Evans, M. (2000). Are recent increases in deliberate self-harm associated with changes in socio-economic conditions? An ecological analysis of patterns of deliberate self-harm in Bristol 1972–3 and 1995–6. *Psychological Medicine* 30, 1197–1203.

Haddon, M. (2003). *The Curious Incident of the Dog in the Night-time.* London: Jonathan Cape.

Hahlweg, K., Goldstein, M., Neuecherterlein, K., *et al.* (1989). Expressed emotion and patient–relative interaction in families of recent onset schizophrenics. *Journal of Consulting and Clinical Psychology* 57, 11–18.

Haines, J. and Williams, C. L. (1997). Coping and problems of self-mutilators. *Journal of Clinical Psychology* 53 (2), 177–186.

Haines, J., Williams, C. L., Brain, K. L. and Wilson, G. V. (1995). The psychophysiology of self-mutilation. *Journal of Abnormal Psychology* 104 (3), 471–489.

Halpern-Felsher, B. L. and Cauffman, E. (2001). Costs and benefits of a decision. Decision-making competence in adolescents and adults. *Applied Developmental Psychology* 22, 257–273.

Hansard (2007). Written answers, House of Commons, 19 July 2007, Column 536W.

Hansson, K., Cederblad, M., Lichtenstein, P., *et al.* (2008). Individual resiliency factors from a genetic perspective: results from a twin study. *Family Process* 47 (4), 537–551.

Happe, F. (1995). The role of age and verbal ability in the theory of mind task performance of subjects with autism. *Child Development* 66, 843–855.

Happe, F., Ehlers, S., Fletcher, P., *et al.* (1996). Theory of mind: in the brain. Evidence from a PET scan study of Asperger's syndrome. *Clinical Neuroscience and Neuropathology* 8, 197–201.

Happe, F., Ronald, A. and Plomin, R. (2006). Time to give up on a single explanation for autism. *Nature Neuroscience* 9 (10), 1218–1220.

Harpin, V. A. (2005). The effect of ADHD on the life of an individual, their family and community from preschool to adult life. *Archives of Diseases in Childhood* 90 (Suppl. 1), 12–19.

Harrington, R. C. (2005). Depression. In: Rutter, M. and Taylor, E. (eds). *Child and Adolescent Psychiatry*, 4th edition. London: Blackwell.

Harrington, R. C., Kerfott, M., Dyer, E., *et al.* (1998). Randomized trial of a home-based family intervention for children who have deliberately poisoned themselves. *Journal of the American Academy of Child and Adolescent Psychiatry* 37 (5), 512–518.

Harris, M. C., Burgess, P. M., Chant, D. C., Pirkis, J. E. and McGorry, P. D. (2008). Impact of a specialized early psychosis treatment programme on suicide. Retrospective cohort study. *Early Intervention in Psychiatry* 2, 11–21.

Harrison, D. and Sharman, J. (2005). *Understanding Self-harm.* London: Mind Publications. Available at http://www.mind.org.uk/Information/.

Harrison, J. E. and Bolton, P. F. (1997). Annotation: tuberous sclerosis. *Journal of Child Psychology and Psychiatry* 38, 603–614.

Harrison, P. J. and Weinberger, D. R. (2005). Schizophrenia genes, gene expression, and neuropathology: on the matter of their convergence. *Molecular Psychiatry* 10, 40–68.

Harrist, A. W. and Waugh, R. M. (2002). Dyadic synchrony: its structure and function in children's development. *Developmental Review* 22, 555–592.

Harter, S. (1990). Self and identity development. In: Feldman, S. and Elder, G. (eds). *At the Threshold: The Developing Adolescent.* Cambridge, MA: Harvard University Press.

Harvey, S. B., Dean, K., Morgan, C., *et al.* (2008). Self-harm in first-episode psychosis. *The British Journal of Psychiatry* 192, 178–184.

Haslam, N., Williams, B., Prior, M., *et al.* (2006). The latent structure of attention deficit/hyperactivity disorder: a taxometric analysis. *Australian and New Zealand Journal of Psychiatry* 40, 639–647.

Hauser, S. and Allen, J. (2006). Overcoming adversity in adolescence: narratives of resilience. *Psychoanalytic Inquiry* 26 (4), 549–576.

Hauser, S. T., Powers, S. I. and Noam, G. G. (1991). *Adolescents and Their Families: Paths of Ego Development.* New York: Free Press.

Hawton, K. and James, A. (2005). ABC of adolescence: suicide and deliberate self harm in young people. *British Medical Journal* 330, 891–894.

Hawton, K., Fagg, J., Simkin, S., Bale, B. and Bond, A. (2000). Deliberate self-harm in adolescents in Oxford, 1985–1995. *Journal of Adolescence* 23, 47–55.

Hawton, K., Hall, S., Simkin, S., Bale, E., Bond, A. and Codd, S. (2003). Deliberate self-harm in adolescents: a study of characteristics and trends. *Journal of Child Psychology and Psychiatry* 44 (8), 1191–1198.

Hawton, K., Rodham, K. and Evans, E. (2006). *By Their Own Young Hand: Deliberate Self-harm and Suicidal Ideas in Adolescents.* London: Jessica Kingsley.

Hawton, K., Rodham, K., Evans, E and Weatherall, R. (2002). Deliberate self harm in adolescents: self report survey in schools in England *BMJ* 325, 1207–11.

Hayes, A. J., Shaw, J. J., Lever-Green, G., Parker, D. and Gask, L. (2008). Improvements to suicide prevention training for prison staff in England and Wales. *Suicide and Life-Threatening Behavior* 38 (6), 708–713.

Hazell, P., O'Connell, D., Heathcoat, D., Roberston, J. and Henry, D. (1995). Efficacy of tricyclic drugs in treating child and adolescent depression: a meta analysis. *British Medical Journal* 10, 897–901.

Hazell, P., O'Connell, D., Heathcote, D. and Henry, D. (2002). Tricyclic drugs for depression in children and adolescents. *Cochrane Database of Systematic Reviews* (Issue 2), Art. No.: CD002317.

Health Advisory Service (1995). *Together We Stand. The Commissioning, Role and Management of Child and Adolescent Mental Health Services.* London: HMSO.

Health Advisory Service (2001). *The Substance of Young Needs: Review 2001.* London: Home Office.

Helliwell, J. F. (2003). How's life: combining individual and national variables to explain subjective well-being. *Economic Modelling* 20, 331–360.

Helliwell, J. F. (2008). *Life Satisfaction and Quality of Development.* National Bureau of Economic Research (NBER Working Paper 14507), University of British Columbia, Canada, November 2008. Available at www.econ.ubc.ca/helliwell/.

Hendricks, C. B. and Bradley, L. J. (2005). Interpersonal theory and music techniques: a case study for a family with a depressed adolescent family. *Journal Counseling and Therapy for Couples and Families* 13 (4), 400–405.

Herrmann-Doig, T., Maude, D. and Edwards, J. (2002). *Systematic Treatment of Persistent Psychosis (STOPP): A Psychological Approach to Facilitating Recovery in Young People with First-Episode Psychosis.* London: Martin Dunitz.

Heyman, I. and Santosh, P. (2005). Pharmacological and other treatments. In: Rutter, M. and Taylor, E. (eds). *Child and Adolescent Psychiatry,* 4th edition. London: Blackwell.

Hindle, D. (1999). *Personality Development: A Psychoanalytic Perspective.* London: Routledge.

HM Government (2003). *Every Child Matters.* Norwich: The Stationery Office.

Hirsch, B. and DuBois, D. (1991). Self-esteem in early adolescence: the identification and prediction of contrasting longitudinal trajectories. *Journal of Youth and Adolescence* 20, 53–72.

Hoath, F. E. and Sanders, M. R. (2002). A feasibility study of Enhanced Group Triple P Positive Parenting Program for parents of children with attention deficit hyperactivity disorder. *Behaviour Change* 19 (4), 191–206.

Hodges, K., Kline, K., Stern, L., Cytryn, L. and McKnew, D. (1982). Diagnostic concordance between the Child Assessment Schedule (CAS) and the Schedule for Affective Disorders and Schizophrenia for school-age children (K-SADS) in an outpatient sample using lay interviewers. *Journal of the American Academy of Child and Adolescent Psychiatry* 26, 654–661.

Hogarty, G. E. (1995). Personal therapy. A disorder relevant psychotherapy for schizophrenia. *Schizophrenia Bulletin* 21, 379–393.

Hogarty, G. E. (2002). *Personal Therapy for Schizophrenia and Related Disorders: A Guide to Individualized Treatment.* London: Guilford Press.

Hogg, C. (2001). Should nurses always intervene when patients self-harm? No. *Nursing Times* 97 (49), 16.

Holmes, J. (1993). *John Bowlby and Attachment Theory.* London: Routledge.

Honig, A., Romme, M., Ensink, B., Escher, S., Pennings, M. and Vevries, M. (1998). Auditory hallucinations: a comparison between patients and nonpatients. *Journal of Mental and Nervous Disease* 186, 646–651.

Horwath, J. (2007). *Child Neglect: Identification and Assessment.* Basingstoke: Palgrave Macmillan.

Horwitz, A. V. and Wakefield, J. C. (2007). *The Loss of Sadness: How Psychiatry Transformed Normal Sorrow into Depressive Disorder.* New York: Oxford University Press.

Hunt, K., Sweeting, H., Keoghan, M. and Platt, S. (2006). Sex, gender role orientation, gender role attitudes and suicidal thoughts in three generations. A general population study. *Social Psychiatry and Psychiatric Epidemiology* 41 (8), 641–647.

Hutchings, J., Bywater, T. and Daley, D. (2007). A pragmatic randomised controlled trial of a parenting intervention in sure start services for pre-school children at risk of developing conduct disorder: How and why did it work? *Journal of Children's Services* 2 (2), 4–14.

Isacsson, G., Holmgren, P. and Ahlner, J. (2005). Selective serotonin reuptake inhibitor antidepressants and the risk of suicide: a controlled forensic database study of 14,857 suicides. *Acta Psychiatrica Scandinavica* 111, 286–290.

Jackson, H. and Birchwood, M. (2006). Trauma and first episode psychosis. In: Larkin, W. and Morrison, A. P. (eds). *Trauma and Psychosis: New Directions for Theory and Therapy*. London: Routledge.

Jackson, H., McGorry, P., Henry, L., *et al.* (2001). Cognitively oriented psychotherapy for early psychosis (COPE): a 1-year follow-up. *British Journal of Clinical Psychology* 40, 57–70.

Jackson, H., McGorry, P., Edwards, J., *et al.* (2005). A controlled trial of cognitively oriented psychotherapy for early psychosis (COPE) with four-year follow-up readmission data. *Psychological Medicine* 35 (9), 1295–1306.

Jacobs, J. E. and Ganzel, A. K. (1993). Decision making in adolescence: Are we asking the wrong question? In: Maehr, M. L. and Pintrich, P. R. (eds). *Advances in Motivation and Achievement, Vol. 8: Motivation in Adolescence*. Greenwich, CT: JAI Press.

Jané-Llopis, E. and Braddick, F. (eds) (2008). *Mental Health in Youth and Education*. Consensus paper. Luxembourg: European Communities. Available at http://ec.europa.eu/health/ph_determinants/life_style/mental/docs/consensus_youth_en.pdf.

Janssen, I., Hanssen, M., Bak, M., *et al.* (2003). Discrimination and delusional ideation. *The British Journal of Psychiatry* 182, 71–76.

Janssen, I., Krabbendam, L., Bak, M., *et al.* (2004). Childhood abuse as a risk factor for psychotic experiences. *Acta Psychiatrica Scandinavica* 109, 38–45.

Jenkins, J. (1998). Diagnostic criteria for schizophrenia and related psychotic disorders: integration and suppression of cultural evidence in DSM-IV. *Transcultural Psychiatry* 35 (3), 357–376.

Jenkins, J. H. and Barrett, R. J. (eds) (2004). *Schizophrenia, Culture and Subjectivity*. Cambridge: Cambridge University Press.

Joa, I., Johannessen, J., Larsen, T. and McGlashan, T. (2008). Information campaigns: 10 years of experience in the Early Treatment and Intervention in Psychosis (TIPS) Study. *Psychiatric Annals* 38 (8), 512–520.

Joa, I., Johannessen, J. O., Langeveld, J., *et al.* (2009). Baseline profiles of adolescent vs. adult-onset first-episode psychosis in an early detection program. *Acta Psychiatrica Scandinavica* 119, 494–500.

Jobes, D. A. (2000). Collaborating to prevent suicide: a clinical-research perspective. *Suicide and Life-Threatening Behavior* 30 (1), 8–17.

Johnsen, E. and Jørgensen, H. A. (2008). Effectiveness of second generation antipsychotics: a systematic review of randomized trials. *BMC Psychiatry* 8, 31.

Johnston, C. and Mash, E. J. (2001). Families of children with attention-deficit/hyperactivity disorder: review and recommendations for future research. *Clinical Child and Family Psychological Review* 4, 183–207.

Johnston, J. R., Campbell, L. E. and Mayes, S. S. (1985). Latency children in post separation and divorce disputes. *Journal of the American Academy of Child Psychiatry* 24, 563–574.

Joiner, T. E and Rudd, M. D. (2000). Intensity and duration of suicidal crises vary as a function of previous suicide attempts and negative life events. *Journal of Consulting and Clinical Psychology* 68, 909–916.

Jones, K., Daley, D., Hutchings, J., Bywater, T. and Eames, C. (2007). Efficacy of the Incredible Years Basic Parent Training Programme as an early intervention for children with conduct problems and ADHD. *Child Care: Health and Development* 33 (6), 749–756.

Jones, P., Rodgers, B., Murray, R. and Marmont, M. (1994). Child development risk factors for adult schizophrenia in the British 1946 birth cohort. *The Lancet* 344, 1398–1402.

Jones, P. B., Barnes, T. R., Davies, L., *et al.* (2006). Randomized controlled trial of effect on quality of life of second- vs first-generation antipsychotic drugs in schizophrenia: Cost Utility of the Latest Antipsychotic Drugs in Schizophrenia Study (CUtLASS 1). *Archives of General Psychiatry* 63, 1079–1087.

Jones, V., Davies, R. and Jenkins, R. (2004). Self-harm by people with learning difficulties: Something to be expected or investigated? *Disability and Society* 19 (5), 487–500.

Jordan, R. (1999). *Autistic Spectrum Disorder: An Introductory Handbook for Practitioners.* London: David Fulton.

Joseph Rowntree Foundation (2008). *What Are Today's Social Evils? The Results of a Web Consultation.* York: Joseph Rowntree Foundation. Available at http://www.jrf .org.uk/sites/files/jrf/social-evils-consultation-report.pdf.

Jureidini, J. N. (2007). Study was not a trial of antidepressants. *British Medical Journal* 335, 221.

Jureidini, J. (2009). How do we safely treat depression in children, adolescents and young adults? *Drug Safety* 32, 275–282.

Jureidini, J. N., Doecke, C. J., Mansfield, P. R., Haby, M. M., Menkes, D. B., Tonkin, A. L. (2004a). Efficacy and safety of antidepressants for children and adolescents. *British Medical Journal* 328, 879–883.

Jureidini, J., Tonkin, A. and Mansfield, P. R. (2004b). TADS study raises concerns. *British Medical Journal* 329, 1343–1344.

Kanner, L. (1943). Autistic disturbances of affective contact. *Nervous Child* 2, 217–250.

Katz, L. Y. and Cox, B. J. (2002). Dialectical behavior therapy for suicidal adolescent inpatients: a case study. *Clinical Case Studies* 1, 81–92.

Katz, L. Y., Cox, B. J., Gunasekara, S. and Miller, A. (2004). Feasibility of dialectical behavior therapy for suicidal adolescent inpatients. *Journal of the American Academy of Child and Adolescent Psychiatry* 43 (3), 276–282.

Keenan, K., Hipwell, A., Duax, J., Stouthamer-Loeber, M. and Loeber, R. (2004). Phenomenology of depression in young girls. *Journal of the American Academy of Child and Adolescent Psychiatry* 42, 1098–1106.

Keinan, G., Meir, E. and Gome-Nemirovsky, T. (1984). Measurement of risk takers' personality. *Psychological Report* 55, 163–167.

Kempe, H., Silverman, E., Steele, B., Droegemuller, W. and Silver, H. (1962). The battered child syndrome. *Journal of American Medical Association* 181, 17–24.

Kemperman, I., Russ, M. J. and Shearin, E. (1997). Self-injurious behaviour and mood regulation in borderline patients. *Journal of Personality Disorders* 11 (2), 146–157.

Kendall, J., Hatton, D., Beckett, A., *et al.* (2003). Children's accounts of attention deficit/ hyperactivity disorder. *Advances in Nursing Science* 26, 114–130.

Kendler, K. S., McGuire, M., Gruenberg, A. M., Spellman, M., O'Hare, A. and Walsh, D. (1993). The Roscommon family study. I: Methods, diagnosis of probands and risk of schizophrenia in relatives. *Archives of General Psychiatry* 50, 527–540.

Kendler, K. S., Neale, M. C. and Walsh, D. (1995). Evaluating the spectrum concept of schizophrenia in the Roscommon Family Study. *The American Journal of Psychiatry* 152, 749–754.

Kendler, K. S., Maclean, C. J., O'Neill, A., *et al.* (1996). Evidence of a schizophrenic vulnerability locus on chromosome 8p in the Irish study of high density schizophrenia families. *The American Journal of Psychiatry* 153 (12), 1534–1540.

Keshavan, M. S., Diwadkar, V. A., Montrose, D. M., Rajarethinam, R. and Sweeney, J. A. (2005). Premorbid indicators and risk for schizophrenia: a selective review and update. *Schizophrenia Research* 79, 45–57.

Keshavan, M. S., Montrose, D. M., Rajarethinam, R., Diwadkar, V., Prasad, K. and Sweeney, J. A. (2008). Psychopathology among offspring of parents with schizophrenia: relationship to premorbid impairments. *Schizophrenia Research* 103, 114–120.

Kessler, R. C., Avenevoli, S. and Ries Merkangas, K. (2001). Mood disorders in children and adolescents: an epidemiological perspective. *Biological Psychiatry* 49, 1002–1014.

Kidd, S. A. (2004). The walls were closing in and we were trapped: a qualitative analysis of street youth suicide. *Youth and Society* 36, 30–55.

Kidd, S. A. (2006). Factors precipitating suicidality among homeless youth: a quantitative follow-up. *Youth and Society* 37, 393–422.

Kidd, S. A. and Carroll, M. (2007). Coping and suicidality among homeless youth. *Journal of Adolescence* 30, 283–296.

Kidwell, J. S., Dunham, R. M., Bacho, R. A., Pastorino, E. and Portes, P. R. (1995). Adolescent identity exploration: a test of Erikson's theory of transitional crisis. *Adolescence* 30, 785–793.

Kim, J. S. (2008). Examining the effectiveness of solution-focused brief therapy: a meta-analysis. *Research on Social Work Practice* 18, 107–115.

King, M., McKeown, E., Warner, J., *et al.* (2003). Mental health and quality of life of gay men and lesbians in England and Wales: controlled, cross-sectional study. *The British Journal of Psychiatry* 183 (6), 552–558.

Kirk, E. (2007). Edges and ledges: young people and informal support at 42nd Street. In: Spandler, H. and Warner, S. (eds). *Beyond Fear and Control: Working with Young People Who Self-harm.* Ross on Wye: PPCS Books.

Kirsch, I. and Sapirstein, G. (1998). Listening to Prozac but hearing placebo: a meta-analysis of antidepressant medication. *Prevention and Treatment* 1, Article 0002a. The American Psychological Association.

Kleber, H. D. (1999). Opioids: detoxification. In: Galanter, M. and Kleber, H. D. (eds). *Textbook of Substance Abuse Treatment,* 2nd edition. Washington, DC: American Psychiatric Press.

Klein, D. N., Lewinsohn, P. M., Seeley, J. R. and Rohde, P. (2001). A family study of major depressive disorder in a community sample of adolescents. *Archives of General Psychiatry* 58, 13–20.

Klohnen, E. C. and Bera, S. (1998). Behavioral and experiential patterns of avoidantly and securely attached women across adulthood: a 31-year longitudinal perspective. *Journal of Personality and Social Psychology* 74, 211–223.

Klonsky, D. E. (2007). The functions of deliberate self-injury: a review of the evidence. *Clinical Psychology Review* 27 (2), 226–239.

Koenig, J. I., Kirkpatrick, B. and Lee, P. (2002). Glucocorticoid hormones and early brain development in schizophrenia. *Neuropsychopharmacology* 27 (2), 309–318.

Korbin, J. (2007). Issues of culture. In: Wilson, K. and James, A. (eds). *The Child Protection Handbook*, 3rd edition. London: Ballière Tindall Elseviere.

Kripalani, M., Gash, A. and Riley, J. (2008). CBT for self-harm: Conclusions Overstated? (9 April 2008). Electronic letters published – response to Slee, N., Garnefski, N., van der Leeden, R., Arensman, E and Spinhoven, P (2008). Cognitive–behavioural intervention for self-harm: randomised controlled trial. The British Journal of Psychiatry 192, 202–211.

Kuczynski, L. (ed) (2003). *Handbook of Dynamics in Parent–Child Relations*. Thousand Oaks, CA: Sage.

Kuhn, D. (1991). *The Skills of Argument*. Cambridge: Cambridge University Press.

Kutcher, S. (1997). The pharmacotherapy of adolescent depression. *Journal of Child Psychology and Psychiatry* 38 (7), 755–767.

LaFromboise, T. (2006). American Indian youth suicide prevention. *Prevention Researcher* 13, 16–18.

LaFromboise, T. and Howard-Pitney, B. (1995). The Zuni life skills development curriculum: description and evaluation of a suicide prevention program. *Journal of Counseling Psychology* 42 (4), 479–486.

Lake, C. R. and Hurwitz, N. (2007). Schizoaffective disorder merges schizophrenia and bipolar disorders as one disease – there is no schizoaffective disorder. *Current Opinion Psychiatry* 20, 365–379.

Lamb, M. E., Thompson, R. A., Gardner, W., Charnov, E. L. and Connell, J. P. (1985). Infant–mother attachment: the origins and developmental significance of individual differences in the strange situation: its study and biological interpretation. *Behavioral and Brain Sciences* 7, 127–147.

Lambert, M., Conus, P., Lubman, D. I., *et al.* (2005). The impact of substance use disorders on clinical outcome in 643 patients with first-episode psychosis. *Acta Psychiatrica Scandinavica* 112 (2), 141–148.

Laming, L. (2003). *The Victoria Climbie Inquiry*. London: HMSO.

Landes, D. S. (1969). Prometheus unbound: technological change and industrial development in Western Europe from 1750 to the present Cambridge University Press. In: Fulcher, J. and Scott, J. (eds) (2007). *Sociology and Anthropology*, 3rd edition. Oxford: Oxford University Press.

Langer, S., Scourield, J. and Fincham, B. (2008). Documenting the quick and the dead: a study of suicide files in a coroner's office. *Sociological Review* 56 (2), 293–308.

Lask, B. and Bryant-Waugh, R. (2007). Overview and management. In: Lask, B. and Bryant-Waugh, R. (eds). *Eating Disorders in Childhood and Adolescence*, 3rd edition. East Sussex: Psychology Press.

Lask, B., Taylor, S. and Nunn, K. (2003). *Practical Child Psychiatry: The Clinician's Guide*. London. BMJ Publishing Group.

Laudet, A. B., Magura, S., Vogel, H. S., Howard, S. and Knight, E. L. (2004). Perceived reasons for substance misuse among persons with a psychiatric disorder. *American Journal of Orthopsychiatry* 74 (3), 365–375.

Laukkanen, E., Rissanen, M., Honkalampi, K., Kylmä, J., Tolmunen, T. and Hintikka, J. (2009). The prevalence of self-cutting and other self-harm among 13- to 18-year-old Finnish adolescents. *Social Psychiatry and Psychiatric Epidemiology* 44 (1), 23–28.

Laurens, K. R., Hodgins, S., Maughan, B., Murray, R. M., Rutter, M. L. and Taylor, E. A. (2007). Community screening for psychotic-like experiences and other putative antecedents of schizophrenia in children aged 9–12 years. *Schizophrenia Research* 90, 130–146.

Lavis, P. (2010). Do parents have a positive impact on children's wellbeing? *Young Minds Magazine* 104, 30.

Lawrence, A. (2004). *Principles of Child Protection: Management and Practice.* Maidenhead: Open University Press.

Layard, R. (2003). *Happiness: Has Social Science a Clue?* Lionel Robbins Memorial Lectures 2002/3, London School of Economics. Available at http://cep.lse.ac.uk/events/lectures/layard/RL030303.pdf.

Layard, R. (2005). *Happiness: Lessons from a New Science.* London: Penguin.

Layard, R. and Dunn, J. (2009). *A Good Childhood. Searching for Values in a Competitive Age.* London: The Children's Society/Penguin.

Le Grange, D. and Schmidt, U. (2005). The treatment of adolescents with bulimia. *Journal of Mental Health* 14 (6), 587–597.

Leccese, M. and Waldron, H. B. (1994). Assessing adolescent substance use: a critique of current measurement instruments. *Journal of Substance Abuse Treatment* 11 (6), 553–563.

Lelliott, P., Audini, B. and Duffett, R. (2001). Survey of patients from an inner-London health authority in medium secure psychiatric care. *The British Journal of Psychiatry* 178, 62–66.

Lerner, R., Lerner, J. and Tubman, J. (1989). Organismic and contextual bases of development in adolescence. In: Adams, G., Montemayor, R. and Gullotta, T. (eds). *Biology of Adolescent Behaviour and Development.* London: Sage.

Lester, D. (1998). Adolescent suicide risk: a paradox. *Journal of Adolescence* 21, 499–503.

Lester, H., Birchwood, M., Bryan, S., England, E., Rogers, H. and Sirvastava, N. (2009). Development and implementation of early intervention services for young people with psychosis: case study. *The British Journal of Psychiatry* 194, 446–450.

Leucht, S., Corves, C., Arbter, D., Engel, R. R., Li, C. and Davis, J. M. (2009). Second-generation versus first-generation antipsychotic drugs for schizophrenia: a metaanalysis. *Lancet* 373 (9657), 31–41.

Lewinsohn, P. M. and Clarke, G. N. (1999). Psychosocial treatments for adolescent depression. *Clinical Psychology Review* 19, 329–342.

Lewis, M. (1997). *Altering Fate: Why the Past Does Not Predict the Future.* New York: The Guilford Press.

Lewis, M., Feiring, C. and Rosenthal, S. (2000). Attachment over time. *Child Development* 71 (3), 707–720.

Lewis, M. D. (2005). Self-organising individual differences in brain development. *Developmental Review* 25, 252–277.

Lieberman, J. A., Scott Stroup, T., McEvoy, J. P., *et al.*, for the Clinical Antipsychotic Trials of Intervention Effectiveness (CATIE) Investigators (2005). Effectiveness of antipsychotic drugs in patients with chronic schizophrenia. *The New England Journal of Medicine* 353 (12), 1209–1223.

Lindsay, W. R. (1999). Cognitive therapy. *The Psychologist* 12, 238–241.

Lindsay, W. R., Howells, L. and Pitcaithly, D. (1993). Cognitive therapy for depression with individuals with intellectual disabilities. *British Journal of Medical Psychology* 66, 135–141.

Linehan, M. (1993a). *Cognitive–Behavioural Treatment of Borderline Personality Disorder.* New York: The Guildford Press.

Linehan, M. (1993b). *Skills Training Manual for Treating Borderline Personality Disorder.* New York: The Guilford Press.

Linehan, M. (2008). Suicide intervention research: a field in desperate need of development. *Suicide and Life-Threatening Behavior* 38 (5), 483–485.

Linehan, M. M., Comtois, K. A., Murray, A. M., *et al.* (2006). Two-year randomized controlled trial and follow-up of dialectical behavior therapy vs therapy by experts for suicidal behaviors and borderline personality disorder. *Archives of General Psychiatry* 63, 757–766.

Lingford-Hughes, A. R., Welch, S. and Nutt, D. J. (2004). Evidence-based guidelines for the pharmacological management of substance misuse, addiction and co morbidity: recommendations from the British Association for Psychopharmacology. *Journal of Psychopharmacology* 18 (3), 293–335.

Lloyd, G., Stead, J. and Cohen, D. (eds) (2006). *Critical New Perspectives on ADHD.* London: Routledge.

London Borough of Brent (1985) *A Child in Trust: The Report of the Panel of Inquiry into the Circumstances Surrounding the Death of Jasmine Beckford.* London: London Borough of Brent.

London Borough of Lambeth (1987). *Whose Child? The Report of the Panel of Inquiry into the Death of Tyra Henry 1987.* London: London Borough of Lambeth.

Lovell, A. (2007). Learning disability against itself: the self-injury/self-harm conundrum. *British Journal of Learning Disabilities* 36 (2), 109–121.

Lucas, A. (2008). *Demystifying Anorexia Nervosa: An Optimistic Guide to Understanding and Healing.* Oxford: Oxford University Press.

Lunsky, Y. and Palucka, A. (2004). Depression in intellectual disability. *Current Opinion in Psychiatry* 17, 359–363.

Lynskey, M. T. and Fergusson, D. M. (1997). Factors protecting against the development of adjustment difficulties in young adults exposed to childhood sexual abuse. *Child Abuse and Neglect* 21 (12), 1177–1190.

Lyon, C. M. (2007). Child protection in the international and domestic civil legal context. In: Wilson, K. and James, A. (eds). *The Child Protection Handbook*, 3rd edition. London: Ballière Tindall Elseviere.

MacDonald, R. and Marsh, J. (2005). *Disconnected Youth? Growing up in Britain's Poor Neighbourhoods.* Basingstoke: Palgrave Macmillan.

Madge, N., Hewitt, A., Hawton, K., *et al.* (2008). Deliberate self-harm within an international community sample of young people: comparative findings from the Child and Adolescent Self-harm in Europe (CASE) Study. *Journal of Child Psychology and Psychiatry* 49 (6), 667–677.

Main, M. and Solomon, J. (1986). Discovery of an insecure-disorganised/disoriented attachment pattern. In: Brazelton, T. B. and Yogman, M. W. (eds). *Affective Development in Infancy.* Norwood, NJ: Ablex.

Main, M., Kaplan, K. and Cassidy, J. (1985). Security in infancy, childhood and adult-hood. A move to the level or representation cited in Bretherton, I. and Waters, E. (eds). Growing points of attachment theory and research. *Monographs of the Society for Research in Child Development* 50, 66–104.

Mangnal, J. and Yurkovich, E. (2008). A literature review of deliberate self-harm. *Perspectives in Psychiatric Care* 44 (3), 175–184.

Mann, J. J., Brent, D. A. and Arango, V. (2001). The neurobiology and genetics of suicide and attempted suicide: a focus on the serotonergic system. *Neuropsychopharmacology* 24, 467–477.

Mann, J. J., Apter, A., Bertolote, J., *et al.* (2005). Suicide prevention strategies: a systematic review. *Journal of American Medical Association* 294, 2064–2067.

Mann, T., Tomiyama, J., Westling, E., Lew, A. M., Samuels, B. and Chatman, J. (2007). Medicare's search for effective obesity treatments: diets are not the answer. *American Psychologist* 62 (3), 220–233.

Marcenko, M. O., Fishman, G. and Friedman, J. (1999). Reexamining adolescent suicidal ideation: a developmental perspective applied to a diverse population. *Journal of Youth and Adolescence* 28, 121–138.

March, J., Silva, S., Petrycki, S., *et al.*, Treatment for Adolescents with Depression Study (TADS) Team. (2004). Fluoxetine, cognitive–behavioral therapy, and their combination for adolescents with depression: Treatment for Adolescents with Depression Study (TADS) randomized controlled trial. *Journal of the American Medical Association* 292 (7), 807–820.

March, J., Silva, S., Benedetto, B., TADS Team (2006). The Treatment for Adolescents with Depression Study (TADS): methods and message at 12 weeks. *Journal of the American Academy of Child and Adolescent Psychiatry* 45, 1393–1403.

March, J. S., Silva, S., Petrycki, S. (2007). The Treatment for Adolescents with Depression Study (TADS): long-term effectiveness and safety outcomes. *Archives of General Psychiatry* 64 (10), 1132–1143.

Marcia, J. E. (1966). Development and validation of ego identity status. *Journal of Personality and Social Psychology* 3, 551–558.

Marcia, J. E. (1980). Identity in adolescence. In: Adelson, J. (ed) (1980). *Handbook of Adolescent Psychology*. New York: Wiley.

Marcia, J. E. (1987). The identity status approach to the study of ego identity development. In: Honess, T. and Yardley, K. (eds). *Self and Identity Perspectives Across the Lifespan*. London: Routledge and Kegan Paul.

Marcia, J. E. (1994). The empirical study of ego identity. In: Bosma, H. A., Graafsma, T. L. G., Grotevant, H. D. and De Levita, D. J. (eds). *Identity and Development*. Newbury Park, CA: Sage.

Marston, G. M., Perry, D. W. and Roy, A. (1997). Manifestations of depression in people with intellectual disabilities. *Journal of Intellectual Disability Research* 41, 476–480.

Martin, S. R., Boekamp, J. R., McConville, D. W. and Wheeler, E. E. (2010). Anger and sadness perception in clinically referred preschoolers: emotion processes and externalizing behavior symptoms. *Child Psychiatry and Human Development* 41 (1), 30–46.

Matsuzawa, J., Matsui, M., Konishi, T., *et al.* (2001). Age-related volumetric changes of brain gray and white matter in healthy infants and children. *Cerebral Cortex* 11, 335–342.

Mazza, J. J. and Reynolds, W. M. (1998). A longitudinal investigation of depression, hopelessness, social support, and major and minor life events and their relation to suicidal ideation in adolescents. *Suicide and Life-Threatening Behavior* 28, 358–374.

McArdle, P. (2004). Substance abuse by children and young people. *Archives of Disease in Childhood* 89, 701–704.

McCann, D., Barrett, A., Cooper, A., *et al.* (2007). Food additives and hyperactive behaviour in 3 year old and 8 to 9 year old children in the community: a randomised, double-blind, placebo-controlled trial. *The Lancet* 3, 1560–1567.

McClellan, J. and McCurry, C. (1998). Neurocognitive pathways in the development of schizophrenia. *Seminars in Clinical Neuropsychiatry* 3 (4), 320–332.

Mcglashan, T. H., Levy, S. T. and Carpenter, W. D. (1975). Integration and sealing over: clinically distinct recovery styles from schizophrenia. *Archives of General Psychiatry* 32, 1269–1272.

McGorry, P. D. (2006). The recognition and optimum management of early psychosis: applying the concept of staging in the treatment of psychosis. In: Johannessen, I. O., Martindale, B. V. and Cullberg, J. (eds). *Evolving Psychosis*. Hove: Routledge.

McGorry, P. D. and Edwards, J. (1997). *The Early Psychosis Training Pack. Early Psychosis Prevention and Intervention Centre*. Melbourne: EPPIC.

McIntyre, R. S. and Jerrell, J. J. (2008). Metabolic and cardiovascular adverse events associated with antipsychotic treatment in children and adolescents. *Archives of Pediatrics & Adolescent Medicine* 162 (10), 929–935.

McKeganey, N. P., McIntosh, J and MacDonald, F. (2003) Young People's Experience of Illegal Drug Use in the Family. *Drugs: Education, Prevention and Policy.* 10(2) 169–184.

McKenna, P. J. (2007). *Schizophrenia and Related Syndromes*, 2nd edition. London: Routledge.

McLaughlin, C. (2007). *Suicide-Related Behaviour: Understanding, Caring and Therapeutic Responses*. Chichester: John Wiley and Sons.

McLean, K., Maxwell, M., Platt, S., Harris, F. and Jepson, R. (2008). *Risk and Protective Factors for Suicide and Suicidal Behaviour: A Literature Review*. Edinburgh: Scottish Government Social Research.

McLeer, S. V., Callaghan, M., Henry, D., *et al.* (1994). Psychiatric disorders in sexually abused children. *Journal of the American Academy of Child and Adolescent Psychiatry* 33, 313–319.

Medical Research Council (MRC) (2001). *Review of Autism Research: Epidemiology and Causes*. London: MRC.

Meeus, W., Iedema, J., Helsen, M. and Vollebergh, W. (1999). Patterns of adolescent identity development: review of literature and longitudinal analysis. *Development Review* 19, 419–461.

Meeus, W., Oosterwegel, A. and Vollebergh, W. (2002). Parental and peer attachment and identity development in adolescence. *Journal of Adolescence* 25, 93–106.

Meins, W. (1993). Prevalence and risk factors for depressive disorders in adults with intellectual disability. *Australia and New Zealand Journal of Developmental Disabilities* 18, 147–156.

Melle, I., Larsen, T. K., Haahr, U., *et al.* (2004). Reducing the duration of untreated first-episode psychosis: effects on clinical presentation. *Archives of General Psychiatry* 61, 143–150.

Melle, I., Haahr, U., Friis, S., *et al.* (2005). Reducing the duration of untreated first-episode psychosis – effects on baseline social functioning and quality of life. *Acta Psychiatrica Scandinavica* 112, 469–473.

Melrose, M., Turner, P., Pitts, J. and Barrett, D. (2007). The impact of heavy cannabis use on young people. *Vulnerability and youth transitions*. Joseph Rowntree Foundation.

Meltzer, H., Gatward, R., Goodman, R. and Ford, T. (2000). *The Mental Health of Children and Adolescents in Britain.* London: Office for National Statistics, Her Majesty's Stationery Office.

Meltzer, H., Harrington, R., Goodman, R. and Jenkins, R. (2001). *Children and Adolescents Who Try to Harm, Hurt or Kill Themselves.* London: National Statistics.

Mental Health Foundation (1999). *Bright Futures: Promoting Children and Young People's Mental Health.* London: Mental Health Foundation.

Mental Health Foundation (2006). *Truth Hurts: Report of the National Inquiry into Self-harm Among Young People.* London: Mental Health Foundation and Camelot Foundation.

Merrell, C. and Tymms, P. (2005). A longitudinal study of the achievements, progress and attitudes of severely inattentive, hyperactive and impulsive young children. Paper Presented at the Annual Conference of the British Educational Research Association. September 2005, University of Glamorgan, UK.

Mesibov, G. B., Shea, V. and Schopler, E. (2004). *The TEACCH Approach to Autism Spectrum Disorders.* New York: Springer.

Messer, J. M. and Fremouw, W. J. (2008). A critical review of explanatory models for self-mutilating behaviors in adolescents. *Clinical Psychology Review* 28, 162–178.

Metha, A., Weber, B. and Webb, D. L. (1998). Youth suicide prevention. A survey analysis of policies and effects in the 50 states. *Suicide and Life-Threatening Behaviour* 28(2), 150–164.

Midence, K. (2006). An introduction to and rationale for psychosocial interventions. In: Gamble, C. and Brennan, G. (eds). *Working with Serious Mental Illness: A Manual for Clinical Practice,* 2nd edition. London: Bailliere Tindall.

Milberger, S., Biederman, J., Faraone, S. V. *et al.* (1997). Pregnancy, delivery and infancy complications and attention deficit hyperactivity disorder: issues of gene–environment interaction. *Biological Psychiatry* 41, 65–75.

Miller, A., Rathus, J. H., Linehan, M., Wetzler, S. and Leigh, E. (1997). Dialectical behaviour therapy adapted for suicidal adolescents. *Journal of Practical Psychiatry and Behavioural Health* 3, 78–86.

Miller, A. L. and Smith, H. L. (2008). Adolescent non-suicidal self-injurious behavior: the latest epidemic to assess and treat. *Applied and Preventive Psychology* 12 (4), 178–188.

Miller, P. J. and Armstrong, M. (2005). The term 'deliberate' is unhelpful (29 April 2005) response to Keith Hawton and Anthony James suicide and deliberate self-harm in young people. *British Medical Journal* 330, 891–894.

Miller, R. and Mason, S. E. (2006). Phase specific treatment for recovery in an early psychosis programme. In: Johannessen, I. O., Martindale, B. V. and Cullberg, J. (eds). *Evolving Psychosis.* Hove: Routledge.

Minuchin, S. (1974). *Families and Family Therapy.* London: Tavistock.

Mitchell, B., Carleton, B., Smith, A., Prosser, R., Brownell, M. and Kozyrskyj, A. (2008). Trends in psychostimulant and antidepressant use by children in 2 Canadian provinces. *Canadian Journal of Psychiatry* 53 (3), 152–159.

Model Health Inquiry (2007). *Fashioning a Healthy Future: The Report of the Model Health Inquiry.* London: Model Health Inquiry.

Moffitt, T., Caspi, A. and Belsky, J. (1992). Family context, girls' behaviour, and the onset of puberty: a test of a sociobiological model. *Child Development* 63, 47–58.

Moor, S., Maguire, A., McQueen, H., *et al.* (2007). Improving the recognition of depression in adolescence: Can we teach the teachers? *Journal of Adolescence* 30, 81–95.

Moore, S. (1995). Girl's understanding and social constructions of menarche. *Journal of Adolescence* 18, 87–104.

Morrell, S., Page, A. and Taylor, R. J. (2007). The decline in Australian young male suicide. *Social Science and Medicine* 64, 747–754.

Morrison, A., Frame, L. and Larkin, W. (2003). Relationships between trauma and psychosis: a review and integration. *British Journal of Clinical Psychology* 42, 331–353.

Morrison, A. P., Renton, J. C., French, P. and Bentall, R. P. (2008). *Think You're Crazy? Think Again: A Resource Book for Cognitive Therapy for Psychosis.* London: Routledge.

Morrison, R. and O'Connor, R. C. (2008). The role of rumination, attentional biases and stress in psychological distress. *British Journal of Psychology* 99, 191–209.

Morriss, R., Gask, L., Webb, R., Dixon, C. and Appleby, L. (2005). The effects on suicide rates of an educational intervention for front-line health professionals with suicidal patients (the STORM project). *Psychological Medicine* 35, 957–960.

MTA Co-operative Group (2004). National Institute of Mental Health Multimodal Treatment Study of ADHD follow-up: changes in effectiveness and growth after the end of the treatment (attention deficit hyperactivity disorder). *Pediatrics* 113 (4), 762–770.

Muehlenkamp, J. J. and Gutierrez, P. M. (2004). An investigation of differences between self-injurious behavior and suicide attempts in a sample of adolescents. *Suicide and Life-Threatening Behavior* 34 (1), 12–23.

Mufson, L., Dorta, K. P., Moreau, D. and Weissman, M. M. (2004a). *Interpersonal Psychotherapy for Depressed Adolescents*, 2nd edition. New York: The Guilford Press.

Mufson, L., Dorta, K., Olfson, M., Weissman, M. and Hoagwood, K. (2004b). Effectiveness research: transporting interpersonal psychotherapy for depressed adolescents (IPT-A) from the lab to school-based health clinics. *Clinical Child and Family Psychology Review* 7 (4), 251–261.

Muise, A., Stein, D. and Arbess, G. (2003). Eating disorders in adolescent boys: a review of the adolescent and young adult literature. *Journal of Adolescent Health* 33, 427–435.

Mukoma, W. and Flisher, A. J. (2004). Evaluations of health promoting schools: a review of nine studies. *Health Promotion International* 19, 357–368.

Mullins, L. L., Fuemmeler, B. F., Hoff, A., Chaney, J. M., Van Pelt, J. and Ewing, C. (2004). The relationship of parental overprotection and perceived child vulnerability to depressive symptomotology in children with type 1 diabetes mellitus: the moderating influence of parenting stress. *Children's Health Care* 33, 21–34.

Muratori, F., Salvadori, F., D'Arcangelo, G., Viglione, V. and Picchi, L. (2005). Childhood psychopathological antecedents in early onset schizophrenia. *European Psychiatry* 20, 309–314.

Murray, M. L., de Vries, C. S. and Wong, I. C. K. (2004). A drug utilisation study of antidepressants in children and adolescents using the General Practice Research Database. *Archives of Disease in Childhood* 89, 1098–1102.

Mussen, P. H. and Jones, M. C. (1957). Self-conceptions, motivations, and interpersonal attitudes of late and early maturing boys. *Child Development* 28, 243–256.

National Autistic Society (2009). *Estimated Population of Autism Spectrum Disorders in the UK*. Available at http://www.nas.org.uk/nas/jsp/polopoly.jsp?d=235&a=3527.

National Equality Panel (2010). *An Anatomy of Economic Inequality in the UK Report of the National Equality Panel*. London: Government Equalities Office. Available at http://www.equalities.gov.uk/national_equality_panel/publications.aspx.

National MAPPA Team (2009). *MAPPA Guidance 2009 Version 3.0*. National Offender Management Service Public Protection Unit: Crown Copyright.

National Self Harm Network (2000). *Cutting the Risk: Self-harm, Self-care, and Risk Reduction*. Bristol: National Self Harm Network.

National Statistics (2006). Suicide trends and geographical variations in the United Kingdom, 1991–2004. *Health Statistics Quarterly* 31, 6–22.

NCCMH (National Collaborating Centre for Mental Health) (2009). *Attention Deficit Hyperactivity Disorder – The NICE Guideline on Diagnosis and Management of ADHD in Children, Young People and Adult*. Commissioned by the National Institute for Health and Clinical Excellence (NICE). London: British Psychological Society and the Royal College of Psychiatrists.

Nelson, E. L., Barnard, M. and Cain, S. (2003). Treating childhood depression over videoconferencing. *Telemedicine Journal and E-Health* 9, 49–55.

Nemtsov, A. (2003). Suicides and alcohol consumption in Russia, 1965–1999. *Drug and Alcohol Dependence* 71, 161–168.

New, A. S., Trestman, R. L., Mitropulou, V. and Benishay, D. S. (1997). Serotonergic function and self-injurious behaviour in personality disorder patients. *Psychiatry Research* 69 (1), 17–26.

Newman, R. S. and Hirt, M. (1983). The psychoanalytic theory of depression: symptoms as a function of aggressive wishes and level of articulation. *Journal of Abnormal Psychology* 92, 42–48.

Newton, E., Larkin, M., Melhuish, R. and Wykes, T. (2007). More than just a place to talk: young people's experiences of group psychological therapy as an early intervention for auditory hallucinations. *Psychology and Psychotherapy: Theory, Research and Practice* 80, 127–149.

NHS Quality Improvement Scotland (QIS) (2006). *Eating Disorders in Scotland: Recommendations for Management and Treatment*. Edinburgh: NHS QIS.

NICE (National Institute for Clinical Excellence) (2004a). *Clinical Guideline 9: Eating Disorders: Core Interventions in the Treatment and Management of Anorexia Nervosa, Bulimia Nervosa and Related Eating Disorders*. London: NICE.

NICE (2004b). *Self-harm: The Short-Term Physical and Psychological Management and Secondary Prevention of Self-harm in Primary and Secondary Care*. London: NICE.

NICE (2005). *Depression in Children and Young People: Identification and Management in Primary, Community and Secondary Care*. NICE Clinical Guideline 28. London: NICE.

NICE (2009). *Schizophrenia: Core Interventions in the Treatment and Management of Schizophrenia in Adults in Primary and Secondary Care*. NICE Clinical Guideline 82. London: NICE.

NICE – National Institute for Health and Clinical Excellence (2006). *Methylphenidate, Atomoxetine and Dexamfetamine for Attention Deficit Hyperactivity Disorder (ADHD) in Children and Adolescent*. Technology Appraisal Guidance No. 98. London: NICE.

NICE – National Institute for Health and Clinical Excellence (2007a). *Drug Misuse: Psychosocial Interventions*. NICE Clinical Guideline 51. London: NICE.

NICE – National Institute for Health and Clinical Excellence (2007b). *Drug Misuse: Opioid Detoxification*. NICE Clinical Guideline 52. London: NICE.

Nicholls, D. (2007). Aetiology. In: Lask, B. and Bryant-Waugh, R. (eds). *Eating Disorders in Childhood and Adolescence*, 3rd edition. Hove: Routledge.

NIMHE (2006). *National Suicide Prevention Strategy for England. Annual Report on Progress 2005.* Care Services Improvement Partnership Leeds: National Institute for Mental Health in England.

Nissen, S. E. (2006). ADHD drugs and cardiovascular risk. *The New England Journal of Medicine* 354 (14), 1445–1448.

Nock, M. K., Borges, G., Bromet, E. J., *et al.* (2008). Cross-national prevalence and risk factors for suicidal ideation, plans and attempts. *The British Journal of Psychiatry* 192, 98–105.

Northern Ireland Government (2006). *Our Children and Young People – Our Pledg. A Ten Year Strategy for Children and Young People 2006–2016.* Belfast: Children and Young People's Unit.

NTA (2007). *Assessing Young People for Substance Misuse.* London: NTA.

Nuffield Foundation (2009). *Time Trends in Parenting and Outcomes for Young People.* London: Nuffield Foundation.

Nylund, D. and Ceske, K. (1997). Voices of political resistance: young women's co-research on anti-depression. In: Smith, C. and Nylund, D. (eds). *Narrative Therapies with Children and Adolescents.* London: The Guilford Press.

O'Carroll, P. W., Berman, A. L., Maris, R., Moscicki, E., Tanney, B. and Silverman, M. (1996). Beyond the Tower of Babel: a nomenclature for suicidology. *Suicide and Life-Threatening Behavior* 26 (3), 237–252.

O'Connor, R. and Sheehy, N. (2000). *Understanding Suicidal Behaviour.* Leicester: BPS Books.

O'Connor, R. C., Rasmussen, S., Miles, J. and Hawton, K. (2009). Deliberate self-harm in adolescents: self-report survey in schools in Scotland. *The British Journal of Psychiatry* 194, 68–72.

Offer, D. (1969). *The Psychological World of the Teenager.* New York: Basic Books.

Offer, D., Ostrov, E., Howard, K. I. and Atkinson, R. (1992). A study of quietly disturbed and normal adolescents in ten countries. In: Schwartzberg, A. Z. (ed). *International Annals of Adolescent Psychiatry* 2, 285–297.

Offord, A., Turner, H. and Cooper, M. (2006). Adolescent inpatient treatment for anorexia nervosa: a qualitative study exploring young adults' retrospective views of treatment and discharge. *European Eating Disorders Review* 14, 377–387.

O'Hagan, M. (2009). *Recovery and Wellbeing: Different Words, Same Agenda.* Scottish Recovery Network, Marking Recovery Real Conference. Available at http://www .scottishrecovery.net/Recovery-films-and-video-clips/making-recovery-real-conference .html.

O'Hara, S. and Smith, K. (2007). Presentations of eating disorders in the news media: What are the implications for patient diagnosis and treatment? *Patient Education and Counseling* 68, 43–51.

Oldershaw, A., Richards, C., Simic, M. and Schmidt, U. (2008). Parents' perspectives on adolescent self-harm: qualitative study. *The British Journal of Psychiatry* 193, 140–144.

Olfson, M., Blanco, C., Liu, L., Moreno, C. and Laje, G. (2006). National trends in the outpatient treatment of children and adolescents with antipsychotic drugs. *Archives of General Psychiatry* 63, 679–685.

Ollendick, T. H., Shortt, A. L. and Sander, J. B. (2005). Internalizing disorders of childhood and adolescence. In: Maddux, J. E. and Winstead, B. A. (eds). *Psychopathology: Foundations for a Contemporary Understanding.* Mahwah, NJ: Lawrence Erlbaum Associates.

Olsen, E. (2006). Failure to thrive: still a problem of definition. *Clinical Pediatrics* 45 (1), 1–6.

Olsen, E., Petersen, J., Skovgaard, A., Weile, B., Jørgensen, T. and Wright, C. (2007). Failure to thrive: the prevalence and concurrence of anthropometric criteria in a general infant population. *Archives of Diseases in Childhood* 92 (2), 109–114.

Orbach, I. (2006). The body–mind of the suicidal person. In: Ellis, T. E. (ed). *Cognition and Suicide: Theory, Research, and Therapy*. Washington, DC: American Psychological Association.

Orbach, S. (2006). *Fat Is a Feminist Issue*. London: Arrow Books.

Owens, C., Lambert, H., Lloyd, K. and Donovan, J. (2008). Tales of biographical disintegration: how parents make sense of their sons' suicides. *Sociology of Health and Illness* 30 (2), 237–254.

Owens, D., Horrocks, J. and House, A. (2002). Fatal and non-fatal repetition of self-harm. Systematic review. *The British Journal of Psychiatry* 181, 193–199.

Owens, G., Crowell, J., Pan, H., Treboux, D., O'Connor, E. and Waters, E. (1995). The prototype hypothesis and the origins of attachment working models: adult relationships with parents and romantic partners. In: Waters, E., Vaughn, B., Posada, G. and Kondo-Ikemura, K. (eds). *Caregiving, Cultural, and Cognitive Perspectives on Secure-Base Behaviour and Working Models: New Growing Points of Attachment Theory and Research*. Chicago, IL: University of Chicago Press.

Palmer, B. A., Pankratz, V. S. and Bostwick, J. M. (2005). The lifetime risk of suicide in schizophrenia: a reexamination. *Archives of General Psychiatry* 62, 247–253.

Palmer, S. (2008). Suicide statistics for the UK and the national suicide prevention strategy. In: Palmer, S. (ed). *Suicide Strategies and Interventions for Reduction and Prevention*. Hove: Routledge.

Palmqvist, R. and Santavirta, N. (2006). What friends are for: the relationships between body image, substance use, and peer influence among Finnish adolescents. *Journal of Youth and Adolescence* 35 (2), 203–215.

Parrish, M. and Tunkle, J. (2005). Clinical challenges following an adolescent's death by suicide: bereavement issues faced by family, friends, schools, and clinicians. *Clinical Social Work Journal* 33 (1), 81–102.

Pascual-Castroviejo, I. and Ruggieri, M. (2008). Lesch Nyhan Syndrome. In: Ruggieri, M., Pascual-Castroviejo, I. and Di Rocco, C. (eds). *Neurocutaneous Disorders Phakomatoses and Hamartoneoplastic Syndromes*. Vienna: Springer.

Patel, N. C., Crismon, M., Shafer, L., *et al*. (2006). Ethnic variation in symptoms and response to risperidone in youths with schizophrenia-spectrum disorders. *Social Psychiatry and Psychiatric Epidemiology* 41 (5), 341–346.

Pattison, S. and Harris, B. (2006). Adding value to education through improved mental health: a review of the research evidence on the effectiveness of counselling for children and young people. *Australian Educational Researcher* 33 (2), 97–121.

Patton, G., Coffey, C., Sawyer, S., *et al*. (2009). Global patterns of mortality in young people: a systematic analysis of population health data. *Lancet* 374 (9693), 881–892.

Paulson, B. L. and Everall, R. D. (2003). Suicidal adolescents: helpful aspects of psychotherapy. *Archives of Suicide Research* 7, 309–321.

Payne, R., Oliver, J. and Bain, M. (2009). Patterns and predictors of re-admission to hospital with self-poisoning in Scotland. *Public Health* 123 (2), 134–137.

Pearce, N. and Hillman, J. (1998). *Wasted Youth*. London: Institute for Public Policy.

Peck, E. and Greatley, A. (1999). *Mental Health Priorities for Primary Care*. London: King's Fund, Centre for Mental Health Services Development.

Peeters, T. and Gillberg, C. (1999). *Autism – Medical and Educational Aspects*, 2nd edition. London: Whurr Publishers.

Pembroke, L. R. (2007). Harm minimisation: limiting the damage of self-injury. In: Spandler, H. and Warner, S. (eds). *Beyond Fear and Control: Working with Young People Who Self-harm*. Ross on Wye: PPCS Books.

Pengelly, N., Ford, B., Blenkiron, P. and Reilly, S. (2008). Harm minimisation after repeated self-harm: development of a trust handbook. *Psychiatric Bulletin* 32, 60–63.

Penn, D. L., Meyer, P. S., Evans, E., Wirth, R. J., Cai, K. and Burchinal, M. (2009). A randomized controlled trial of group cognitive–behavioral therapy vs. enhanced supportive therapy for auditory hallucinations. *Schizophrenia Research* 109, 52–59.

Pepper, S. C. (1942). *World Hypotheses: A Study in Evidence*. Berkeley: University of California Press.

Perälä, J., Suvisaari, J., Saarni, S. I., *et al.* (2007). Lifetime prevalence of psychotic and bipolar I disorders in a general population. *Archives of General Psychiatry* 64, 19–28.

Petersen, L., Jeppesen, P., Thorup, A., *et al.* (2005). A randomised multicentre trial of integrated versus standard treatment for patients with a first episode of psychotic illness. *British Medical Journal* 331 (7517), 602.

Peterson, A. C. and Crockett, L. J. (1985). Pubertal timing and grade effects on adjustment. *Journal of Youth and Adolescence* 14, 191–206.

Pfeffer, C., Jiang, H. and Kakuna, T. (2000). Child–Adolescent Suicidal Potential Index (CASPI): a screen for early onset suicidal behaviour. *Psychological Assessment* 12, 304–318.

Pfeffer, C., Jiang, H., Kakuma, T., Hwang, J. and Metsch, M. (2002). Group intervention for children bereaved by the suicide of a relative. *Journal of the American Academy of Child and Adolescent Psychiatry* 41, 505–513.

Pharoah, F. M., Rathbone, J., Mari, J. and Steiner, D. (2003). *Family Intervention for Schizophrenia (Cochrane Review)*. The Cochrane Library (Issue 3) Oxford: Update Software.

Piaget, J. (1952). *The Origins of Intelligence in Children* (Cook, M., Trans.). New York: International Universities Press.

Pierce, D. (1977). Suicide intent in self-injury. *The British Journal of Psychiatry* 130, 377–385.

Pinhas, L., Steinegger, C. and Katzman, D. (2007). Clinical assessment and physical complications. In: Lask, B. and Bryant-Waugh, R. (eds). *Eating Disorders in Childhood and Adolescence*, 3rd edition. London: Routledge.

Pitschel-Walz, G., Leucht, S., Bäuml, J., Kissling, W. and Engel, R. R. (2001). The effect of family interventions on relapse and rehospitalization in schizophrenia – a meta-analysis. *Schizophrenia Bulletin* 27 (1), 73–92.

Plomin, R., Owen, M. J. and McGuffin, P. (1994). The genetic basis of complex human behaviours. *Science* 264 (5166), 1733–1739.

Polanczyk, G., Silva de Lima, M., Horta, B. H., *et al.* (2007). The worldwide prevalence of ADHD: a systematic review and meta-regression analysis. *The American Journal of Psychiatry* 164, 942–948.

Poulton, R., Caspi, A., Moffitt, T. E., Cannon, M., Murray, R. and Harrington, H. (2000). Children's self-reported psychotic symptoms and adult schizophreniform disorder: a 15-year longitudinal study. *Archives of General Psychiatry* 57, 1053–1058.

Priest, H. and Gibbs, M. (2004). *Mental Health Care for People with Learning Disabilities*. London: Churchill Livingstone.

Proctor, G. (2007). Disordered boundaries? A critique of borderline personality disorder. In: Spandler, H. and Warner, S. (eds). *Beyond Fear and Control: Working with Young People Who Self-harm*. Ross on Wye: PPCS Books.

Pryor, J. and Rogers, B. (2001). *Children in Changing Families: Life After Parental Separation*. Oxford: Blackwell Publishers.

Puckering, C. (2004). Mellow parenting, an intensive intervention to change relationships. *Signal (Bulletin of the World Association for Infant Mental Health)* 12, 1–5.

Puckering, C. (2007). What every baby needs. Children in Scotland May, 18–19.

Puffett, N. (2009). Prison self-harm levels revealed. Children and Young People Now February, 1.

Puig-Antich, J. and Chambers, W. (1978). *The Schedule for Affective Disorders and Schizophrenia for School-Age Children*. Unpublished interview schedule, New York State Psychiatric Institute, New York.

Puura, K., Almqvist, F., Tamminen, T., *et al.* (1998). Children with symptoms of depression – What do the adults see? *Journal of Child Psychology & Psychiatry* 39 (4), 577–585.

Radke-Yarrow, M. and Sherman, T. (1990). Hard growing: children who survive. In: Rolf, J., Masten, A., Cicchetti, D., Nuechterlein, K. and Weintraub, S. (eds). *Relationships Within Families: Mutual Influences*. Cambridge: Cambridge University Press.

Raghavan, R. and Patel, P. (2005). *Learning Disabilities and Mental Health: A Nursing Perspective*. Oxford: Blackwell Publishing.

Rankin, J. L., Lane, D. J., Gibbons, F. X. and Gerrard, M. (2004). Adolescent self-consciousness: longitudinal age changes and gender differences in two cohorts. *Journal of Research on Adolescence* 14, 1–21.

Read, J. (2004). Does schizophrenia exist? Reliability and validity. In: Read, J., Mosher, L. R. and Bentall, R. P. (eds). *Models of Madness*. Hove: Routledge.

Read, J., van Os, J., Morrison, A. P. and Ross, C. A. (2005). Childhood trauma, psychosis and schizophrenia: a literature review with theoretical and clinical implications. *Acta Psychiatrica Scandinavica* 112, 330–350.

Reading, B. and Birchwood, M. (2005). Early intervention in psychosis: rationale and evidence for effectiveness. *Disease Management and Health Outcome* 13, 53–63.

Rector, N. A. and Beck, A. T. (2002). A clinical review of cognitive therapy for schizophrenia. *Current Psychiatry Reports* 4, 284–292.

Reichert, A., Kreiker, S., Mehler-Wex, C. and Warnke, A. (2008). The psychopathological and psychosocial outcome of early-onset schizophrenia: preliminary data of a 13-year follow-up. *Child and Adolescent Psychiatry and Mental Health* 2, 6.

Ribbens-McCarthy, J. and Jessop, J. (2005). *Young People, Bereavement and Loss: Disruptive Transitions*. UK: National Children's Bureau.

Ricciardelli, L. A., Marita, P., McCabe, J. L. and Thomas, K. (2006). A longitudinal investigation of the development of weight and muscle concerns among preadolescent boys. *Journal of Youth and Adolescence* 35 (2), 177–188.

Richards, M. H., Boxer, A. W., Peterson, A. C. and Albrecht, R. (1990). Relation of weight to body image in pubertal girls and boys from two communities. *Developmental Psychology* 26, 313–321.

Richardson, A. J. (2004). Clinical trials of fatty acid treatment in ADHD, dyslexia, dyspraxia and the autistic spectrum. *Prostaglandins, Leukotrienes and Essential Fatty Acids* 70 (4), 383–390.

Richardson, A. J. and Puri, B. K. (2000). The potential role of fatty acids in attention deficit/hyperactivity disorder. *Prostaglandins, Leukotrienes and Essential Fatty Acids* 63 (1/2), 79–87.

Richardson, J. and Joughin, C. (2002). *Parent-Training Programmes for the Management of Young Children with Conduct Disorders. Findings from Research*. London: Gaskell.

Ringham, R., Klump, K., Kaye, W., *et al.* (2006). Eating disorder symptomatology among ballet dancers. *International Journal of Eating Disorders* 39 (6), 503–506.

Roberts, C., Kane, R., Thomson, H., Bishop, B. and Hart, B. (2003). The prevention of depressive symptoms in rural school children: a randomised controlled trial. *Journal of Consulting and Clinical Psychology* 71 (3), 622–628.

Roberts, C., Kane, R., Bishop, B., Matthews, H. and Thomson, H. (2004). The prevention of depressive symptoms in rural school children: a follow-up study. *The International Journal of Mental Health Promotion* 6, 4–16.

Robinson, J., Harris, M., Harrigan, S., *et al.* (2010). Suicide attempt in first-episode psychosis: a 7.4 year follow-up study. *Schizophrenia Research* 116 (1), 1–8.

Robinson, S. M. and Alloy, L. B. (2003). Negative inferential style and stress-reactive rumination: interactive risk factors in the aetiology of depression. *Cognitive Therapy and Research* 27, 275–291.

Rodham, K., Hawton, K. and Evans, E. (2004). Reasons for deliberate self-harm: comparison of self-poisoners and self-cutters in a community sample of adolescents. *Journal of the American Academy of Child and Adolescent Psychiatry* 43, 80–87.

Rodham, K., Gavin, J. and Miles, M. (2007). I hear, I listen and I care: a qualitative investigation into the function of a self-harm message board. *Suicide and Life-Threatening Behavior* 37 (4), 422–430.

Roe, E. and Becker, J. (2005). Drug prevention with vulnerable young people: a review. *Drugs: Education, Prevention and Policy* 12 (2), 85–99.

Rojahn, J., Matson, J. L., Lott, D., Esbensen, A. J. and Smalls, Y. (2002). The behaviour problems inventory: an instrument for the assessment of self-injury, stereotypical behaviour and aggression/destructive behaviour in individuals with developmental disorders. *Journal of Autism and Developmental Disorders* 31, 577–588.

Romme, M. (1998). Listening to the voice hearers. *Journal of Psychosocial Nursing and Mental Health Services* 36, 40–44.

Romme, M. and Escher, D. (2000). *Making Sense of Voices: A Guide for Professional Who Work with Voice Hearers*. London: MIND Publications.

Romme, M. and Escher, S. (1993). *Accepting Voices*. London: MIND Publications.

Romme, R. and Morrison, M. (2007). The harmful concept of schizophrenia. *Mental Health Nursing* 27 (2), 7–11.

Rooney, R., Pike, L., Roberts, C., Snowball, S., Rudge, L. and Mullen, A. (2000). *The Positive Thinking Program: Prevention Manual*. Perth, Australia: Curtin University of Technology.

Rooney, R., Roberts, C., Kane, R., *et al.* (2006). The prevention of depression in 8- to 9-year-old children: a pilot study. *Australian Journal of Guidance and Counselling* 16 (1), 76–90.

Rose, A. J. (2002). Co-rumination in the friendships of girls and boys. *Child Development* 73, 1830–1843.

Rosenberg, M. (1965). *Society and the Adolescent Self-image*. Princeton, NJ: Princeton University Press.

Rosenberg, S. D., Lu, W., Mueser, K. T., Jankowski, M. K. and Cournos, F. (2007). Correlates of adverse childhood events among adults with schizophrenia spectrum disorders. *Psychiatric Services* 58 (2), 245–253.

Rowe, F., Stewart, D. and Patterson, C. (2007). Promoting school connectedness through whole school approaches. *Health Education* 107 (6), 524–542.

Rowling, L. (2006). Adolescence and emerging adulthood (12–17 years and 18–24 years). In: Cattan, M. and Tilford, S. (eds). *Mental Health Promotion: A Lifespan Approach*. Maidenhead: Open University Press, McGraw Hill Education.

Rubenstein, J. L., Heeren, T., Houseman, D., Rubin, C. and Stechler, G. (1989). Suicidal behaviour in 'normal' adolescents: risk and protective factors. *American Journal of Orthopsychiatry* 59, 59–71.

Rudd, M., Joiner, T. and Rajab, H. (1996). Relationships among suicidal ideators, attempters and multiple attempters in a young adult sample. *Journal of Abnormal Psychology* 105, 541–550.

Rudd, M. D. and Joiner, T. E., Jr. (1998). An integrative conceptual framework for assessing and treating suicidal behaviour in adolescents. *Journal of Adolescence* 21, 473–488.

Rugino, T. A. and Janvier, Y. M. (2005). Aripiprazole in children and adolescents: clinical experience. *Journal of Child Neurology* 20, 603–610.

Russell, A. T. (1992). Schizophrenia. In: Hooper, S. R., Hynd, G. W. and Mattison, R. E. (eds). *Assessment and Diagnosis of Child and Adolescent Psychiatric Disorders: Current Issues and Procedures*. Hillside, NJ: Lawrence Erlbaum.

Russell, P. (2006). *A Matter of Substance?* Stirling: Aberlour Child Care Trust.

Rutter, M. (1996). Connections between child and adult psychopathology. *European Child Adolescent Psychology* 5 (Suppl. 1), 4–7.

Rutter, M. (2005). Aetiology of autism: findings and questions. *Journal of Intellectual Disability Research* 49 (4), 231–238.

Rutter, M. (2006). The promotion of resilience in the face of adversity. In: Clarke-Stewart, A. and Dunn, J. (eds). *Families Count: Effect on Child and Adolescent Development*. Cambridge, UK: Cambridge University Press.

Rutter, M. and O'Connor, T. G. (2004). Are there biological programming effects for psychological development? Findings from a study of Romanian adoptees. *Developmental Psychology* 40, 81–94.

Rutter, M. and Smith, D. J. (1995). *Psychosocial Disorders in Young People: Time, Trends and Their Causes*. Chichester: John Wiley and Sons Ltd.

Rutter, M., Cox, A., Tupling, C., *et al.* (1975). Attainment and adjustment in two geographical areas. I: The prevalence of psychiatric disorder. *The British Journal of Psychiatry* 126, 493–509.

Salokangas, R. K., Vaahtera, K., Pacriev, S., Sohlman, B. and Lehtinen, V. (2002). Gender differences in depressive symptoms. An artefact caused by measurement instruments? *Journal of Affective Disorders* 68 (2–3), 215–220.

Sameroff, A. (2006). Identifying risk and protective factors for healthy child development. In: Clarke-Stewart, A. and Dunn, J. (2006). *Families Count: Effect on Child and Adolescent Development*. Cambridge, UK: Cambridge University Press.

Sanders, M., Markie-Dadds, C. and Turner, K. (2003). Theoretical, scientific and clinical foundations of the Triple-P Positive Parenting Program: a population approach to the promotion of parenting competence. *Parenting Research and Practice Monograph No 1*. University of Queensland, Parenting and Family Support Centre.

Santonastaso, P. (1998). Impulsive and compulsive self-injurious behaviour in bulimia nervosa: prevalence and psychological correlates. *Journal of Nervous and Mental Disease* 186 (3), 157–165.

Sato, M. (2006). Renaming schizophrenia: a Japanese perspective. *World Psychiatry* 5 (1), 53–55.

Schmidt, U. and Davidson, K. (2004). *Life After Self-Harm: A Guide to the Future.* Hove: Brunner-Routledge.

Schmidtke, A. and Schaller, S. (2000). The role of mass media in suicide prevention. In: Hawton, K. and van Heeringen, K. (eds). *The International Handbook of Suicide and Attempted Suicide.* New York: Wiley.

Schneider, M. J., Bijam-Schulte, A. M., Janssen, C. G. C. and Stolk, J. (1996). The origins of self-injurious behaviour of children with mental retardation. *British Journal Development Disabilities* 2, 136–148.

Schreier, A., Wolke, D., Thomas, K., *et al.* (2009). Prospective study of peer victimization in childhood and psychotic symptoms in a nonclinical population at age 12 years. *Archives of General Psychiatry* 66 (5), 527–536.

Scott, J. and Hill, M. (2006). *The Health Needs of Looked After and Accommodated Children and Young People in Scotland: Messages from Research.* Edinburgh: Scottish Executive.

Scottish Executive (2002a). *It's Everyone's Job to Make Sure I'm Alright. Report of the Child Protection Audit and Review.* Edinburgh: The Stationary Office. Available at http://www.scotland.gov.uk/Publications/2002/11/15820/14009.

Scottish Executive (2002b). *Choose Life: A National Action Plan and Strategy to Prevent Suicide in Scotland.* Edinburgh: Scottish Executive.

Scottish Executive (2002c). *Drug Treatment Services for Young People. A Research Review.* Edinburgh: The Stationery Office.

Scottish Executive (2003). *National Programme for Improving Mental Health and Well-being.* Edinburgh: Scottish Executive.

Scottish Executive (2006). *Rights, Relationships and Recovery: The Report of the National Review of Mental Health Nursing in Scotland: National Review of Mental Health Nursing in Scotland.* Edinburgh: Scottish Executive.

Scottish Government (2009). *Towards a Mentally Flourishing Scotland: Policy and Action Plan 2009–2011.* Edinburgh: Scottish Government.

Scottish Intercollegiate Guidelines Network (SIGN) (2001). *Attention Deficit and Hyperkinetic Disorders in Children and Young People: A National Clinical Guideline.* SIGN Publication No. 52. Edinburgh: SIGN. Available at www.sign.ac.uk.

Scottish Intercollegiate Guidelines Network (SIGN) (2008). *Autism Spectrum Disorders: Booklet for Young People.* NHS Evidence website. Available at http://www.evidence.nhs.uk/default.aspx.

Scottish Public Health Observatory (2007). *Obesity in Scotland: An Epidemiology Briefing.* Edinburgh: Scottish Public Health Observatory. Available at www.scotpho.org.uk.

Scourfield, J., Roen, K. and McDermott, E. (2008). Lesbian, gay, bisexual and transgender young people's experience of distress: resilience, ambivalence and self-destructive behaviour. *Health and Social Care in the Community* 16 (3), 329–336.

Selman, R. L. (1980). *The Growth of Interpersonal Understanding.* New York: Academic Press.

Sergeant, J. A., Geurts, H. and Oosterlaan, J. (2002). How specific is a deficit of executive functioning for attention deficit/hyperactivity disorder? *Behavioural Brain Research* 130, 3–28.

Sewell, R. A., Ranganathan, M. and D'Souza, D. C. (2009). Cannabinoids and psychosis. *International Review of Psychiatry* 21 (2), 152–162.

Shaffer, D. and Craft, L. (1999). Methods of adolescent suicide prevention. *Journal of Clinical Psychiatry* 60, 70–74.

Shaffer, D., Fisher, P., Dulcan, M. K., *et al.* (1996a). The NIMH Diagnostic Interview Schedule for Children Version 2.3 (DISC-2.3): Description, acceptability, prevalence rates, and performance in the MECA Study. Methods for the Epidemiology of Child and Adolescent Mental Disorders Study. *Journal of the American Academy of Child and Adolescent Psychiatry* 35, 865–877.

Shaffer, D., Garland, A., Vieland, V., Underwood, M. M and Busner, C. (1991). The impact of curriculum-based suicide prevention program for teenagers. *J Am Acad Child Adolesc Psychiatry* 30, 588–596.

Shaffer, D., Gould, M. S., Fisher, P., *et al.* (1996b). Psychiatric diagnosis in child and adolescent suicide. *Archives of General Psychiatry* 53, 339–348.

Shattock, P., Whiteley, P. and Savery, D. (2001). *Autism as a Metabolic Disorder: Guidelines for Gluten and Casein-Free Dietary intervention (Revised)*. University of Sunderland, UK: Autism Research Unit.

Shaw, C. and Shaw, T. (2007). A dialogue of hope and survival. In: Spandler, H. and Warner, S. (eds). *Beyond Fear and Control: Working with Young People Who Self-harm*. Ross on Wye: PPCS Books.

Shaw, T. (2007). *Historical Abuse Systematic Review: Residential Schools and Children's Homes in Scotland 1950 to 1995*. Edinburgh: The Scottish Government.

Shayer, M., Kuchemann, D. E. and Wylam, H. (1976). The distribution of Piagetian stages of thinking in British middle and secondary school children. *British Journal of Educational Psychology* 46, 164–173.

Shearer, M. C. and Bermingham, S. L. (2008). The ethics of paediatric anti-depressant use: eErring on the side of caution. *Journal of Medical Ethics* 34 (10), 710–714.

Sheitman, B. B., Lieberman, J. A., Lee, H. and Strauss, R. (1997). The evaluation and treatment of first-episode psychosis. *Schizophrenia Bulletin* 23 (4), 653–661.

Sheridan, M. S. (2003). The deceit continues: an updated literature review of Munchausen syndrome by proxy. *Child Abuse and Neglect* 27 (4), 431–451.

Shevlin, M., Dorahy, M. and Adamson, G. (2007). Childhood traumas and hallucinations: an analysis of the National Comorbidity Survey. *Journal of Psychiatric Research* 41, 222–228.

Shiwach, R. S. (1998). Auto-nucleation a culture specific phenomenon. A case series and review. *Comprehensive Psychiatry* 39 (5), 318–322.

Shulman, S. and Scharf, M. (2000). Adolescent romantic behaviors and perceptions: age-related differences and links with family and peer relationships. *Journal of Research on Adolescence* 10, 99–118.

Silbereisen, R. and Kracke, B. (1993). Variation in maturational timing and adjustment in adolescence. In: Jackson, S. and Rodriguez-Tome, H. (eds). *The Social Worlds of Adolescence*. Hove: Erlbaum.

Silverman, M. M., Berman, A. L., Sanddal, N. D., *et al.* (2007). Rebuilding the Tower of Babel: a revised nomenclature for the study of suicide and suicidal behaviors. Part 1: Background, rationale, and methodology. *Suicide and Life-Threatening Behavior* 37, 248–263.

Simmons, R. G. and Blyth, D. A. (1987). *Moving into Adolescence*. Hawthorne, NY: Aldine.

Simpson, S. A., Rhodes, W. S. and Nelligan, J. S. (1992). Support-seeking and support-giving within couple members in anxiety-provoking situation: the role of attachment styles. *Journal of Personality and Social Psychology* 62, 434–446.

Singh, I. and Rose, N. (2006). Social and cultural issues in ADHD diagnoses and psychostimulant treatment. ADHD Consensus Conference to the NICE Guidelines Development Group, October 2006, in NICE (2009). *Attention Deficit Hyperactivity Disorder*.

Sinton, M. M. and Birch, L. L. (2006). Individual and sociocultural influences on pre-adolescent girls' appearance schemas and body dissatisfaction. *Journal of Youth and Adolescence* 35 (2), 165–176.

Slee, N., Arensman, E., Garnefski, N. and Spinhoven, P. (2007). Cognitive behavioural therapy for deliberate self harm crisis. *The Journal of Crisis Intervention and Suicide Prevention* 28 (4), 175–182.

Slee, N., Garnefski, N., van der Leeden, R., Arensman, E. and Spinhoven, P. (2008). Cognitive–behavioural intervention for self-harm: randomised controlled trial. *The British Journal of Psychiatry* 192, 202–211.

Smetana, J., Metzger, A., Gettman, D. C. and Campione-Barr, N. (2006). Disclosure and secrecy in adolescent–parent relationships. *Child Development* 77, 201–217.

Smith, A., Shenton, O. and Rice, J. (1996). *Accelerated Learning in the Classroom*. Stafford: Network Educational Press.

SNAP (2000). *Mental Health Promotion Among Young People*. Glasgow: Office for Public Health in Scotland.

Sonuga-Barke, E. J. S. (1998). Categorical model in child psychopathology: a conceptual and empirical analysis. *The Journal of Child Psychology and Psychiatry* 39, 15–133.

Sonuga-Barke, E. J. S. (2006). Categorical models of attention deficit/hyperactivity disorder: a conceptual and empirical analysis. ADHD Consensus Conference, October 2006, in NICE (2009). Appendix 16, *Attention Deficit Hyperactivity Disorder*.

Southgate, L., Tchanturia, K. and Treasure, J. (2005). Building a model of the aetiology of eating disorders by translating experimental neuroscience into clinical practice. *Journal of Mental Health* 14 (6), 553–566.

Spandler, H. (1996). *Who's Hurting Who? Young People Self Harm and Suicide*. Manchester: 42nd Street.

Spencer, M. B., Dupree, D. and Hartmann, T. (1997). A phenomenological variant of ecological systems theory (PVEST): a self-organization perspective in context. *Development and Psychopathology* 9 (4), 817–833.

Spitz, R. (1945). Hospitalism: an inquiry into the genesis of psychiatric conditions in early childhood. *Psychoanalytical Study of the Child* 1, 53–74.

Stack, S. (2005). Suicide in the media: a quantitative review of studies based on non-fictional stories. *Suicide and Life-Threatening Behavior* 35 (2), 121–133.

Stain, H., Sartore, G. M., Andrews, D. and Kelly, B. (2008). First-episode psychosis in rural, coastal and remote Australian communities. *Australasian Psychiatry* 16 (2), 119–124.

Stallard, P. (2002). Cognitive behaviour therapy with children and young people: a selective review of key issues. *Behavioural and Cognitive Psychotherapy* 30 (3), 297–309.

Stallard, P. (2005). *A Clinician's Guide to Think Good-Feel Good: Using CBT with Children and Young People*. Available at http://www.myilibrary.com/Browse/open.asp?ID=28757.

Standing Conference on Drug Abuse (SCODA) and The Children's Legal Centre (CLC) (1999). *Young People and Drugs: Policy Guidance for Drug Interventions*. London: Drugscope.

Stanley, B., Gameroff, M. J., Michalsen, V. and Mann, J. J. (2001). Are suicide attempters who self-mutilate a unique population? *The American Journal of Psychiatry* 158 (3), 427–432.

Steele, M. and Doey, T. (2007). Suicidal behaviour in children and adolescents. Part 1: Etiology and risk factors. *Canadian Journal of Psychiatry* 52 (6), 21S–33S.

Steer, C. R. (2005). Managing attention deficit/hyperactivity disorder: unmet needs and future directions. *Archives of Diseases in Childhood* 90 (Suppl. 1), 19–25.

Stefanis, N. C., Delespaul, P., Henquet, C., Bakoula, C., Stefanis, C. N. and Van Os, J. (2004). Early adolescent cannabis exposure and positive and negative dimensions of psychosis. *Addiction* 99, 1333–1341.

Stein, J. H. and Reiser, L. W. (1994). A study of white middle class adolescent boys' responses to 'semenarche' (the first ejaculation). *Journal of Youth and Adolescence* 23, 373–384.

Steinberg, L. (1989). Pubertal maturation and parent–adolescent distance: an evolutionary perspective. In: Adams, G., Montemayor, R. and Gullotta, T. (eds). *Advances in Adolescent Development*, Vol. 1, pp. 71–97. Beverly Hills, CA: Sage.

Steinberg, L. (2001). We know some things: adolescent–parent relationships in retrospect and prospect. *Journal of Research into Adolescence* 11, 1–19.

Steinberg, L. D. (1988). Reciprocal relation between parent–child distance and pubertal maturation. *Developmental Psychology* 24, 122–128.

Steinberg, L. D. (1990). Interdependence in the family: autonomy, conflict, and harmony in the parent–adolescent relationship. In: Feldman, S. S. and Elliott, G. R. (eds). *At the Threshold*. Cambridge, MA: Harvard University Press.

Stepp, S., Morse, J., Yaggi, K., Reynolds, S., Reed, L. and Pilkonis, P. (2008). The role of attachment styles and interpersonal problems in suicide-related behaviors. *Suicide and Life-Threatening Behavior* 38 (5), 592–607.

Stevens, S. E., Sonuga-Barke, E. J., Kreppner, J. M., *et al.* (2008). Inattention/overactivity following early severe institutional deprivation: presentation and associations in early adolescence. *Journal of Abnormal Child Psychology* 36, 385–398.

Stevenson, D. T. and Romney, D. M. (1984). Depression in learning disabled children. *Journal of Learning Disabilities* 17 (10), 579–582.

Stoelb, M. and Chiriboga, J. (1998). A process model for assessing adolescent risk for suicide. *Journal of Adolescence* 21, 397–406.

Stoep, A., McCauley, E., Flynn, C. and Stone, A. (2009). Thoughts of death and suicide in early adolescence. *Suicide and Life-Threatening Behavior* 39 (6), 599–613.

Stone, M., Laughren, T., Jones, M. L., *et al.* (2009). Risk of suicidality in clinical trials of antidepressants in adults: analysis of proprietary data submitted to US Food and Drug Administration. *British Medical Journal* 339, b2880.

Straub, R. E., MacLean, C. J., O'Neill, F. A., Welsh, D. and Kendler, K. S. (1997). Support for a possible schizophrenia vulnerability locus in region 5q22–31 in Irish families. *Molecular Psychiatry* 2, 148–155.

Street, C. and Herts, B. (2005). *Putting Participation into Practice. A Guide for Practitioners Working in Services to Promote the Mental Health of and Well-being of Young People*. London: YoungMinds. Available at http://www.youngminds.org.uk/publications.

Strong, M. (2000). *A Bright Red Scar: Self-mutilation and the Language of Pain*. London: Virago.

Sundquist, K., Frank, G. and Sundquist, J. (2004). Urbanisation and incidence of psychosis and depression. Follow-up study of 4.4 million women and men in Sweden. *The British Journal of Psychiatry* 184, 293–298.

Suominen, K., Isometsä, E., Martunnen, M., Ostamo, A. and Lönnqvist, J. (2004). Health care contacts before and after attempted suicide among adolescent and young adult versus older suicide attempters. *Psychological Medicine* 34 (2), 313–321.

Sutton, A. (1998). Psychodynamics of self-directed destructive behaviours in adolescence. *Advances in Psychiatric Treatment* 4, 31–38.

Sutton, J. (2007). *Healing the Hurt Within: Understanding Self-injury and Self-harm and Heal the Emotional Wounds*. Oxford: How to Books.

Sutton, J. and Martinson, S. (2003). Self-injury and related issues. Retrieved 1 May 2007, from http://www.siari.co.uk cited in Sutton, J. (2007) *Healing the Hurt Within: Understanding Self-injury and Self-harm and Heal the Emotional Wounds*. Oxford: How to Books.

TADS (Treatment for Adolescents with Depression Study) (2004). Fluoxetine, cognitive–behavioral therapy, and their combination for adolescents with depression: Treatment for Adolescents with Depression Study (TADS) randomized controlled trial. *Journal of American Medical Association* 18 (292), 807–820.

Tamplin, A., Goodyer, I. M. and Herbert, J. (1998). Family functioning and parent general health in families of adolescents with major depressive disorder. *Journal of Affective Disorders* 48 (1), 1–13.

Tandon, R., Keshavan, M. and Nasrallah, H. (2008). Schizophrenia, 'just the facts' what we know in 2008. 2. Epidemiology and etiology. *Schizophrenia Research* 102 (1), 1–18.

Tarrier, N., Taylor, K. and Gooding, P. (2008). Cognitive–behavioral interventions to reduce suicide behavior: a systematic review and meta-analysis. *Behavior Modification* 32 (1), 77–108.

Taylor, E., Doepfner, M., Sergeant, J., *et al.* (2004). European clinical guidelines for hyperkinetic disorder – first upgrade. *European Child and Adolescent Psychiatry* 13 (1), 17–30.

Thapar, A., Fowler, T., Rice, F., *et al.* (2003). Maternal smoking during pregnancy and attention deficit hyperactivity disorder symptoms in offspring. *The American Journal of Psychiatry* 160, 1985–1989.

The European Network of Schizophrenia Networks for the Study of Gene–Environment Interactions (EU-GEI) (2008). Schizophrenia aetiology: Do gene–environment interactions hold the key? *Schizophrenia Research* 102, 21–26.

Thompson, E. A., Eggert, L. L. and Herting, J. R. (2000). Mediating effects of an indicated prevention program for reducing youth depression and suicide behaviours. *Suicide and Life-Threatening Behavior* 30 (3), 252–271.

Thompson, E. A., Eggert, L. L., Randell, B. P. and Pike, K. C. (2001). Evaluation of indicated suicide risk prevention approaches for potential high school dropouts. *American Journal of Public Health* 91 (5), 742–752.

Thompson, N. and Bhugra, D. (2000). Rates of deliberate self-harm in Asians: findings and models. *International Review of Psychiatry* 12, 37–43.

Thornicroft, G., Brohan, E., Rose, D., Sartorius, N. and Leese, M. (2009). Global pattern of experienced and anticipated discrimination against people with schizophrenia: a cross-sectional survey. *Lancet* 373, 408–415.

Tick, N. T., van der Ende, J. and Verhulst, F. C. (2008). Ten-year trends in self-reported emotional and behavioural problems of Dutch adolescents. *Social Psychiatry and Psychiatric Epidemiology* 43, 349–355.

Tien, A. Y. (1991). Distributions of hallucinations in the population. *Social Psychiatry and Psychiatric Epidemiology* 26 (6), 287–292.

Tienari, P., Wynne, L. C., Läksy, K., *et al.* (2003). Genetic boundaries of the schizophrenia spectrum: evidence from the Finnish Adoptive Family Study. *The American Journal of Psychiatry* 160, 1587–1594.

Tilford, S. (2006). Infancy and childhood (0–5 years and 6–12 years). In: Cattan, M. and Tilford, S. (eds). *Mental Health Promotion: A Lifespan Approach.* Maidenhead: Open University Press, McGraw Hill Education.

Timimi, S. (2004). *Childhood Depression? A Paper in Response to the NICE Scope for Clinical Guideline on Depression in Children.* Available at http://www.critpsynet .freeuk.com/childdepression.htm.

Timimi, S. (2005). *Naughty Boys Anti-social Behaviour, ADHD and the Role of Culture.* Basingstoke: Palgrave Macmillan.

Timimi, S. (2006). Arguments against the use of the concept of ADHD in clinical practice. ADHD Consensus Conference, October 2006, in NICE (2009). Appendix 16, *Attention Deficit Hyperactivity Disorder.*

Timimi, S. (2007). The medicalisation of childhood. *Healthcare Counselling and Psychotherapy Journal* 7 (1), 7–9.

Timimi, S. and 33 Co-endorsers (2004). A critique of the international consensus statement on ADHD. *Clinical Child and Family Psychology Review* 7, 59–63.

Tishler, C. L., Reiss, N. S. and Rhodes, A. R. (2007). Suicidal behavior in children younger than twelve: a diagnostic challenge for emergency department personnel. *Academic Emergency Medicine* 14 (9), 810–818.

Tobin-Richards, M. H., Boxer, A. M. and Peterson, A. C. (1983). The psychological significance of pubertal change: sex differences in perceptions of self during early adolescence. In: Brooks-Gunn, J. and Peterson, A. C. (eds). *Girls at Puberty: Biological and Psychosocial Perspectives.* New York: Plenum.

Tolmac, J. and Hodes, M. (2004). Ethnicity and adolescent psychiatric admission for psychotic disorders. *The British Journal of Psychiatry* 184, 428–431.

Tonge, B. (2007). The psychopathology of children with intellectual disabilities. In: Bouras, N. and Holt, G. (eds). *Psychiatric and Behavioural Disorders in Intellectual and Developmental Disabilities,* 2nd edition. Cambridge: Cambridge University Press.

Tonge, B. J. and Einfeld, S. L. (2003). Psychopathology and intellectual disability. The Australian child to adult longitudinal study. In: Glidden, L. M. (ed). *International Review of Research in Mental Retardation,* Vol. 26, pp. 61–91. CA: Academic Press.

Torrey, E. F., Miller, J., Rawlings, R. and Yolken, R. H. (1997). Seasonality of births in schizophrenia and bipolar disorder: a review of the literature. *Schizophrenia Research* 28, 1–38.

Treasure, J. (2007). Getting beneath the phenotype of anorexia nervosa: the search for viable phenotypes and genotypes. *La Revue Canadienne de Psychiatrie* 52 (4), 212–219.

Treasure, J., Smith, G. and Crane, A. (2007). *Skills-Based Learning for Caring for a Loved One with an Eating Disorder: The New Maudsley Method.* London: Routledge.

Trevarthen, C. and Aitken, K. (2001). Infant intersubjectivity: research, theory, and clinical applications. *Journal of Child Psychology and Psychiatry* 42 (1), 3–48.

Trowell, J., Joffe, I., Campbell, J., *et al.* (2007). Childhood depression: a place for psychotherapy. An outcome study comparing individual psychodynamic psychotherapy and family therapy. *European Child & Adolescent Psychiatry* 16 (3), 157–167.

Tsapakis, E., Soldani, F., Tondo, L. and Baldessarini, R. J. (2008). Efficacy of antidepressants in juvenile depression: meta-analysis. *The British Journal of Psychiatry* 193, 10–17.

Tucker, P. (2009). Intervention is of value in improving outcomes. *Australasian Psychiatry: Bulletin of Royal Australian and New Zealand College of Psychiatrists* 17 (4), 291–294.

Turner, R. M. (2000). Naturalistic evaluation of dialectical behavior therapy-oriented treatment for borderline personality disorder. *Cognitive and Behavioral Practice* 7, 413–419.

Tyrer, P. and Kendall, T. (2009). The spurious advance of antipsychotic drug therapy. *The Lancet* 373, 4–5.

UNICEF (2003). *A League Table of Child Maltreatment Deaths in Rich Nations*. Innocenti Report Card 5, Florence, Italy: UNICEF Innocenti Research Centre. Available at http://www.unicef-irc.org/publications/pdf/repcard5e.pdf.

UNICEF (2007). *Child Poverty in Perspective: An Overview of Child Well-being in Rich Countries*. Innocenti Report Card 7, Florence, Italy: UNICEF Innocenti Research Centre. Available at http://www.unicef.org.uk/publications/pdf/rc7_eng.pdf.

United Nations (1989). *Convention on the Rights of the Child*. London: HMSO.

United Nations (2007). *Human Development Report 2007/2008*. New York: United Nations Development Programme (UNDP).

Usala, T., Clavenna, A., Zuddas, A. and Bonati, M. (2008). Randomised controlled trials of selective serotonin reuptake inhibitors in treating depression in children and adolescents: a systematic review and meta-analysis. *European Neuropsychopharmacology: The Journal of the European College of Neuropsychopharmacology* 18 (1), 62–73.

Vajani, M., Annest, J. L., Crosby, A. E., Alexander, J. D. and Millet, L. M. (2007). Nonfatal and fatal self-harm injuries among children aged 10–14 years – United States and Oregon, 2001–2003. *Suicide and Life-Threatening Behavior* 37 (5), 493–506.

Valicenti-McDermott, M. R. and Demb, H. (2006). Clinical effects and adverse reactions of off-label use of aripiprazole in children and adolescents with developmental disabilities. *Journal of Child and Adolescent Psychopharmacology* 16, 549–560.

van Hoeken, D., Seidall, J. and Hoek, H. (2005). Epidemiology. In: Treasure, J., Schmidt, U. and van Furth, E. (eds). *The Essential Handbook of Eating Disorders*. Chichester: John Wiley and Sons Ltd.

Van Ijzendoorn, M. H. (1995). Adult attachment representations, parental responsiveness, and infant attachment: a meta-analysis of the predictive validity of the adult attachment interview. *Psychological Bulletin* 117 (3), 387–403.

Van Os, J. and Poulton, R. (2008). Environmental vulnerability and genetic environmental interactions. In: Jackson, H. and McGorry, P. (eds). *The Recognition and Management of Early Psychosis: A Preventive Approach*, 2nd edition. Cambridge: Cambridge University Press.

Veling, W., Susser, E., van Os, J., Mackenbach, J. P., Selten, J. P. and Hoek, H. W. (2008). Ethnic density of neighborhoods and incidence of psychotic disorders among immigrants. *The American Journal of Psychiatry* 165, 66–73.

Velleman, R. (2001). *Counselling for Alcohol Problems.* London: Sage Publications.

Viner, R. M. and Taylor, B. (2007). Adult outcomes of binge drinking in adolescence: findings from a UK cohort. *Journal of Community Health* 61, 902–907.

Waaktaar, T., Borge, A. I. H., Fundingsrud, H. P., Christie, H. J. and Torgersen, S. (2004). The role of stressful life events in the development of depressive symptoms in adolescence – a longitudinal community study. *Journal of Adolescence* 27, 153–163.

Wakefield, A. J., Murch, S. H., Anthony, A., *et al.* (1998). Ileal-lymphoid-nodular hyperplasia, non-specific colitis, and pervasive developmental disorder in children. *Lancet* 351 (9103), 637–641.

Waldrop, A., Hanson, R., Resnick, H., Kilpatrick, D., Naugle, A. and Saunders, B. (2007). Risk factors for suicidal behavior among a national sample of adolescents: implications for prevention. *Journal of Traumatic Stress* 20 (5), 869–887.

Walker, L. and Taylor, J. H. (1991). Family interactions and the development of moral reasoning. *Child Development* 62, 264–283.

Walsh, F. (1993). Conceptualisation of normal family processes. In: Walsh, F. (ed). *Normal Family Processes*, 2nd edition. New York: Guildford Press.

Walsh, F. (2003). Changing families in a changing world: reconstructing family normality. Chapter 1. In: Walsh, F. (ed). *Normal Family Processes*, 3rd edition. New York/London: The Guildford Press.

Wannan, G. and Fombonne, E. (1998). Gender differences in rates and correlates of suicidal behaviour amongst child psychiatric outpatients. *Journal of Adolescence* 21, 371–382.

Waska, R. T. (1998). Self-mutilation, substance abuse, and the psychoanalytic approach: four cases. *American Journal of Psychotherapy* 52 (1), 18–27.

Watanabe, N., Hunot, V., Omori, I. M., Churchill, R. and Furukawa, T. A. (2007). Psychotherapy for depression among children and adolescents: a systematic review. *Acta Psychiatrica Scandinavica* 116, 84–95.

Waters, E., Merrick, S., Treboux, D., Crowell, J. and Albersheim, L. (2000). Attachment security in infancy and early adulthood: A twenty-year longitudinal study. *Child Development* 71 (3), 684–689.

Webster-Stratton, C. (1992). *The Incredible Years: A Trouble-Shooting Guide for Parents of Children Aged 3–8.* Toronto: Umbrella Press. Available at www.incredibleyears.com.

Webster-Stratton, C. (1998). *How to Promote Children's Social and Emotional Competence.* London: Paul Chapman Publishing.

Webster-Stratton, C. and Herbert, M. (1994). *Troubled Families, Problem Children.* London: Wiley.

Webster-Stratton, C. and Reid, M. J. (2008). Strengthening social and emotional competence in socioeconomically disadvantaged young children: preschool and kindergarten school-based curricula. In: Brown, W. H., Odom, S. L. and McConnell, S. R. (eds). *Social Competence of Young Children: Risk, Disability, and Intervention.* Baltimore: Paul H. Brookes Publishing Co.

Weinfield, N. S., Sroufe, A. and Egeland, B. (2000). Attachment from infancy to early adulthood in a high risk sample: continuity, discontinuity, and their correlates. *Child Development* 71 (3), 695–702.

Weissman, M. M., Prusoff, B. A. and DiMascio, A. (1979). The efficacy of drugs and psychotherapy in the treatment of acute depressive episodes. *The American Journal of Psychiatry* 136, 555–558.

Weissman, M. M., Markowitz, J. C. and Klerman, G. L. (2000). IPT for depressed adolescent (IPTA). In: Weissman, M. M., Markowitz, J. C. and Klerman, G. L. (eds). *Comprehensive Guide to Interpersonal Psychotherapy*. New York: Basic Books.

Weissman, M. M., Wickramaratne, P., Nomura, Y., *et al*. (2005). Families at high and low risk for depression: a 3-generation study. *Archives of General Psychiatry* 62, 29–36.

Weisz, J. R., McCarthy, C. A. and Valeri, S. M. (2006). Effects of psychotherapy for depression in children and adolescents: a meta-analysis. *Psychological Bulletin* 132, 132–149.

Wekerle, C. and Wolfe, D. (2003). Child maltreatment. In: Mash, E. and Barkley, R. (eds). *Child Psychopathology*, 2nd edition. New York: Guildford.

Weller, E. and Weller, R. (2000). The serious nature of teenage 'blues'. *Journal of Affective Disorders* 61 (Suppl. 1), S1.

Weller, E. B., Kloos, A., Kang, J. and Weller, R. A. (2006a). Depression in children and adolescents: Does gender make a difference? *Current Psychiatry Reports* 8 (2), 108–114.

Weller, E. B., Kloos, A., Kang, J. and Weller, R. A. (2006b). Mood disorders. In: Dulcan, M. K. and Wiener, J. M. (eds). *Essentials of Child and Adolescent Psychiatry*. Washington, DC: American Psychiatric Publishing.

Werry, J. S. (1992). Child and adolescent schizophrenia. *Journal of Autism and Developmental Disorders* 22, 601–624.

Werry, J. S. and Taylor, E. (1994). Schizophrenic and allied disorders. In: Rutter, M., Taylor, E. and Hersov, L. (eds). *Child and Adolescent Psychiatry, Modern Approaches*. Abingdon: Blackwell Science.

West, P. and Sweeting, H. (2003). Fifteen, female and stressed: changing patterns of psychological distress over time. *Journal of Child Psychology and Psychiatry* 44 (3), 399–411.

Wheeler, B. W., Gunnell, D., Chris Metcalfe, C., Stephens, P. and Martin, R. M. (2008). The population impact on incidence of suicide and non-fatal self-harm of regulatory action against the use of selective serotonin reuptake inhibitors in under 18s in the United Kingdom: ecological study. *British Medical Journal* 336 (7643), 542–545.

White, M. (1993). Deconstruction and therapy. In: Gilligan, S. and Price, R. (eds). *Therapeutic Conversations*. New York: WW Norton and Company.

White, M. (2007). *Maps of Narrative Practice*. New York: WW Norton.

White, M. and Epston, D. (1990). *Narrative Means to Therapeutic Ends*. New York: Norton. Available at www.dulwichcentre.com.au.

Whitehead, R. E. and Douglas, H. (2005). Health visitors' experiences of using the Solihull approach. *Community Practitioner* 78 (1), 20–23.

Whitfield, C. L., Dubeb, S. R., Felitti, V. J. and Anda, R. F. (2005). Adverse childhood experiences and hallucinations. *Child Abuse and Neglect* 29, 797–810.

Whitlock, J. (2009). *The Cutting Edge: Non-suicidal Self-injury in Adolescence*. Ithaca, New York: ACT for Youth Center of Excellence.

Whittington, C. J., Kendall, T., Fonagy, P., Cottrell, D., Cotgrove, A. and Boddington, E. (2004). Selective serotonin reuptake inhibitors in childhood depression: systematic review of published versus unpublished data. *Lancet* 363, 1341–1345.

WHO (World Health Organization) (1992). *The International Classification of Diseases, 10th edition (ICD-10). Classification of Mental and Behavioural Disorders: Clinical Descriptions and Diagnostic Guidelines*, pp. 75 and 76. Geneva: WHO.

WHO (2000). *Multisite Intervention on Suicidal Behaviours – SUPRE-MISS: Components and Instruments*. Geneva: WHO.

WHO (2002). *Prevention of Suicidal Behaviours: A Task for All*. Geneva: WHO.

WHO (2004a). *Distribution of Suicide Rates by Gender and Age 2000*. Available at http://www.who.int/mental_health/prevention/suicide/suicidecharts/en/.

WHO (2004b). *Promoting Mental Health: Concepts – Emerging Evidence, Practice*. Report of the World Health Organization, Department of Mental Health and Substance Abuse in collaboration with the Victorian Health Promotion Foundation and the University of Melbourne. Edited by Herrman, H., Saxena, S and Moodie, R Geneva: World Health Organization. Available at http://www.who.int/mental_health/evidence/MH_Promotion_Book.pdf.

WHO (2005). *Child and Adolescent Mental Health: Policies and Plans*. Geneva: WHO.

WHO (2008a). *Suicide and Suicide Prevention in Asia*. Geneva: WHO Document Production Services.

WHO (2008b). *The Global of Burden of Disease: 2004 Update*. Switzerland WHO Library Cataloguing-in-Publication Data. Available at http://www.who.int/healthinfo/global_burden_disease/GBD_report_2004update_full.pdf.

WHO (2008c). *Number of Suicides by Age Group and Gender. United Kingdom of Great Britain and Northern Ireland, 2005*. Available at http://www.who.int/mental_health/media/unitkingd.pdf.

WHO (2009a). *Mental Health: Depression – What Is Depression?* Available at http://www.who.int/mental_health/management/depression/definition/en/.

WHO (2009b). *Suicide Risk High for Young People*. Available at http://www.who.int/mediacentre/multimedia/podcasts/2009/suicide_prevention_20090915/en/.

WHO (2009c). *Number of Suicides by Age Group and Gender*. United Kingdom of Great Britain and Northern Ireland, 2007 Available at http://www.who.int/mental_health/media/unitkingd.pdf.

WHO (2010). *SUPRE Prevention of Suicidal Behaviours: A Task for All*. Available at http://www.who.int/mental_health/prevention/suicide/information/en/index.html.

Whyte, D. A. (ed) (1997). *Explorations in Family Nursing*. London: Routledge.

Wichstrøm, L. (2000). Predictors of adolescent suicide attempts: a nationally representative longitudinal study of Norwegian adolescents. *Journal of the American Academy of Child and Adolescent Psychiatry* 39, 603–610.

Williams, D. (1992). *Nobody Nowhere*. London: Corgi Books.

Winchel, R. M. and Stanley, M. (1991). Self-injurious behavior: a review of the behavior and biology of self-mutilation. *The American Journal of Psychiatry* 148, 306–317.

Wing, L. (1981). Asperger syndrome: a clinical account. *Psychological Medicine* 11 (1), 115–129.

Wing, L. and Gould, J. (1979). Severe impairments of social interaction and associated abnormalities in children: epidemiology and classification. *Journal of Autism and Developmental Disorders* 9, 11–29.

Wing, L., Leekham, S. R., Libby, S. J., Gould, J. and Larcombe, M. (2002). The diagnostic interview for social and communication disorders: background, inter-rater reliability and clinical use. *Journal of Child Psychology and Psychiatry* 43, 307–325.

Winters, K. C. and Stinchfield, R. D. (1995). Current issues and the future needs in the assessment of adolescent drug abuse. In: Rahdert, E. and Czechowicz, D. (eds). *Adolescent Drug Abuse: Clinical Assessment and Therapeutic Interventions*. Rockville: United States Department of Health and Human Services.

Winterstein, A. G., Gerhard, T., Shuster, J., *et al.* (2007). Cardiac safety of central nervous system stimulants in children and adolescents with attention deficit hyperactivity disorder. *Pediatrics* 120 (6), 1494–1501.

Wisely, J., Hare, D. J. and Fernandez-Ford, L. (2002). A study of the topography and nature of self-injurious behaviour in people with learning disabilities. *Journal of Intellectual Disabilities* 6, 61–71.

Wolpert, M., Fuggle, P., Cottrell, D., *et al.* (2006). *Drawing on the Evidence: Advice for Mental Health Professionals Working with Children and Adolescents*, 2nd edition. London: CAMHS Publications.

Wood, A., Harrington, R. and Moore, A. (1996). Controlled trial of a cognitive–behavioural intervention in adolescent patients with depressive disorder. *Journal of Child Psychology and Psychiatry* 37, 737–746.

Wood, A., Trainor, G., Rothwell, J., Moore, A. and Harrington, R. (2001). Randomized trial of a group therapy for repeated deliberate self-harm in adolescents. *Journal of the American Academy of Child and Adolescent Psychiatry* 40 (11), 1246–1253.

Woodberry, K. A. and Popenoe, E. J. (2008). Implementing dialectical behaviour therapy with adolescents and their families in a community outpatient clinic. *Cognitive and Behavioral Practice* 15 (3), 277–286.

Woods, J. (2006). The self-report of Andi. *Clinical Child Psychology and Psychiatry* 11, 283–292.

World Psychiatric Association (2002). *Schizophrenia – Open the Doors, the WPA Global Programme Against Stigma and Discrimination Because of Schizophrenia*. New York: World Psychiatric Association. Available at http://www.openthedoors.com/english/media/Training_8.15.05.pdf.

Wragg, J. A. and Whitehead, R. E. (2004). CBT for adolescents with psychosis: investigating the feasibility and effectiveness of early intervention using a single case design. *Behavioural and Cognitive Psychotherapy* 32, 313–329.

Wright, L. M. and Leahey, M. (2000). *Nurses and Families: A Guide to Family Assessment and Intervention*. Philadelphia, PA: FA Davis.

Wu, P., Bird, H. R., Liu, X., *et al.* (2006). Childhood depressive symptoms and early onset of alcohol use. *Pediatrics* 118 (5), 1907–1915.

Wykes, T., Hayward, P., Thomas, N., *et al.* (2005). What are the effects of group cognitive behaviour therapy for voices? A randomised control trial. *Schizophrenia Research* 77, 201–210.

Wykes, T., Steel, C., Everitt, B. and Tarrier, N. (2008). Cognitive behavior therapy for schizophrenia: effect sizes, clinical models, and methodological rigor. *Schizophrenia Bulletin* 34, 523–537.

Yates, T. M. (2004). The developmental psychopathology of self-injurious behavior: compensatory regulation in posttraumatic adaptation. *Clinical Psychology Review* 24, 35–74.

Young, J. F., Mufson, L. and Davies, M. (2006). Efficacy of interpersonal psychotherapy-adolescent skills training: an indicated preventive intervention for depression. *Journal of Child Psychology and Psychiatry* 47 (12), 1254–1262.

Young, R., Van Beinum, M., Sweeting, H. and West, P. (2007). Young people who self-harm. *The British Journal of Psychiatry* 191, 44–49.

YoungMinds (2006). *Looking After Looked After Children: Sharing Emerging Practice*. London: YoungMinds.

Youniss, J. and Smoller, S. (1985). *Adolescent Relations with Mothers, Fathers and Friends*. Chicago, IL: University of Chicago Press.

Youth Justice Board (2006). *Asset*. London: Youth Justice Board.

Zammit, S., Horwood, J., Thompson, A., *et al.* (2008). Investigating if psychosis-like symptoms (PLIKS) are associated with family history of schizophrenia or paternal age in the ALSPAC birth cohort. *Schizophrenia Research* 104, 279–286.

Zenere, F. K. and Lazarus, P. J. (1997). The decline of youth suicidal behaviour in an urban multicultural public school system following the introduction of a suicidal prevention and intervention programme. *Suicide and Life-Threatening Behavior* 27 (4), 387–402.

Zimmerman, M. A., Copeland, L. A., Shope, J. T. and Dielman, T. E. (1991). A longitudinal study of self-esteem: implications for adolescent development. *Journal of Youth and Adolescence* 26 (2), 117–141.

Zipfel, S., Lowe, B. and Herzog, W. (2005). Medical complications. In: Treasure, J., Schmidt, U. and Furth, E. (eds). *The Essential Handbook of Eating Disorders*. Chichester: John Wiley and Sons Ltd.

Zito, J. M., Safer, D. J., DosReis, S., *et al.* (2003). Psychotropic practice patterns for youth: a 10-year perspective. *Archives of Pediatrics and Adolescent Medicine* 157, 17–25.

Zito, J. M., Safer, D. J., de Jong-van den Berg, L. T. W., *et al.* (2008). A three-country comparison of psychotropic medication prevalence in youth. *Child and Adolescent Psychiatry and Mental Health* 2, 26.

Zubin, J. and Spring, B. (1977). Vulnerability: a new view on schizophrenia. *Journal of Abnormal Psychology* 86, 103–126.

INDEX

adolescence, 15, 21, 51–60, 81, 105, 110, 156, 182, 204, 206, 240, 241, 252
  brain development in, 58–59
  egocentrism in, 58
  family, 35
  imaginary audience, 56
  mental health problems in, 19
  personal fable, 56–57
  reasoning, 55–56
AESCHI working group, 131
anorexia, 70, 113, 149–164
Applied Suicide and Intervention Skills Training (ASIST), 120
Asperger, H, 218
Asperger's syndrome, 218, 219, 220, 221, 222, 227, 229, 230, 231, 232, 233, 234, 236
ASYLUM, 190
attachment, 11, 15, 26, 30, 38, 41, 42, 47–51, 72, 92, 114, 137, 138, 202, 245, 254
  critics of, 50
  insecure attachment, 15, 48–49, 69, 73
  internal working model, 49–51
  secure attachment, 48, 138
  secure base, 26, 41–42, 44
  synchrony, 48
Attention Deficit Hyperactivity Disorder (ADHD), 18, 113, 191–217, 219, 244, 249
  gender differences, 193, 195, 198, 202, 204
Autistic Spectrum Disorder (ASD), 196, 201, 217–238
  gender differences, 223
  psychological abnormalities, 221, 223, 224, 227–229
  risk factors, 223–226

  sensory motor dysfunction, 226–227
  The TEACCH (Treatment and Education of Autistic and Communications-Handicapped Children), 235, 236
  theory of mind, 227–228
  weak central coherence, 228–229
autonomy, 7, 38, 111

Barnardos, 148
battered baby syndrome, 132
Beat/beating eating disorders, 164
behaviour modification, 43, 206, 207
behavioural family therapy (BFT), 187
binge eating disorder (BED), 150
body image, 52, 57, 58, 111, 153, 156
  vulnerability to suicide, 111
body mass index (BMI), 150, 151, 154, 160, 161, 163
boundaries, 38
Bowlby, J, 41, 49, 50, 51
bulimia, 150, 151, 152, 153, 156, 158, 159, 160, 162
bullying, 92, 98, 113, 169

cannabis, 170, 176, 242, 243, 252
Carter, and McGoldrick, 33–37
Centre for Economic Performance (CEP), 6–7
child abuse, 15, 69, 70, 75, 92, 93, 111, 112, 113, 119, 132–148, 156, 169, 198, 254
  assessment, 139–143
  Child Protection Legislation in the United Kingdom, 20, 142–143
  child protection register, 136, 141, 146
  incidence and prevalence, 136
  intervention, 142, 143, 145, 146

child abuse (*continued*)
  prevention, 144–145
  risk factors, 137–138
childhood autism (Kenner's syndrome)
    217, 219, 220, 221, 223, 234
child protection inquiries, 132
Child Poverty Action Group (CPAG), 10,
    12, 20
Children Act, 142, 251
Children 1st, 148
Children's Society, 8, 11, 27, 28
chooselife, 109, 110, 120, 129, 130, 131
Cognitive Behaviour Therapy (CBT), 76,
    81, 82, 99, 100, 102, 103, 123, 124,
    161–162, 174, 181, 182, 183, 186,
    206
  ADHD, 206
  depression, 99, 100, 102, 103
  eating disorders, 161–162
  psychosis, 174, 181, 182, 183, 186
  self harm, 76, 81, 82
  suicide, 123, 124
Cognitive Psychotherapy in Early
    Psychosis (COPE), 183
Cognitive Therapy-Based to Promote
    Adjustment and Recovery following
    a First Episode of Psychosis (CARF),
    184
Collaborative Assessment and Manage-
    ment of Suicidality (CAMS), 121,
    131
Compassionate Friends, 129
Conners Rating Scales, 204
CRUSE, 130
culturally sensitive treatment, 21, 114,
    130, 175, 199, 253

delusions, 169, 171, 172, 175, 179, 180,
    181, 183
depression, 6, 17, 18, 54, 57, 75, 87–107,
    111, 112, 113, 114, 115, 118,
    123, 124, 125, 126, 156, 172,
    183, 184, 185, 193, 200, 201,
    202, 203, 207, 222, 229, 234,
    241, 243, 244, 249, 253
  definition, 88–89
  diagnosis, 88–90, 94–95
  prevalence, 87, 90–91
  resilience, 98–99
  symptoms, 95–97, 102, 104, 105, 106

vulnerability to depression, 91–92, 106
Determinants (of health), 14, 21, 22, 23,
    24, 27
Dialectical Behaviour Therapy, 76, 81–82,
    124, 162
  eating disorders, 162
  self harm, 76, 81–82
DSM-IV-R, 89, 90, 95, 167, 194, 195, 204,
    219, 233
dieting, 150, 158,
dissociation, 71, 75
dysphagia, 150

eating disorders, 18, 57, 66, 76, 149–164,
    186, 230, 244
  beliefs, 150, 161, 162, 163
  body mass index (BMI), 150, 151, 154,
    160, 161, 163
  co-existing mental health problems,
    156–157
  continuum, 149
  function of, 156
  gender differences, 153
  intervention, 161–162
  resilience, 158–159
  vulnerability, 154–156
eating disorder not otherwise specified
    (EDNOS), 151–152
education, 7–11, 69, 105, 126, 202, 205,
    207, 208, 210, 234, 235, 236, 237,
    239, 245, 253
  literacy, 11
  numeracy, 11
emotional abuse, 92, 93, 113, 133, 134,
    136, 145
engagement, 42, 65, 76, 99, 100, 105, 121,
    122, 174, 175, 176, 177, 178, 179,
    187, 188, 221, 235, 246
Erikson, E, 46, 52
  identity formation, 51–54
  criticisms of, 51
Every Child Matters, 20, 43
executive function, 197, 228
expressed emotion (EE), 186, 187

family, 11–12, 14, 15, 17, 18 , 19, 23–25,
    29–45, 50, 52, 72, 78, 112, 115, 123,
    124, 127–128, 149, 157, 159, 160,
    162, 163, 164, 186–188, 193, 195,
    200, 202, 203, 205, 207, 209, 222,

233, 235, 237, 242, 245, 246, 247, 248, 250, 251, 252, 253
function and dysfunction, 30–31
processes, 30
life cycle, 31–37
multigenerational life cycle model, 31, 33
myth of traditional family, 31
structure, 37
subsystems, 38–39
systems, 37–39
    generic, 37
    idiosyncratic, 37
transactional patterns, 37, 39
family therapy, 37–42, 81, 105, 186–188, 207, 253
attachment, 41–42
narrative approaches, 39–40
substance misuse, 253
fictitious or induced Illness, 133
formulation, 25
fragile x, 229, 234
Freud, S, 47

Good Childhood Inquiry, 8
globalisation, 4, 5–7
groups, 68, 69, 77, 78, 82, 83, 98, 99, 101, 104, 114–115, 126, 181–182, 183, 207, 209

happiness, 6
Hawton, K, 65, 66, 67, 69, 74, 75, 80, 83, 110
Health Advisory Service (HAS), 13, 240
Health and Safety, 9, 11
health inequalities, 22
Helliwell, J, 7
hyperactivity, 192, 194, 195, 198, 212, 213

identity formation in adolescence, 13, 22, 46, 51–53, 57, 58, 60, 111, 245
impulsivity, 192, 194, 195, 213
inattention, 192, 194, 195, 208, 213
individualism, 4, 7, 22
Informed consent, 26
Internal working model, 46, 49–51
International Classification of Diseases, 18, 89, 90, 94, 95, 167, 194, 195, 218, 240
inter-subjectivity, 235, 236

Interpersonal Therapy - Adolescent Skills Training (IP-AST), 76, 98

Joseph Rowntree Foundation (JRF), 7
Jureidini, J, 102, 103, 106

Kanner, L, 218, 219, 220, 221, 237

Layard, R, 6, 7, 8, 10, 11, 12, 22, 23, 27
Learning disability, 65, 69, 77, 78, 90, 91, 94, 95, 96, 99, 100, 106, 168, 176, 177, 178, 182, 202, 205, 219, 223
depression, 90, 91, 94, 95, 96, 99, 100, 106
psychosis, 168, 177, 178, 182,
self harm, 65, 69, 77, 78
legal definition of child, 142
Lesbian, Bisexual, Gay, and Transgender (LBGT) young people, 69, 112, 115, 119
self harm, 69
suicide, 69, 112, 115, 119
Linehan, M, 81, 82, 123
looked after or accommodated children and young people, 19, 20, 23, 42, 69, 85, 115, 245
self harm, 69, 85
substance misuse, 245
loss, 15, 23, 26, 33, 41, 49, 50, 69, 90, 92, 127, 181, 184, 187, 244

maintaining factors, 5, 14–16, 20, 21, 23
March, J, 102, 106, 124
Marcia, J, 51, 52–53
McGorry, P, 167, 172, 179, 185, 188, 189
media, 7, 31, 57, 112, 113, 125, 149, 157
medication, 101–105, 124, 162–163, 165, 172, 173, 177, 178–180, 185, 186, 203–204, 209–213, 251–253
antidepressants, 101–105, 162–163
Dexamfetamine, 210, 212
first generation antipsychotics, 178–180
Methylphenidate, 200, 210
second generation (atypical) antipsychotic, 165, 178–180
SSRIs, 101–105
substance misuse, 251–253

mental health, 13–17, 29, 48, 52
  definition, 13, 14
  positive, 17, 22
mental disorders, 5, 13, 14, 17–21
  definition, 18
  prevalence, 18, 19
Minnesota 12 steps programme, 253
Minuchin, S, 37–39
Model Health Inquiry, 157
motivational interviewing, 161, 163,
  253–254

narrative therapies, 94, 104
National Centre For Suicide Research And
  Prevention, 131
National Health Service, Quality
  Improvement Scotland (NHS-QIS),
  159, 160, 162, 163
National Institute of Clinical Evidence
  (NICE), 83, 84, 104, 105, 162, 163,
  164, 182, 194, 200, 201, 212, 241,
  245, 250, 253
  ADHD, 194, 200, 201, 212
  eating disorders, 162, 163, 164
  psychosis, 182
  substance misuse, 245, 250
  self-harm, 83, 84
National Registry of Evidence-Based
  Programs and Practices (Nrepp), 130
National Society for the Prevention of
  Cruelty to children, 132, 148
non-organic failure to thrive, 135

Omega 3 and 6, 174, 198, 213
Organisation for Economic Cooperation
  and Development (OECD),
  8, 9, 11, 20
organismic and mechanistic models of
  development, 47, 51, 62

PAPYRUS, 129
parental control, 54, 113
parenting support and education, 42–44,
  78, 207, 237, 250
  aims, 42–44
participation, 5, 25
Partnership and the No Order Principle,
  143
Penn Prevention Program (PPP), 98

pervasive development disorder, 218, 222,
  234
Phenomenological Variant of Ecological
  Systems Theory (PVEST) 60–62
  goal seeking processes, 62
  proximal processes, 61
  reorienting processes, 62
  secondary coping processes, 61–62
physical abuse, 49, 92, 113
Piaget, J, 47, 56
picture exchange communication system,
  235
poverty, 7, 8, 10, 14, 92, 111, 113, 115, 168,
  174, 244, 253
  families, 32, 34
  UK, Ireland, USA, Czech Republic, 7, 10
  relationship to GDP, 10
precipitating factors, 5, 14, 15, 16
protective factors (against developing
  mental health problems), 5, 14–17,
  20, 21, 25
psychodynamic therapy, 47, 51, 76, 81, 82,
  103–104
psychosis, 65, 75, 112, 113, 114, 165–190,
  243, 249
  assessment, 174–177
  culture, 175
  early intervention, 165, 173–174
  family, 186–188
  interventions, 173–188
  Stress Vulnerability model, 170
  very early onset psychosis, 171
  vulnerability, 168–171
psychotic-like symptoms (PLIKS), 168
Psychosis sucks, 190
puberty, 47, 55, 57, 58, 88, 91, 96, 112, 155

recovery, 20, 21, 25, 30, 31–32, 34, 36, 84,
  154, 172, 173, 246
resilience, 13, 17, 21, 22, 50, 59, 61, 69, 70,
  71, 98–99, 115–116, 138, 158, 159,
  184–185, 200–201, 244–246
rethink, 189
risk factors (for developing mental health
  problems), 5, 14–17, 21, 22, 27
Romme, M, 166, 181, 182, 189
Royal College of Paediatrics and Child
  Health, 148
Royal College of Psychiatrists, 167

Rutter, M, 6, 17, 19, 21, 196, 198, 199, 223, 224, 225, 226, 229, 231

Sally - Anne test, 227–228
Scottish Eating Disorders Interest Group, SEDIG, 164
secure base, 41, 42, 47, 48
Seishin Bunretsu Byo (mind-split-disease), 166
self concept, 52, 55
self-esteem, 14, 54–55, 71, 73, 92, 97, 112, 126, 150, 157, 158, 183, 184, 194, 195, 207, 213, 244
self-harm, 64–86, 97, 109, 113, 115, 119, 124, 160, 163, 243, 244, 249
    assessment, 74–75
    definition, 64, 65–66, 67, 76
    intervention, 76–84
    models of, 71–73
    parental views, 73–74
    personal impact on working alongside, 83–84
    reasons for, 70, 74, 75, 83
    resilience, 69–70
    vulnerability, 68–69
sexual abuse, 48, 49, 52, 56, 57, 70, 71, 92, 93, 111, 113, 119
SIGN, 190, 195, 212, 237
    ADHD, 195, 212
    ASD, 237
    psychosis, 190
Skills-based Training on Risk Management (STORM), 121
social capital, 22
social learning theory, 206
substance misuse, 15, 32, 75, 76, 92, 95, 96, 97, 111, 112, 113, 114, 119, 130, 156, 169, 170, 175, 176, 177, 183, 185, 195, 203, 239–254
    assessment, 246–249
        parental involvement, 247–248
    definition, 241
    dependence, 240, 241, 245, 248
    intervention, 249–254
    prevalence, 241–242
    resilience, 244–246
    vulnerability, 244–246
        vulnerability to suicide, 112, 113, 114, 119

suicide, 65, 69, 70, 74, 76, 79, 82, 83, 95, 96, 97, 102, 103, 104, 108–131, 243
    assessment, 117–125
    classification, 109
    definition, 109
    gender differences, 110, 111, 116, 117, 126
    intervention, 116, 118–124
    postvention, 127–128
    prevalence, 109–111
    prevention, 120, 123, 125–127
    resilience, 115–116
    vulnerability, 111–115
Suicide Prevention Programme (SUPRE), 108, 125
SureStart, 43
Systematic Targeting of Prolonged Psychosis (STOPP), 184

TEACCH (Treatment and Education of Autistic and Communications-Handicapped Children), 235, 236
The Positive Thinking Program, 98
therapeutic relationship, 5, 26–27, 104, 193, 247
TIPS, 173, 190
Togo Snitch Sho (integration disorder), 166
trauma, 47, 69, 72, 93, 156, 169, 170, 183, 184, 189, 197, 203, 244, 254
Treatment of Adolescent Depression Study (TADS), 102, 106
triad of impairments, 219, 224
trust, 7, 22, 26, 27, 47, 69, 160, 179

UNICEF, 7, 8, 9, 10, 12, 13, 23, 28
    Report card, 10–13
    report on welfare of children, 10–13
        Canada, 9, 12
        Poland, 9, 11, 12
        UK, 9–12
        USA, 9–12
United Nations Convention on the Rights of the Child, 5, 6, 8, 13, 25, 142

Walsh, F, 30–33
Webster-Stratton, C, 43, 70, 78, 207
well-being, 12–14, 29, 31, 32
    Indicators UNICEF, 10–13
    behaviours and risks, 12

well-being (*continued*)
    educational, 9, 11
    material well being, 9, 10
    monitoring, 10
    subjective well-being, 9, 12–13
  mental health, 13–17
    definition of good mental health, 13
Whitaker, C, 30
Wing, L, 219, 224, 233, 236, 238
WHO, 87, 89, 108, 110, 111, 125, 131,
    167, 188, 194, 218, 219, 233, 234,
    240, 241

ASD, 234
depression, 87, 89
psychosis, 167, 188
stigma, 167
substance misuse, 241
suicide, 108, 110, 111, 125, 131
working alongside, 76, 83, 118, 123, 177

ZUNI Life Skills Development curriculum,
    121